Early Diagnosis of
Diabetic Kidney Disease

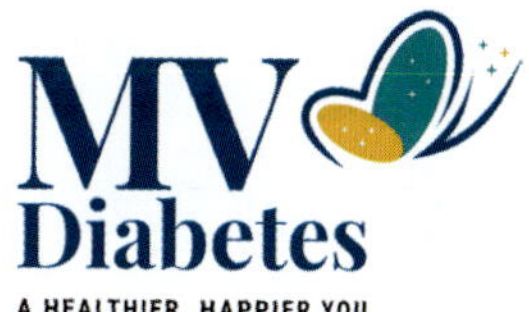

Early Diagnosis of
Diabetic Kidney Disease

Editor-in-Chief

Vijay Viswanathan

MD PhD FRCP(London, Glasgow)

Head and Chief Physician, MV Diabetes
Department of Diabetology
President, Prof M Viswanathan Diabetes Research Centre
Chennai, Tamil Nadu, India

Co-Editor

Sivashankari Selva Elavarasan

MDS Advanced PG Diploma in Clinical Research

Senior Research Officer
Department of Diabetic Kidney Disease
Prof M Viswanathan Diabetes Research Centre
Chennai, Tamil Nadu, India

Foreword

Shyam B Bansal

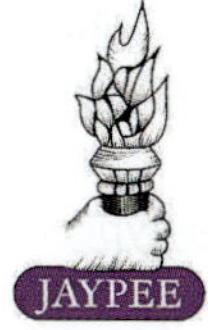

JAYPEE BROTHERS MEDICAL PUBLISHERS
The Health Sciences Publisher
New Delhi | London

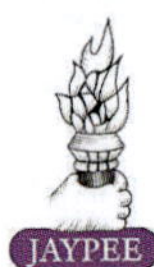

Jaypee Brothers Medical Publishers (P) Ltd

Headquarters
EMCA House, 23/23-B
Ansari Road, Daryaganj
New Delhi 110 002, India
Landline: +91-11-23272143, +91-11-23272703
+91-11-23282021, +91-11-23245672
e-mail: jaypee@jaypeebrothers.com

Corporate Office
4838/24, Ansari Road, Daryaganj
New Delhi 110 002, India
Phone: +91-11-43574357
Fax: +91-11-43574314
e-mail: jaypee@jaypeebrothers.com

Overseas Office
JP Medical Ltd.
83, Victoria Street, London
SW1H 0HW (UK)
Phone: +44-20 3170 8910
e-mail: info@jpmedpub.com

EU GPSR Authorised Representative
Logos Europe, 9 rue Nicolas Poussin
17000, La Rochelle, France
Phone: +33 (0) 6 67 93 73 78
e-mail: contact@logoseurope.eu

Website: www.jaypeebrothers.com
Website: www.jaypeedigital.com

Inquiries for bulk sales may be solicited at: jaypee@jaypeebrothers.com

Early Diagnosis of Diabetic Kidney Disease

First Edition: **2026**

ISBN: 978-93-7202-353-4

Printed at: Samrat Offset Pvt. Ltd.

CONTRIBUTORS

Arutselvi Devarajan MSc PhD
Research Scientist
Department of Epidemiology
Prof M Viswanathan Diabetes
Research Centre
Chennai, Tamil Nadu, India

Manisha Jadaun MBBS
MS(General Surgery) PhD(General
Surgery) FIAGES
Consultant Limb Salvage
Surgeon
Department of General Surgery
Gwalior Diabetes and Foot Care
Center
Gwalior, Madhya Pradesh, India

Manjula Arunraj MSc
MPhil(Applied Psychology) PGD in
Counseling and Psychotherapy
Psychologist
Department of Psychology
MV Diabetes and
Prof M Viswanathan Diabetes
Research Centre
Chennai, Tamil Nadu, India

Patricia Trueman MSc PhD
Consultant DSMES (Diabetes
Self-Management Education
and Support)
Diet Department
MV Diabetes
Chennai, Tamil Nadu, India

Prashanth Arun MD(General
Medicine) PG D.Diab(UK)
Senior Physician and
Diabetologist
Department of Diabetology
MV Diabetes
Chennai, Tamil Nadu, India

Rajeshwar Singh Jadaun
MD(Medicine) Diabetologist
Fellowship in Diabetes
Director
Department of General Surgery
Gajra Raja Medical College
Gwalior Diabetes and Foot Care
Gwalior, Madhya Pradesh, India

Reshma Mirshad MSc PhD
Medical Associate
Prof M Viswanathan Diabetes
Research Centre
Chennai, Tamil Nadu, India

Rizwana Parveen MSc
Research Associate
Department of Primary
Prevention of Diabetes
Prof M Viswanathan Diabetes
Research Centre
Chennai, Tamil Nadu, India

Satyavani Kumpatla MSc MTech
PhD
Senior Research Scientist
Diabetes Research Department
Prof M Viswanathan Diabetes
Research Centre
Chennai, Tamil Nadu, India

**Sivashankari Selva
Elavarasan** MDS Advanced PG
Diploma in Clinical Research
Senior Research Officer
Department of Diabetic Kidney
Disease
Prof M Viswanathan Diabetes
Research Centre
Chennai, Tamil Nadu, India

T Navaneethan MBBS
MD(General Medicine)
DM(Nephrology)
Consultant Nephrologist
Department of Nephrology
MV Diabetes
Chennai, Tamil Nadu, India

Udyama Juttada MSc PhD
Scientist
Department of Molecular
Biology and Biochemistry
Prof M Viswanathan Diabetes
Research Centre
Chennai, Tamil Nadu, India

Vaishnavi Vijay MSc(Clinical
Psychology)
Head, Mind and Wellness Clinic
and Clinical Psychologist
Department of Psychology
MV Hospital for Diabetes and
Prof M Viswanathan Diabetes
Research Centre
Chennai, Tamil Nadu, India

Vijay Viswanathan MD PhD
FRCP(London and Glasgow)
Head and Chief Physician, MV
Diabetes
Department of Diabetology
President, Prof M Viswanathan
Diabetes Research Centre
Chennai, Tamil Nadu, India

FOREWORD

Diabetes mellitus has emerged as one of the greatest public health challenges of our time, and diabetic kidney disease (DKD) remains the leading cause of chronic kidney disease and end-stage kidney failure worldwide. The burden of DKD is particularly profound in low- and middle-income countries, where rising prevalence of diabetes, late presentation, and limited access to specialized care continue to increase morbidity and mortality.

Over the past two decades, our understanding of DKD has evolved remarkably. What was once viewed as an inexorable and uniform complication of diabetes is now recognized as a heterogeneous disease process influenced by genetic susceptibility, metabolic milieu, hemodynamic factors, inflammation, and fibrosis. Advances in pathophysiology, diagnostics, and therapeutics—especially the advent of renoprotective agents such as SGLT2 inhibitors, nonsteroidal mineralocorticoid receptor antagonists, and GLP-1 receptor agonists—have transformed the clinical landscape, offering renewed hope for prevention and disease modification.

Despite these advances, significant gaps persist in the translation of evidence into routine clinical practice. Early detection remains suboptimal, multidisciplinary care is inconsistently implemented, and awareness among healthcare providers and patients alike continues to lag behind the growing burden of disease. In this context, a comprehensive, evidence-based, and clinically relevant resource on DKD is both timely and essential.

This book *"Early Diagnosis of Diabetic Kidney Disease"* brings together an outstanding group of clinicians and researchers, who have combined their expertise to address DKD in a structured and pragmatic manner. The chapters span the spectrum from epidemiology and pathogenesis to contemporary diagnostic approaches, individualized risk stratification, and state-of-the-art management strategies. Special emphasis on India-specific challenges, real-world practice, and preventive nephrology enhances the relevance of this text for practicing clinicians.

I am confident that this book will serve as a valuable reference for nephrologists, endocrinologists, internists, postgraduate trainees, and allied healthcare professionals involved in the care of patients with diabetes and kidney disease.

I congratulate Dr Vijay Viswanathan and other contributors for their scholarly effort and commend them for producing a book that bridges science with clinical practice. I wish this publication every success and hope that it will make a meaningful contribution to the fight against diabetic kidney disease.

Shyam B Bansal
DM FRCP FASN FISN
Director and Head, Department of Nephrology
Medanta – The Medicity
Gurugram, Haryana, India
Secretary, Indian Society of Nephrology

PREFACE

Diabetic kidney disease (DKD) remains one of the most common and serious microvascular complications of diabetes mellitus, contributing substantially to morbidity, mortality, and healthcare burden worldwide. Early identification and timely intervention are critical in altering the natural course of the disease, preventing progression to end-stage kidney disease, and improving long-term patient outcomes. Despite advances in understanding and management, gaps persist in early diagnosis, risk stratification, and integrated care, particularly in resource-constrained settings.

The book *"Early Diagnosis of Diabetic Kidney Disease"* has been conceptualized to provide a comprehensive, evidence-based, and clinically relevant overview of DKD, with a clear focus on early detection and prevention. Beginning with the epidemiology and burden of DKD, the chapters systematically address pathogenesis, risk factors, and current standards for assessment using eGFR, albuminuria, and KDIGO guidelines. Emerging genetic markers and biomarkers for early detection are discussed alongside the psychological dimensions of living with DKD, highlighting the need for holistic patient-centered care.

The volume also explores recent therapeutic advances, nutritional strategies, management of comorbidities and complications, and models of comprehensive care. Special emphasis is placed on prevention strategies and the Indian experience, reflecting regional realities and practices. Practical guidance on diabetic foot complications, referral to nephrology services, and renal replacement therapy ensures clinical applicability across levels of care.

Authored by experienced clinicians and researchers, this book is intended for diabetologists, nephrologists, physicians, trainees, nurses, dietitians, postgraduate students, and allied healthcare professionals involved in diabetes and kidney care. We hope this work will serve as a valuable resource to promote early diagnosis, informed decision-making, and improved outcomes for individuals at risk of or living with DKD.

Vijay Viswanathan

PREFACE

ACKNOWLEDGMENTS

We would like to express our heartfelt gratitude to all those who have contributed to the successful completion of this book, "*Early Diagnosis of Diabetic Kidney Disease*". This volume is the result of collective academic effort, guidance, and sustained support from numerous individuals and institutions.

We sincerely thank our senior mentors and academic leaders for their valuable guidance, encouragement, and unwavering support throughout the conceptualization and compilation of this book. Their vision and commitment to advancing knowledge in diabetic kidney disease have been a constant source of inspiration.

We are deeply grateful to all the contributing authors for sharing their expertise, clinical experience, and scholarly insights. Their dedication and timely contributions have greatly enriched the scientific content and clinical relevance of this book.

We would like to acknowledge *Dr Sivashankari Selva Elavarasan (Co-Editor)* for her sincere and relentless efforts in meticulous writing, scientific editing, and comprehensive compilation for the successful completion of this book. We would also like to thank *Ms Meera Vijay (Librarian)* for her systematic compilation of the abstracts for the section on Key Research Takeaway. We also acknowledge the invaluable support and encouragement extended by our respective institutions, which facilitated the successful completion of this academic endeavor.

Our sincere appreciation is extended to the team at M/s Jaypee Brothers Medical Publishers (P) Ltd, New Delhi, India, for their professionalism, meticulous editorial support, and continued cooperation throughout the publishing process. We especially thank Mr Ankit Vij (Managing Director), Mr Sabyasachi Hazra (Director—PG and PNR Content), and Mr Akhilesh Saxena (Development Editor) for their dedicated efforts in bringing this book to fruition.

Finally, we thank all colleagues, trainees, and healthcare professionals whose commitment to improving the early diagnosis and management of diabetic kidney disease continues to motivate and guide our work.

Vijay Viswanathan

CONTENTS

1

Epidemiology and Burden of Diabetic Kidney Disease

Vijay Viswanathan, Sivashankari Selva Elavarasan

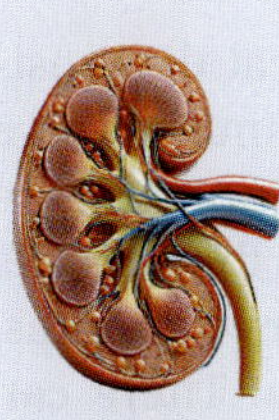

- Diabetic kidney disease: Introduction and definition
- Diabetic nephropathy and diabetic kidney disease
- Epidemiology of DKD in the World
- Epidemiology of DKD in India
- Global burden of DKD and CKD
- Burden of DKD and CKD in India
- Early diagnosis of DKD

Abstract

Diabetic kidney disease (DKD) is one of the major serious complications of diabetes mellitus that affects 30–40% of people living with diabetes. DKD is a clinical diagnosis characterized by persistent albuminuria and a decreased estimated glomerular filtration rate (eGFR) <60 mL/min/1.73 m^2. It becomes the need of the hour to study the global burden of DKD due to the high mortality rates associated with the disease, which is responsible for a significant social and economic burden on the healthcare system. A recent multicentric nationwide study estimated the prevalence of chronic kidney disease (CKD) among people with type 2 diabetes to be 32%. It remains a major global challenge to tackle the burden of CKD in a resource-limited setting like India because the treatment rendered is costly and requires long-term consistent management. This review highlights the important epidemiological findings of DKD and the substantial burden of the disease on the healthcare system in India and around the globe. Nationwide screening of people with DKD remains the key to identifying and treating them before they develop further complications.

Keywords: Chronic kidney disease, epidemiology, India, burden, type 2 diabetes.

INTRODUCTION

Diabetes mellitus (DM) is a chronic, debilitating, devastating, and serious metabolic disease that is also considered a major health problem worldwide. It can cause a significant burden to the healthcare system of the entire nation due to its inconceivable complications. It has been estimated that 589 million people aged between 20 and 79 years are affected globally by the disease, which represents 11% of the world population. These numbers are expected to increase to 853 million by 2050. In the Southeast Asian region, 1.1 billion people are affected by diabetes, with India leading the list of top five countries with nearly 90 million people with diabetes in the age group between 20 and 79 years. India accounts for one in every seven people who are affected by diabetes globally.[1] According to a study by the Indian Council of Medical Research – India Diabetes (ICMR-INDIAB), the overall prevalence of diabetes in India was 11.4% with approximately 101 million people affected by the disease.[2] These numbers are expected to increase rampantly over the years with the alarming increase in the population.

Diabetes is also associated with significant micro as well as macro complications because it can affect the eyes, nerves, kidneys, heart, and feet. These complications can even be life-threatening and can affect the social and physical quality of life. One of the most common long-term and important complications of diabetes seems to be diabetic kidney disease (DKD) which can affect 30–40% of all the people affected by diabetes.[3] Globally, the incidence of chronic kidney disease (CKD) due to diabetes increased by 74%, which was about 1.4 million in 1990 to 2.4 million in 2017.[4] Among the adults living worldwide, diabetes remains the leading cause of end-stage kidney disease (ESKD).[5] This condition is characterized by failure of the kidneys to function normally and they require dialysis or transplantation for their survival. It has also been predicted that only 27–53% of the people with ESKD have access to renal replacement therapy (RRT), leaving middle and low-income countries with limited access to the various treatment modalities.[6]

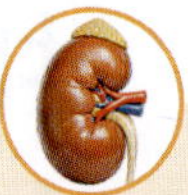

Diabetic kidney disease affects 30–40% of all the people affected by diabetes. Globally, the incidence of CKD due to diabetes increased by 74%, which was about 1.4 million in 1990 to 2.4 million in 2017. Among the adults living worldwide, diabetes remains the leading cause of ESKD.

DEFINITION OF DIABETIC KIDNEY DISEASE

Diabetic kidney disease is a clinical diagnosis characterized by persistent albuminuria and a decreased estimated glomerular filtration rate (eGFR) <60 mL/min/1.73 m^2. When the patient's urine tests positive for albumin for >3 months, it is called persistent albuminuria. There can also be a persistent increase in the albumin-creatinine ratio (ACR ≥30 mg/g). A decline in eGFR and an increase in albuminuria can both have undesirable consequences such as ESKD and eventually death.

Albuminuria can be divided into three categories based on Kidney Disease Improving Global Outcomes (KDIGO) 2012 **(Fig. 1)**.[7]

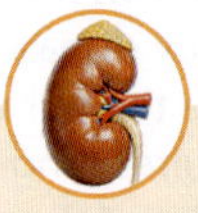

Diabetic kidney disease is a clinical diagnosis characterized by persistent albuminuria and a decreased estimated glomerular filtration rate (eGFR) <60 mL/min/1.73 m^2.

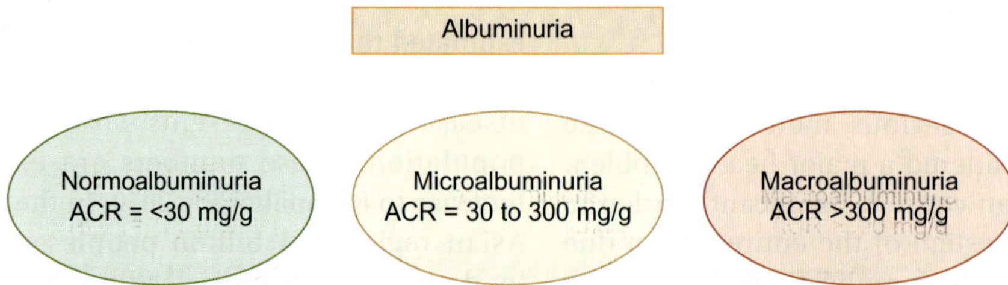

FIG. 1: The different categories of albuminuria based on Kidney Disease Improving Global Outcomes (KDIGO).[7]

DIABETIC NEPHROPATHY AND DIABETIC KIDNEY DISEASE

Diabetic nephropathy (DN) is a classic term that refers to specific functional and structural damages that can occur to the kidneys of people with diabetes. It refers to a standard pattern of glomerular disease. Proteinuria is usually accompanied by hypertension and retinopathy along with a decline in kidney function. However, in some cases, DN is not accompanied by diabetic retinopathy and that does not always exclude its diagnosis.[8] This term eventually evolved into a more generic term called DKD due to the diversity and complexity involved in the pathogenesis of renal impairment among people living with diabetes. This could be the most possible reason for considering DKD as a syndrome rather than a single disease.[9] There is no distinct pathological entity involved in DKD. There can be a variety of reasons for the same namely any unspecified acute kidney injury or hypertensive nephrosclerosis.

According to KDIGO, DN was exclusively used to refer to the histological diagnosis seen in a renal biopsy which includes thickening of the glomerular basement membrane, mesangial expansion accompanied with/without nodular lesions typically described as Kimmelstiel–Wilson lesion, any disruption of the endothelium or loss of podocytes. These changes can ultimately result in the loss of nephron. However, DKD is rather a clinical diagnosis that refers to CKD among people with diabetes.[10]

Mogensen classified DN into five stages based on the natural history of the disease.[11] The five classic stages of DN are illustrated in **Table 1**.

TABLE 1: Shows the classification of DN into five stages by Mogensen.[11]	
Stage 1	Hyperfiltration and hypertrophy
Stage 2	Silent nephropathy
Stage 3	Incipient nephropathy
Stage 4	Overt nephropathy
Stage 5	End-stage renal failure

There are five stages in the development of DN which can be depicted in **Figure 2**.[12]

Diabetic kidney disease is a relatively new term established by the Kidney Disease Outcomes Quality Initiative (KDOQI) in the year 2007, it was previously known as diabetic nephropathy.[13] DKD is also recognized as the most common cause of ESKD and keeping in mind the magnitude of the problem, ESKD can be rightly described as "a medical catastrophe of worldwide dimension".[14] Despite the novel biomarkers and approaches for the diagnosis of DKD, its accuracy without a renal biopsy remains questionable, especially in clinical settings.

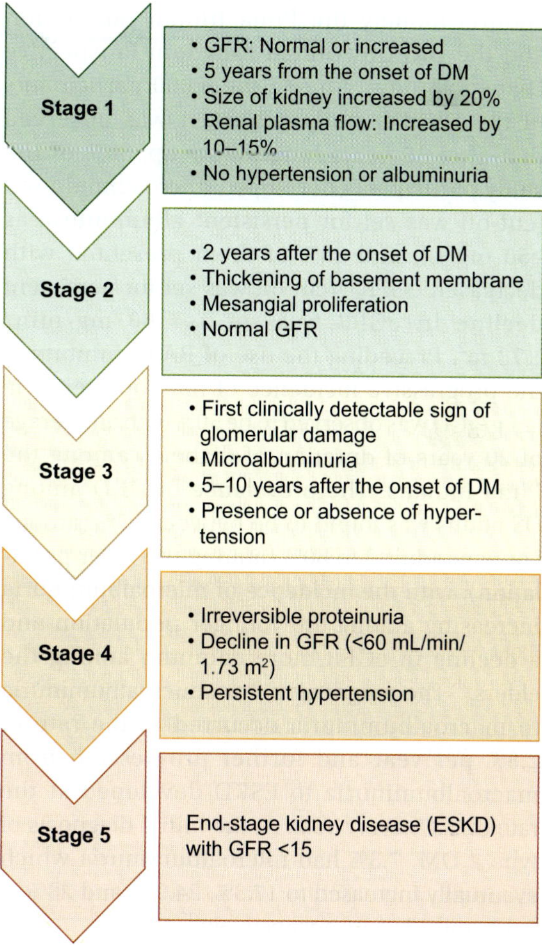

FIG. 2: Shows the five stages of diabetic nephropathy.[12]

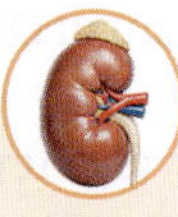

Diabetic nephropathy (DN) is a classic term that refers to specific functional and structural damages that can occur to the kidneys of people with diabetes. According to KDIGO, DN was exclusively used to refer to the histological diagnosis seen in a renal biopsy. DKD is a clinical diagnosis that refers to CKD among people with diabetes.

EPIDEMIOLOGY OF DIABETIC KIDNEY DISEASE IN THE WORLD

There are two best type 2 diabetes long-term cohorts namely the Pima Indian population and the UKPDS (United Kingdom Prospective Diabetic Study). Among the 5,000 participants in the UKPDS study cohort, it was observed that after 15 years long follow-up, 38% of the study participants developed microalbuminuria (cut-off was set for persistent albuminuria as ≥50 mg/L), and 29% of them presented with decreased eGFR[15] (cut off was set for persistent decline in eGFR was set as ≤60 mg/min/ 1.73 m². Preceding the use of RAAS inhibitors, the progressive incidence of macroproteinuria (≥1 g/gCr) was observed to be 50% with an average of 20 years of duration of diabetes among the Pima Indians. The prevalence of DKD among US adults was found to be between 25% (among younger adults) to 50% (among the older population), with the incidence of microalbuminuria increasing among the younger population and a decline in eGFR more common among the elders.[16] The progression from microalbuminuria to macroalbuminuria occurred at the rate of 2.8% per year and further progression from macroalbuminuria to ESKD developed at the rate of 2.3% every year. At the initial diagnosis of type 2 DM, 7.3% had microalbuminuria which eventually increased to 17.3%, 24.9%, and 28% at 5, 10, and 15 years, respectively.[17]

In a cross-sectional study conducted among 32,208 people with T2D across 33 countries, the prevalence of micro- and macroalbuminuria was found to be 38.8% and 9.8%, respectively.[18] The prevalence of micro- and macroalbuminuria among different races can be best illustrated in **Figure 3**.

According to Parving, Asians, and Hispanics recorded the highest prevalence of microalbuminuria (43.2% and 43.8%) as well as macroalbuminuria (12.3% and 10.3%) as depicted in the figure.[19] Similarly, the lowest prevalence of micro as well as macroalbuminuria was reported among Caucasians (33.3% and 7.6% respectively). Among the Japanese population, the prevalence of decreased GFR (<60 mL/min/1.73 m²) and microalbuminuria was 10.5% and 31.6% respectively.[20] Among the people living with diabetes in Egypt, Jordan, and Libya, the prevalence of diabetic nephropathy was observed to be 42%, 33%, and 25% respectively.

The worldwide prevalence of DKD and non-diabetic kidney disease (NDKD) is best illustrated in the **Table 2** below. Among the various countries, China, India, and the United States seem to be leading in the prevalence of DKD **(Table 2)**.[21]

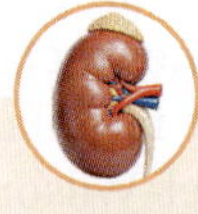

Asians and Hispanics recorded the highest prevalence of microalbuminuria (43.2% and 43.8%) and macroalbuminuria (12.3% and 10.3%). Among the various countries, China, India, and the United States seem to be leading in the prevalence of DKD.

EPIDEMIOLOGY OF DIABETIC KIDNEY DISEASE IN INDIA

In India, DKD is a serious major public health problem imposing a huge burden on the society as well as on the nation. The pattern of renal disease in India was studied by MK Mani who stated that there were no peculiar renal diseases that were prevalent among the Indians. The most common reasons for which the patients visited a renal unit were identified as chronic renal failure (CRF) (43%) and nephrotic syndrome (14.8%). Diabetic

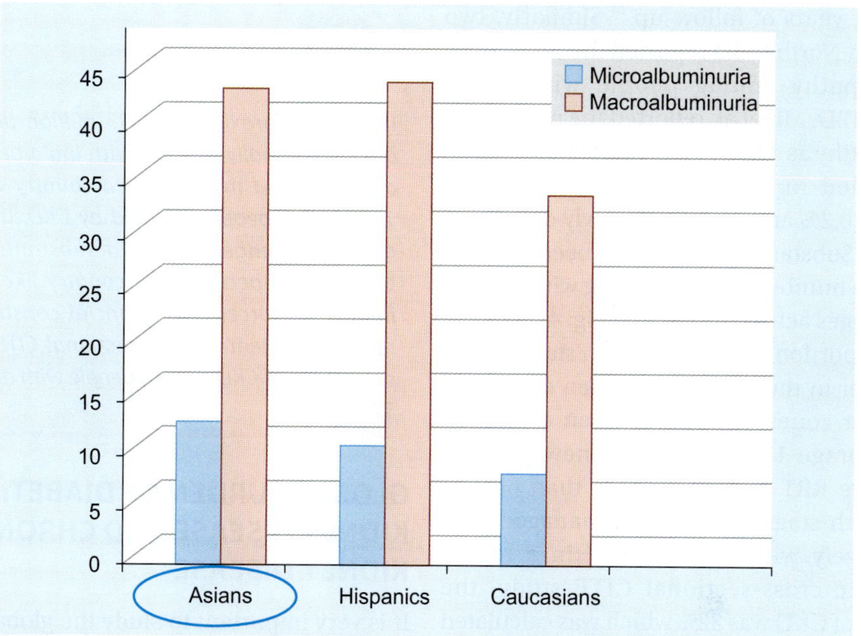

FIG. 3: Illustrates the prevalence of both micro as well as macroalbuminuria among the different races.[19]

Continent/Country	Prevalence of DKD (in %)	Prevalence of NDKD (in %)
China	6–74	16–64
USA	28–63	19–53
India	35–56	23–50
Europe	34–85	14–62
Africa	24–55	44–69

TABLE 2: Shows the prevalence of diabetic kidney disease (DKD) and nondiabetic kidney disease (NDKD) across the major countries and continents.[21]

nephropathy, chronic interstitial nephritis, and chronic glomerulonephritis were the various common causes considered responsible for CRF. Among them, diabetic nephropathy (30.3%) was the most common cause of CRF. In a country like India where we have more lean diabetics who are at a greater risk of developing proteinuria and the kidney function declines more rapidly when compared to their counterparts who are obese and diabetic. In a survey conducted by Mani et al. among the rural population, 7.5% of the people were identified to be at risk of developing CRF.[22]

In 2017, approximately 697 million people were affected globally by CKD, with India being ranked as the second most affected country with nearly 115 million people affected by CKD.[23] In a population-based survey conducted in two major cities Delhi and Chennai in India, the prevalence of CKD and albuminuria was found to be 8.7% and 7.1% respectively.[24] According to Chennai Urban Rural Epidemiology Study 45 (CURES 45), the prevalence of overt nephropathy and microalbuminuria was 2.2% and 26.9% respectively among urban Asian Indians.[25] Similarly in another study from India by Vijay et al., proteinuria was found in approximately one-third of the people with noninsulin dependent diabetes mellitus (NIDDM) and it was also reported that the risk of nephropathy increased along with duration of diabetes.[26] It was also reported in a 12-year observational study by Viswanathan et al. that around 44.1% of people living with T2D developed proteinuria during the subsequent years of follow-up.[27] Similarly, two studies from North India reported the prevalence of nephropathy among people with newly diagnosed T2D. Mir et al. reported the prevalence of nephropathy as 32.9%,[28] and microalbuminuria was recorded in 24.7% and proteinuria was reported in 6.2% among people newly diagnosed with T2D.[29] Substantial efforts have been taken to compile the number of people living with DKD in different stages across the nation **(Fig. 4)**.

The proportion of participants in stages 4 and 5 was higher in the North zone when compared to the other zones. It has also been estimated that on average 170,000–250,000 new patients may require RRT annually. More than 60% of patients with stage 5 CKD were managed only conservatively without dialysis.[30] In a recent multicentric cross-sectional CITE study, the prevalence of CKD was 32% which was calculated using the data of 3,325 patients from 28 centers all over India for a period of 3 months. In this real-world observational study, the various risk factors associated with CKD among people with diabetes was also analyzed.[31] It remains a major challenge to treat a substantial number of people, especially in a country like India with limited resources and financial constraints.

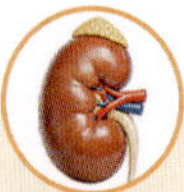

In 2017, approximately 697 million people were affected globally by CKD, with India being ranked as the second most affected country with nearly 115 million people affected by CKD. It remains a major challenge to treat a substantial number of people, especially in a country like India with limited resources and financial constraints. In a recent multicentric cross-sectional CITE study, the prevalence of CKD among people with diabetes was 32%.

GLOBAL BURDEN OF DIABETIC KIDNEY DISEASE AND CHRONIC KIDNEY DISEASE

It is very important to study the global burden of DKD due to the high mortality rates associated with the disease which in turn is responsible for a significant social and economic burden on the healthcare system. A multinational collaborative study was conducted by Global Burden of Disease in 2019 which was used to measure the burden of 369 diseases across 204 countries around the globe which also included the trends

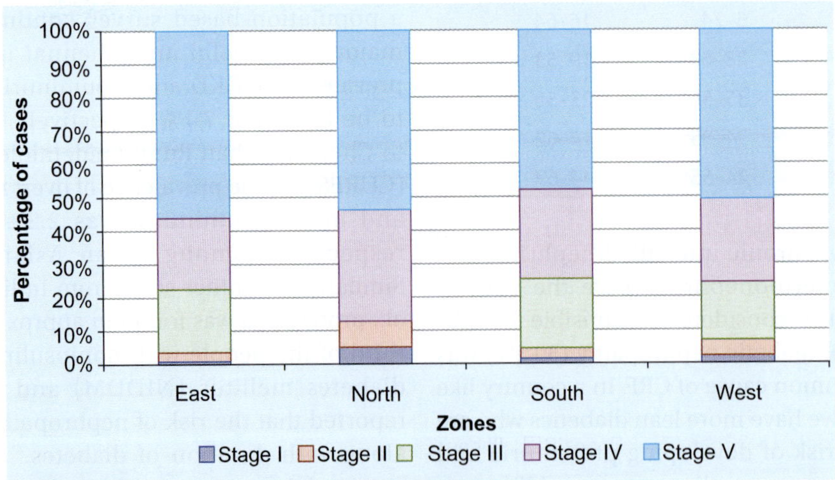

FIG. 4: Shows the percentage of people living with diabetic kidney disease (DKD) in different zones such as East, West, North, and South regions in India.[30]

in various diseases from 1990 to 2019. In this chapter, the global epidemiological characteristics of people living with DKD are enumerated. In the year 2019, approximately 2,500,000 cases were reported worldwide and they also estimated that there was a 21.8% increase in the number of cases since 1990. The number of deaths that were recorded was 406,000, the global incidence as well as the death rates increased with age, with the highest peak in the number of deaths recorded in the age group between 75 and 79 years.[32] There is an alarming increase in the age-standardized death rates for people aged between 20 and 59 years and living with DKD worldwide **(Fig. 5)**.

In 2010, nearly 2.3 million people died due to lack of access to renal replacement therapy (RRT). This is more common, especially in low-income countries in Africa as well as Asia. Globally, the prevalence of RRT is expected to rise to 5.4 million by 2030 and in Asia, it is expected to increase to 2 million from the present 1 million.[33] The lack of national screening programs and the unavailability of a unified CKD registry worldwide to track cases before ESKD are among the challenges faced by healthcare professionals that contribute further to the burden of DKD.[34] However, in 2005, a CKD registry was established in India to collect data and maintain a record of patients' demographics, etiology, analyze the differences in patterns of practice, as well as study regional variations across India.

People living with DKD are considered to be at a greater risk for cardiovascular diseases which is also responsible for the substantial economic burden. Many countries across the globe do not have the appropriate patient care facilities for people affected by DKD with a significant impact on the quality of life. The annual direct cost associated with CKD management increased dramatically with the increasing stages of CKD.[35] There is an urgent need to tackle the disease in its early stages to prevent its progression to advanced stages which can in turn contribute to the substantial economic burden.

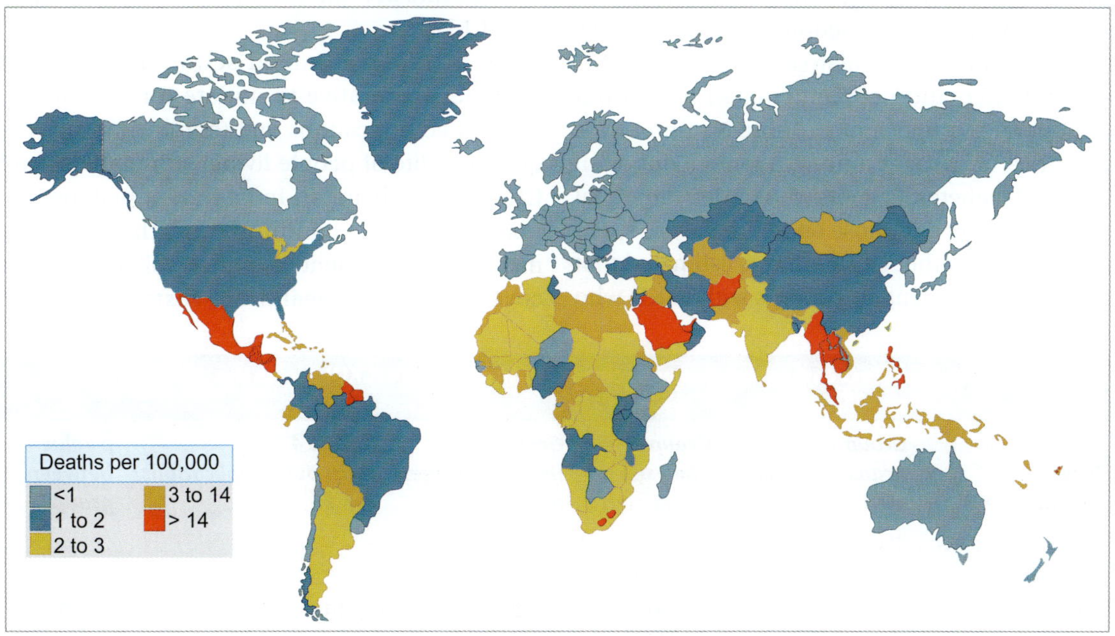

FIG. 5: Shows the age-standardized death rates recorded among people with diabetic kidney disease (DKD) aged between 20 and 59 years per 1,00,000 population in the year 2019 globally.[32]

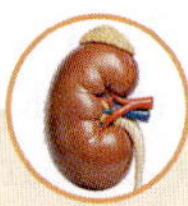

Globally, the prevalence of RRT is expected to rise to 5.4 million by 2030 and in Asia, it is expected to increase to 2 million from the present 1 million. The lack of national screening programs and the unavailability of a CKD registry to keep an account of cases before ESKD are some of the challenges faced by healthcare professionals that contribute further to the burden of DKD.

BURDEN OF DIABETIC KIDNEY DISEASE AND CHRONIC KIDNEY DISEASE IN INDIA

It remains a major global challenge to tackle the burden of CKD in India because the treatment rendered is very expensive and also requires long-term consistent management. A study by Satyavani et al. was done to assess the direct cost of the treatment of hospitalized people living with diabetes and CKD. Participants were classified into four groups namely, people who underwent renal transplantation, people living with CKD, diabetes, and on hemodialysis, people with CKD before ESKD, and people living with T2D but without any complications. **Table 3** summarizes the direct cost spent among people living with CKD and diabetes. Patients who underwent renal transplantation and those on hemodialysis spent more than the other groups. It was estimated that the cost of treatment for patients with ESKD who underwent dialysis and for those who underwent transplantation was found to be ₹500,000 (US $10,753) and ₹345,000 (US $7,419), respectively. Similarly, patients who were not on dialysis spent ₹100,000 (US $2150) in 2 years **(Table 3)**. People with diabetes spend four times more money when compared to people before the ESKD stage. The direct costs calculated included days spent during their hospitalization, total expenditure toward medicine, transportation, consultation fees, laboratory expenses, and the amount of money spent during their hospitalization. Approximately 70% of the patients in the dialysis group underwent dialysis almost eight times in a month. They had to undergo 12 sessions in a month. However, some patients could not afford to spend for all the sessions and were forced to skip them due to financial reasons. The source of funding for these patients was mostly from their savings (46%).[36]

This study made a huge impact because the direct cost associated with CKD in India was studied for the first time. However, this study did not take into account the indirect costs associated with CKD.

In a resource-limited setting like India, it becomes imperative to initiate intervention to prevent complications and thereby improve the quality of life of people living with diabetes and CKD. People living in India have a high out-of-pocket (OOP) expenditure and there are not many reimbursement insurance policies that can cover their entire healthcare costs. There were

TABLE 3: Shows the direct cost associated with chronic kidney disease (CKD) across the different study groups.[36]					
Total expenditure (₹)	**Group 1 (transplantation) n = 12**	**Group 2 (dialysis) n = 45**	**Group 3 (I–IV CKD stages) n = 66**	**Group 4 (without complications) n = 86**	**p value between groups**
Transplantation or hemodialysis	360,000 (774 US $)	49,500 (1,064 US $)	–	–	
Diabetes	30,200 (649 US $)	14,400 (310 US $)	12,700 (273 US $)	3214 (69 US $)	<0.001
Total expenditure for previous 2 years	345,000 (77,419 US $)	500,000 (10,753 US $)	100,000 (2,150 US $)	30,000 (645 US $)	<0.001

a few studies where the OOP was found to be US $7,881 in patients with CKD and undergoing renal transplantation[37] and Suja et al. reported the cost of hemodialysis in people with ESKD for 6 months was projected to be US $4,759.[38] Another study suggests that the annual average costs for patients on hemodialysis along with medication were estimated to be ₹2,13,144 (US $3181).[39] It is thus of paramount importance to establish new dialysis centers, especially in public health centers across the nation to reduce the direct expenditure associated with CKD. It also becomes indispensable to increase the number of centers that can provide such facilities in different regions thereby helping in reducing the indirect expenditure for the patients. The limited awareness about DKD among the general public, the availability of resources as well as affordability to treat the disease can be attributed to neglected treatment for the disease, thereby paving the way to complications that can ultimately result in the death of the patients.

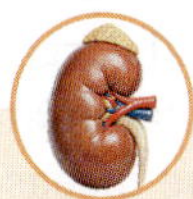

People living in India have a high out-of-pocket (OOP) expenditure and there are not many reimbursement insurance policies that can cover their entire healthcare costs. It remains a major global challenge to tackle the burden of CKD in India because the treatment rendered is very expensive and also requires long-term consistent management.

EARLY DIAGNOSIS OF DIABETIC KIDNEY DISEASE

Prevention is always considered better than cure. Nation-wide screening of people with DKD remains the key to identifying and treating them before they develop further complications. An annual screening of people living with diabetes to evaluate their eGFR and their albuminuria

must be conducted nationwide. There is a need to design nationwide multicentric studies to assess the burden of the disease because there is a paucity of data on the epidemiology of DKD in India. All people with diabetes should undergo an annual screening for CKD. The gold standard for assessing the glomerular filtration rate is to use mGFR. However, in resource-limited settings like India, we can use the CKD-EPI formula to calculate eGFR using age, sex and serum creatinine which is very simple and inexpensive. Urine albumin creatinine ratio (UACR) can be checked in a sample of spot urine for the assessment of albuminuria **(Table 4)**. Persistent albuminuria for 2 or 3 months indicates damage to the kidneys.

TABLE 4: Shows the assessments done for the early diagnosis of diabetic kidney disease (DKD) in India.[40]	
Assessments for the early diagnosis of DKD in India	*Description of the assessment*
Screening	Regular screening for early diagnosis of DKD
Calculation of eGFR	Using CKD-EPI (S cr.) equation to calculate eGFR using age, sex, and serum creatinine
Assessment of albuminuria (UACR)	• UACR is estimated in spot urine to assess albuminuria • If UACR ≥30 mg/g, it indicates microalbuminuria • If UACR ≥300 mg/g, it indicates macroalbuminuria
Monitoring for evaluation of complications	Regular screening for other complications related to diabetes such as neuropathy, retinopathy, and assessment of cardiovascular risk factors
Regular assessment and follow-up	Regular monitoring of blood pressure, blood sugar, eGFR, and UACR to assess the progression of DKD

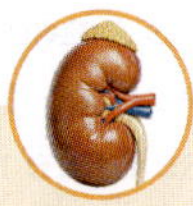

Prevention is always considered better than cure. Nationwide screening of people living with DKD remains the key to identifying and treating them before they develop further complications. An annual screening of people living with diabetes to evaluate their eGFR and assess their albuminuria has to be conducted across the nation.

SUMMARY

Diabetic nephropathy (DN) is a classic term that refers to specific functional and structural damages that can occur to the kidneys of people with diabetes. This term eventually evolved into a more generic term called diabetic kidney disease (DKD) due to the diversity and complexity involved in the pathogenesis of renal impairment among people living with diabetes. DKD is characterized by persistent albuminuria and a decreased estimated glomerular filtration rate (eGFR) <60 mL/min/1.73 m^2. Asians and Hispanics recorded the highest prevalence of microalbuminuria. In a resource-limited setting like India, it becomes imperative to initiate intervention to prevent complications and thereby improve the quality of life of people living with diabetes and CKD. There is an urgent need to tackle the disease in its early stages to prevent its progression to advanced stages, which in turn, can contribute to the substantial economic burden. An annual screening of people living with diabetes to evaluate their eGFR and their albuminuria must be conducted across the nation.

CONCLUSION

Diabetic kidney disease is a heterogeneous and multifactorial disease with a diverse and complex pathogenesis. It has a significant socioeconomic impact on the quality of life of the patients, which can prove catastrophic due to the devastating and debilitating conditions that can arise if not treated appropriately. It is thus imperative to establish cost-effective and multidirectional strategies to prevent the development as well as progression of DKD. Early diagnosis and initiation of the most appropriate treatment can help reduce the global burden of the disease. Despite initiatives by the government of India to establish hemodialysis units and the launch of the National Organ Transplant Program to promote and facilitate renal transplantation, the burden of the disease remains unprecedented. Thus, early screening, lifestyle modifications, and prompt treatment become the need of the hour to prevent or slow the development and progression of DKD.

TAKE HOME MESSAGES

- ❑ Diabetic kidney disease is an emerging major public health problem.
- ❑ The recent trends in urbanization, increase in life-expectancy along with the alarming increase in the number of people affected by diabetes globally can be attributed to the increasing prevalence of DKD across the globe.
- ❑ Screening and early initiation of treatment can alleviate the burden of the disease and help prevent complications.

REFERENCES

1. International Diabetes Federation. (2025). IDF Diabetes Atlas, 11th edition. Brussels, Belgium: 2025. [online] Available from https://www.diabetesatlas.org [Last accessed March 2026].

2. Anjana RM, Unnikrishnan R, Deepa M, Pradeepa R, Tandon N, Das AK, et al. ICMR-INDIAB Collaborative Study Group. Metabolic non-communicable disease health report of India: the ICMR-INDIAB national

cross-sectional study (ICMR-INDIAB-17). Lancet Diabetes Endocrinol. 2023;11(7):474-89.

3. Diabetesatlas.org. (2023). International Diabetes Federation Atlas reports 2023. [online] Available from https://diabetesatlas.org/idfawp/resource-files/2023/11/IDF1040-Atlas-Diabetes-and-Kidney-Disease-Report-V4.pdf [Last accessed March 2026].

4. Li H, Lu W, Wang A, Jiang H, Lyu J. Changing epidemiology of chronic kidney disease as a result of type 2 diabetes mellitus from 1990 to 2017: estimates from global burden of disease 2017. J Diabetes Investig. 2021;12(3):346-56.

5. Couser WG, Remuzzi G, Mendis S, Tonelli M. The contribution of chronic kidney disease to the global burden of major noncommunicable diseases. Kidney Int. 2011;80(12):1258-70.

6. Bharati J, Jha V, Levin A. The global kidney health atlas: Burden and opportunities to improve kidney health worldwide. Ann Nutr Metab. 2020;76 (Suppl 1):25-30.

7. Kidney Disease: Improving Global Outcomes Diabetes Work Group. KDIGO 2012 clinical practice guideline for the evaluation and management of chronic kidney disease. Kidney Int Suppl. 2013;3:1-150.

8. Martínez-Castelao A, Navarro-González JF, Górriz JL, De Alvaro F. The Concept and the Epidemiology of Diabetic Nephropathy Have Changed in Recent Years. J Clin Med. 2015;4(6):1207-16.

9. Piccoli GB, Grassi G, Cabiddu G, Nazha M, Roggero S, Capizzi I, et al. Diabetic Kidney Disease: A Syndrome Rather Than a Single Disease. Rev Diabet Stud. 2015;12(1-2):87-109.

10. De Boer IH, Caramori ML, Chan JCN, Heerspink HJ, Hurst C, Khunti K, et al. Executive summary of the 2020 KDIGO Diabetes Management in CKD Guideline: Evidence-based advances in monitoring and treatment. Kidney Int. 2020;98:839-48.

11. Angelika B, Jolanta M, Edyta Z. Cardiovascular risk in chronic kidney disease - what is new in the pathogenesis and treatment?. Postgrad Med. 2018;130.

12. Gheith O, Farouk N, Nampoory N, Halim MA, Al-Otaibi T. Diabetic kidney disease: world wide difference of prevalence and risk factors. J Nephropharmacol. 2015;5(1):49-56.

13. KDOQI clinical practice guidelines and clinical practice recommendations for diabetes and chronic kidney disease. Am J Kidney Dis. 2007;49:S12-S154.

14. Ritz E, Rychlik I, Locatelli F, Halimi S. End-stage renal failure in type 2 diabetes: a medical catastrophe of worldwide dimensions. Am J Kidney Dis. 1999;34:795-808.

15. Retnakaran R, Cull CA, Thorne KI, Adler AI, Holman RR. Risk factors for renal dysfunction in type 2 diabetes: UK Prospective diabetes study 74. Diabetes. 2006;55:1832-9.

16. Pavkov ME, Knowler WC, Bennett PH, Looker HC, Krakoff J, Nelson RG. Increasing incidence of proteinuria and declining incidence of end-stage renal disease in diabetic Pima Indians. Kidney Int. 2006;70:1840-6.

17. Adler AI, Stevens RJ, Manley SE, Bilous RW, Cull CA, Holman RR. Development and progression of nephropathy in type 2 diabetes: the United Kingdom Prospective Diabetes Study (UKPDS 64) Kidney Int. 2003;63:225-32.

18. Pavkov ME, Bennett PH, Knowler WC, Krakoff J, Sievers ML, Nelson RG. Effect of youth-onset type 2 diabetes mellitus on incidence of end-stage renal disease and mortality in young and middle-aged Pima Indians. JAMA. 2006;296:421-6.

19. Parving HH, Lewis JB, Ravid M, Remuzzi G, Hunsicker LG; DEMAND investigators. Prevalence and risk factors for microalbuminuria in a referred cohort of type II diabetic patients: a global perspective. Kidney Int. 2006;69(11):2057-63.

20. Yokoyama H, Sone H, Oishi M, Kawai K, Fukumoto Y, Kobayashi M. Japan Diabetes Clinical Data Management Study Group Prevalence of albuminuria and renal insufficiency and associated clinical factors in type 2 diabetes: the Japan Diabetes Clinical Data Management study (JDDM15). Nephrol Dial Transplant. 2009;24:1212-9.

21. Fu H, Liu S, Bastacky SI, Wang X, Tian XJ, Zhou D. Diabetic Kidney Diseases Revisited: A New Perspective for A New Era. Mol Metab. 2019;30:250-63.

22. Mani MK. Patterns of renal disease in indigenous populations in India. Nephrology. 1998;4:S4-7.

23. Collaboration GCKD. Global, regional, and national burden of chronic kidney disease, 1990-2017: a systematic analysis for the Global Burden of Disease Study 2017. Lancet 2020;395:709-33.

24. Anand S, Shivashankar R, Ali MK, Kondal D, Binukumar B, Montez-Rath ME, et al. Prevalence of chronic kidney disease in two major Indian cities and projections for associated cardiovascular disease. Kidney Intern. 2015;88(1)178-85.

25. Unnikrishnan R, Rema M, Pradeepa R, Deepa M, Shanthirani CS. Prevalence and Risk Factors of Diabetic Nephropathy in an Urban South Indian Population: The Chennai Urban Rural Epidemiology Study (CURES 45). Diabetes Care. 2007;30(8):2019-24.

26. Vijay V, Snehalatha C, Ramachandran A, Viswanathan M. Prevalence of proteinuria in non-insulin dependent diabetes. J Assoc Physicians India. 1994;42:792-4.

27. Viswanathan V, Tilak P, Kumpatla S. Risk factors associated with the development of overt

nephropathy in type 2 diabetes patients: a 12 years observational study. Indian J Med Res. 2012;136:46-53.

28. Mir SR, Bhat MH, Misgar RA, Bashir MI, Wani AI, Malik MI. Prevalence of microalbuminuria in newly diagnosed T2DM patients attending a tertiary care hospital in North India and its association with various risk factors. Int J Contemp Med Res. 2019;6:D9-D13.

29. Kanakamani J, Ammini AC, Gupta N, Dwivedi SN. Prevalence of microalbuminuria among patients with type 2 diabetes mellitus--a hospital-based study from north India. Diabetes Technol Ther. 2010;12:161-6.

30. Rajapurkar MM, John GT, Kirpalani AL, Abraham G, Agarwal SK, Almeida AF, et al. What do we know about chronic kidney disease in India: first report of the Indian CKD registry. BMC Nephrol. 2012;13:10.

31. Kumar A, Mazumdar A, Bhattacharjee AK, Gupta A, Dasgupta A, Sinha B, et al. Risk factors associated with Indian type 2 diabetes patients with chronic kidney disease: CITE study, a cross-sectional, real-world, observational study. BMC Nephrol. 2025;26(1):245.

32. Xie D, Ma T, Cui H, Li J, Zhang A, Sheng Z, et al. Global burden and influencing factors of chronic kidney disease due to type 2 diabetes in adults aged 20-59 years, 1990-2019. Sci Rep. 2023;13(1):20234.

33. Liyanage T, Ninomiya T, Jha V, Neal B, Patrice HM, Okpechi I, et al. Worldwide access to treatment for end-stage kidney disease: A systematic review. Lancet. 2015;385(9981):1975-82.

34. Thomas B. The Global Burden of Diabetic Kidney Disease: Time Trends and Gender Gaps. Curr Diab Rep. 2019;19(4):18.

35. Jha V, Al-Ghamdi SMG, Li G, Wu MS, Stafylas P, Retat L, et al. Global Economic Burden Associated with Chronic Kidney Disease: A Pragmatic Review of Medical Costs for the Inside CKD Research Programme. Adv Ther. 2023;40(10):4405-20.

36. Satyavani K, Kothandan H, Jayaraman M, Viswanathan V. Direct costs associated with chronic kidney disease among type 2 diabetic patients in India. Indian J Nephrol. 2014;24(3):141-7.

37. Ramachandran R, Jha V. Kidney transplantation is associated with catastrophic out of pocket expenditure in India. PLoS One. 2013;8:e67812.

38. Suja A, Anju R, Anju V, Neethu J, Peeyush P, Saraswathy R. Economic evaluation of end stage renal disease patients undergoing hemodialysis. J Pharm Bioallied Sci. 2012;4:107-11.

39. Ahlawat R, Tiwari P, D'Cruz S. Direct Cost for Treating Chronic Kidney Disease at an Outpatient Setting of a Tertiary Hospital: Evidence from a Cross-Sectional Study. Value Health Reg Issues. 2017;12:36-40.

40. Upadhye KS, Patidar H. Decoding Diabetic Kidney Disease: In-Depth Analysis of Prevalence, Risk Factors, Biomarkers, and Management Strategies. J Med Sci Health. 2024;10(2):204-12.

Key Research Takeaway

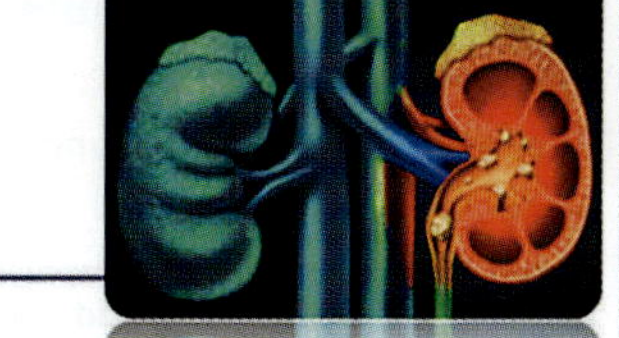

Original Article

Direct costs associated with chronic kidney disease among type 2 diabetic patients in India

K. Satyavani, H. Kothandan, M. Jayaraman, V. Viswanathan

Department of Diabetology, M.V. Hospital for Diabetes and Prof. M. Viswanathan Diabetes Research Centre (WHO Collaborating Centre for Research, Education and Training in Diabetes), Royapuram, Chennai, Tamil Nadu, India

ABSTRACT

The aim of this study was to estimate the direct costs of medical care among hospitalized type 2 diabetic patients with chronic kidney disease (CKD). A total of 209 (M:F, 133:76) patients were divided into groups based on the severity of kidney disease. Group 1 subjects had undergone renal transplantation ($n = 12$), group 2 was CKD patients on hemodialysis ($n = 45$), group 3 was patients with CKD, prior to end-stage renal disease (ESRD) ($n = 66$), and group 4 ($n = 86$) consisted of subjects without any complications. Details about expenditure per hospitalization, length of stay during admission, direct medical and nonmedical cost, expenditure for the previous two years, and source of bearing the expenditure were recorded in a questionnaire. Diabetic patients with CKD prior to ESRD spend more per hospitalization than patients without any complications. [Median □ 12,664 vs. 3,214]. The total median cost of CKD patients on hemodialysis was significantly higher than other CKD patients (INR 61,170 vs. 12,664). The median cost involved in kidney transplantation was □ 392,920. The total expenditure for hospital admissions in two years was significantly higher for dialysis than transplantation. Patients on hemodialysis or kidney transplantation tend to stay longer as inpatient admissions. The source of funds for the expenditure was mainly personal savings (46%). The expenditure on hospital admissions for CKD was considerably higher, and so, there is a need to develop a protocol on a cost-effective strategy for the treatment of CKD.

Nephrol Dial Transplant (1999) 14: 2805–2807

Type 2 diabetes and diabetic nephropathy in India— magnitude of the problem

Vijay Viswanathan

Diabetes Research Centre and M. V. Hospital for Diabetes, Madras, India

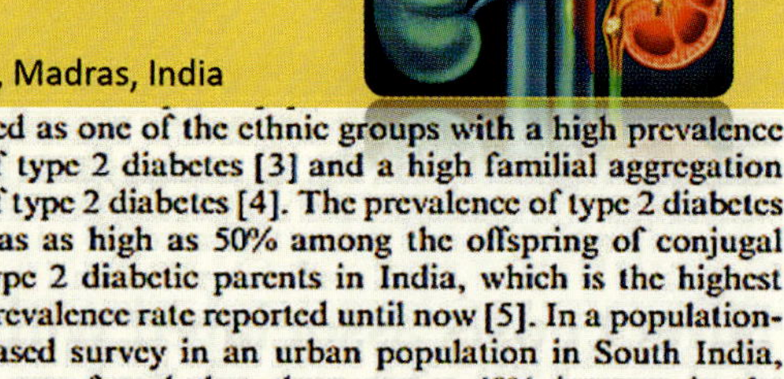

It has been predicted that world wide the prevalence of diabetes in adults would increase to 5.4% by the year 2025 from the prevalence rate of 4.0% in 1995. Consequently the number of adults with diabetes in the world would rise from 135 million in 1995 to 300 million in the year 2025 [1]. It is expected that much of this increase in prevalence rate will occur in developing countries. While a 42% increase is expected in developed countries, a 170% increase is expected in the developing countries. In the latter, most of the diabetic patients are in the age range of 45–64 years, while in developed countries most of them are $\geqslant 65$ years. Therefore diabetic patients in developing countries are even more vulnerable to develop the microvascular complications of diabetes including diabetic nephropathy.

Type 2 diabetes in Asian-Indians: differences from the West

Studies from the UK have found that type 2 diabetes is three to four times more common in South Asians

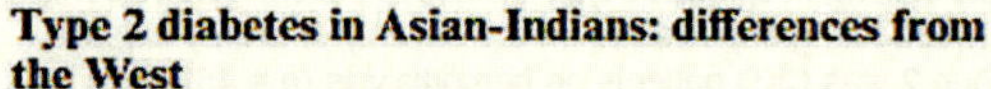

Correspondence and offprint requests to: Dr Vijay Viswanathan, Diabetes Research Centre, No. 4, Main Road, Royapuram, Madras, 600 013, India.

fied as one of the ethnic groups with a high prevalence of type 2 diabetes [3] and a high familial aggregation of type 2 diabetes [4]. The prevalence of type 2 diabetes was as high as 50% among the offspring of conjugal type 2 diabetic parents in India, which is the highest prevalence rate reported until now [5]. In a population-based survey in an urban population in South India, it was found that there was a 40% increase in the age—standardized prevalence of diabetes over a period of 6 years, from 8.2% in 1988–1989 to 11.6% in 1994–1995 [6].

High prevalence of maturity-onset diabetes of the young (MODY)

MODY refers to a type of non-insulin dependent diabetes in which the patients develop diabetes at <25 years of age and have clinical characteristics similar to type 2 diabetes. The prevalence of MODY in a cohort of 4560 patients was found to be 4.8% in South India [7].

Although the prevalence of obesity is less among Asian-Indians than Caucasians, the former have an increased upper body adiposity as measured by the waist to hip ratio (WHR) which is an independent risk factor for type 2 diabetes [8].

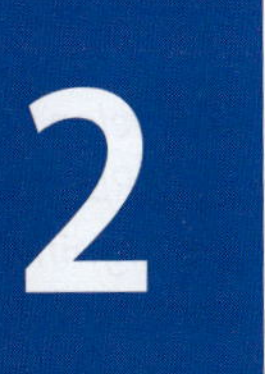

2

Pathogenesis and Risk Factors for the Development and Progression of Diabetic Kidney Disease

Satyavani Kumpatla

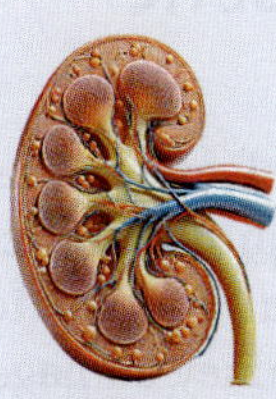

- ➤ Pathophysiology of DKD
- ➤ Risk factors of DKD
- ➤ Non-modifiable risk factors of DKD
- ➤ Modifiable risk factors of DKD
- ➤ Environmental risk factors of DKD
- ➤ Chronic kidney disease of unknown etiology

Abstract

Diabetic kidney disease (DKD) is one of the leading microvascular complications of type 2 diabetes mellitus (T2DM). Globally, it remains one of the principal causes of chronic kidney disease (CKD) and end-stage renal disease (ESRD). Around 30–40% of the people living with diabetes mellitus (DM) are affected by DKD. The structural and functional alterations in the kidneys can be attributed to four major factors, namely metabolic, hemodynamic, and inflammatory and fibrotic, which are involved in the development and progression of DKD. There is a complex interplay of metabolic disturbance, hemodynamic stress, chronic inflammation, and fibrosis. In people with T2DM, chronic hyperglycemia can trigger glomerular hypertrophy and hyperfiltration, which can cause inflammation and fibrosis through advanced glycation end products (AGEs) and oxidative stress. These factors can induce sclerotic changes in the kidneys and also cause a decline in their function. There are several modifiable and nonmodifiable risk factors involved in the onset and progression of CKD. Poor glycemic control, uncontrolled hypertension, dyslipidemia, obesity, and increased intake of salt or protein are the various modifiable risk factors. The nonmodifiable factors like genetic predisposition to CKD, age, and sex can also contribute to the risk of DKD. Thus, a comprehensive intervention that understands the multirisk profile of people with CKD and targets optimum glycemic and blood pressure (BP) control, along with lifestyle interventions like adequate salt and protein intake, weight reduction, and cessation of smoking, can play a crucial role in the early detection and management of people living with CKD and T2DM. These measures can delay the onset and the progression of DKD and also help prevent complications like ESRD.

Keywords: DKD, pathogenesis, risk factors, type 2 diabetes mellitus, ESRD.

INTRODUCTION

The recently released International Diabetes Federation (IDF) Diabetes Atlas confirms that diabetes mellitus (DM) is one of the fastest-growing global health emergencies of the 21st century. In 2024, it was estimated that 589 million adults aged 20–79 years were living with DM and it is projected to reach 853 million by 2050. It is estimated that 95% of the increase in the number of people with DM by 2050 will occur in low- and middle-income countries. India ranks second in terms of DM burden, with 89.8 million living with DM in 2024 and is expected to rise to 156.7 million in 2050.[1] Nearly 30–40% of people with DM will develop diabetic kidney disease (DKD).[2] DKD accounts for about 50% of cases of end-stage renal disease (ESRD) and is the leading cause of death among people living with type 2 diabetes mellitus (T2DM).[3,4] The impact of DM and its complications, such as DKD, leads to a huge economic burden on society in a developing country like India. The direct healthcare costs of hospital admissions for treating chronic kidney disease (CKD) are considerably greater than for those without any complications.[5]

The global upsurge in this disease is mainly due to the increase in the prevalence of traditional risk factors associated with its development, including DM, hypertension, and obesity.[6,7] The concept of "diabetic nephropathy" (DN), defined by a rise in urinary albumin excretion followed by a progressive decline in renal function and traditionally classified in five stages,[8] has been changed to the term "diabetic kidney disease", including all possible renal abnormalities occurring in DM.[9] A comprehensive approach to managing DKD depends on modifying and reducing risk factors, such as combining targeted therapies for hyperglycemia, hypertension, albuminuria, and hyperlipidemia, as well as utilizing renoprotective agents.[10] Identification and efficient management of these modifiable risk factors may improve the prognosis of people with DM at risk of developing DKD. This chapter explores the pathophysiology and risk factors associated with the development and progression of DKD and the latest research on how T2DM might increase the risk of developing DKD.

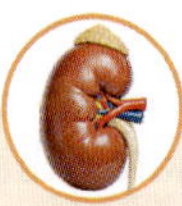

- *India ranks second in DM burden, with 89.8 million cases in 2024, projected to rise to 156.7 million by 2050.*

- *Around 30–40% of people with DM develop DKD, which accounts for nearly 50% of ESRD and is a major cause of death, posing a significant economic burden in developing countries.*
- *The rising rates of DKD are driven by the increasing prevalence of DM, hypertension, and obesity.*
- *The term "diabetic nephropathy" has now been replaced by "diabetic kidney disease", which encompasses all renal abnormalities associated with DM.*

PATHOPHYSIOLOGY OF DIABETIC KIDNEY DISEASE

The pathophysiology of DKD involves various pathological pathways, like hemodynamic, metabolic, and inflammatory and fibrotic pathways that lead to progressive kidney damage and finally ESRD. These pathways produce lesions in the glomeruli, tubuli, interstitium, and vasculature of the kidneys. A series of molecules, receptors, enzymes, and transcription factors are involved in the early stages of kidney disease and later lead to an enlarged kidney with hypertrophy, expanded extracellular matrix, glomerulosclerosis, vascular hyalinosis, interstitial fibrosis, tubular atrophy, and loss of function leading to ESRD. In the pathogenesis of DKD, severe hyperglycemia initiates the changes in the kidney. Uncontrolled levels of blood glucose lead to hyperfiltration, which is followed by metabolic, hormonal, hemodynamic, inflammatory, and epigenetic modifications. The above alterations lead to podocyte injury, glomerulosclerosis, mitochondrial injury, and tubular atrophy.

Metabolic Pathway

The metabolic pathway includes the polyol pathway, hexosamine pathway, advanced glycation end products (AGEs), and protein kinase C (PKC) pathway.[11] The central pathological event in DKD is chronic hyperglycemia, which initiates a cascade of molecular and cellular dysfunction. Hyperglycemia-induced kidney damage mediates through the hemodynamic pathway by enhancing the formation of AGEs, PKC activation, and diacylglycerol synthesis.[12] Activation of each of these pathways can cause injury to the kidneys. Additionally, AGEs have been demonstrated to bind to the membrane receptor RAGE, causing oxidative stress, inflammation, and an increase in reactive oxygen species (ROS) formation induced by hyperglycemia through activation of the electron transport chain, considered as the initiators in the development of DM complications.[13] Hyperglycemia undoubtedly plays a central role; hyperinsulinemia and insulin resistance also may initiate pathogenic mechanisms. Hyperglycemia can induce damage in the cells by the activation of the polyol pathway through the enzyme aldose reductase within the cells. The rate-limiting enzyme glutamine fructose-6-phosphate amidotransferase in the hexosamine pathway is expressed in the glomerulus, suggesting a pathophysiological role. This pathway requires

higher transforming growth factor 1 (TGF-1) expression and stronger PKC activation. In DM, diacylglycerol (DAG) production is increased and can lead to activation of the PKC pathway. PKC can also be activated by ROS and AGEs. The metabolic pathway involved in the pathogenesis of DKD is depicted in the **Flowchart 1**.

Hemodynamic Pathway

Hemodynamic pathway involves glomerular hyperfiltration and hypertension caused by the imbalance between the afferent and efferent arterioles. Hyperfiltration is present in the early stages of DM. Intraglomerular pressure can increase either by an increase in efferent arteriolar tone or a reduction in afferent arteriolar tone. Increase in efferent arteriolar resistance can result from an increase in the concentration of angiotensin II, endothelin 1, and ROS. Reduction

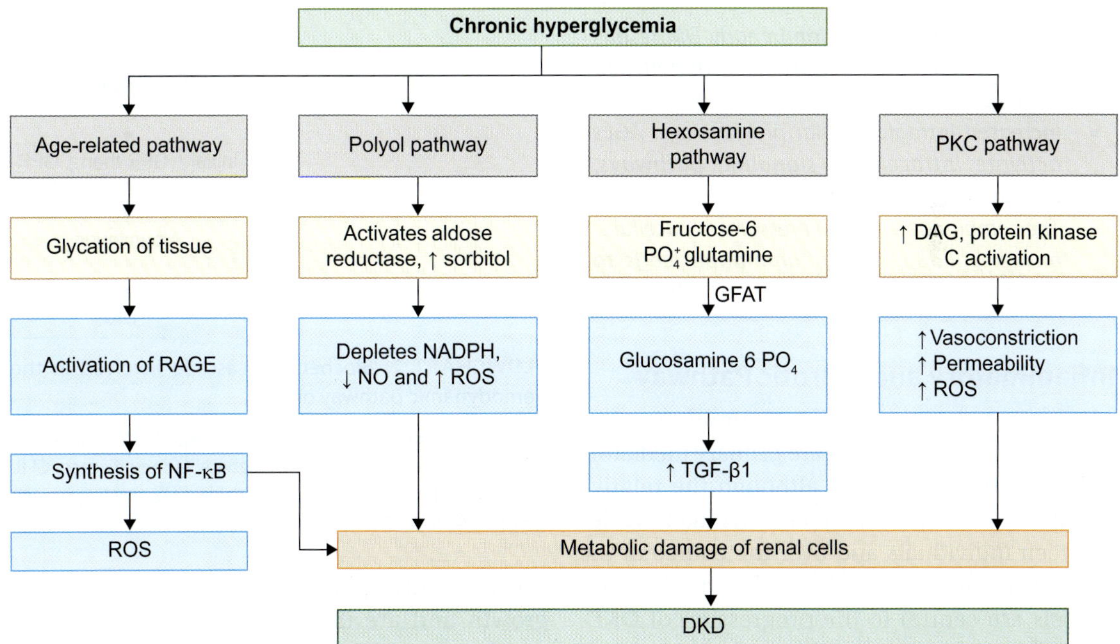

FLOWCHART 1: Metabolic pathway involved in DKD.

(AGE: advanced glycation end products; DAG: diacylglycerol; DKD: diabetic kidney disease; GFAT: glutamine:fructose-6-phosphate amidotransferase; NADPH: nicotinamide adenine dinucleotide phosphate hydrogen; NF-κB: nuclear factor kappa B; NO: nitric oxide; PKC: protein kinase C; PO_4: phosphate; RAGE: receptor for advanced glycation end products; ROS: reactive oxygen species; TGF-β1: transforming growth factor beta 1)

in afferent arteriolar resistance can occur by a reduction in nitric oxide bioavailability. Insulin also reduces afferent arteriolar tone directly and causes hyperfiltration.[14,15] The increased pressure and AGEs activate intracellular signaling molecules. The combination of increased pressure, extracellular matrix deposition in the glomerulus, tubulointerstitium, and inflammation causes structural damage leading to DKD. The hemodynamic pathway is diagrammatically represented in **Flowchart 2**.

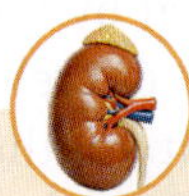

- *Key metabolic pathways involved in DKD: Polyol pathway, hexosamine pathway, AGEs pathway, and PKC pathway.*
- *Hyperglycemia leads to kidney damage through hemodynamic changes and increased AGEs formation, PKC activation, and DAG synthesis.*
- *Activation of these pathways contributes to kidney injury.*
- *Glomerular hyperfiltration in early DM results from an imbalance between afferent and efferent arteriolar tone.*
- *Increased intraglomerular pressure and AGEs activate intracellular signaling pathways, contributing to kidney injury.*
- *The combination of high pressure, extracellular matrix buildup, and inflammation leads to structural damage and progression to DKD.*

Inflammatory and Fibrotic Pathway

Alterations in glomerular hemodynamics, inflammation, and fibrosis are primary mediators of kidney tissue damage, although the relative contribution of these mechanisms likely varies between individuals and over the course of the natural history of DKD.[14,16] Inflammation and fibrosis are central to the progression of DKD, contributing to irreversible kidney damage. Vascular endothelial growth factor (VEGF) is triggered early and promotes vascular expansion, which may contribute to hyaline arteriosclerosis and hypertension-related kidney changes.[17]

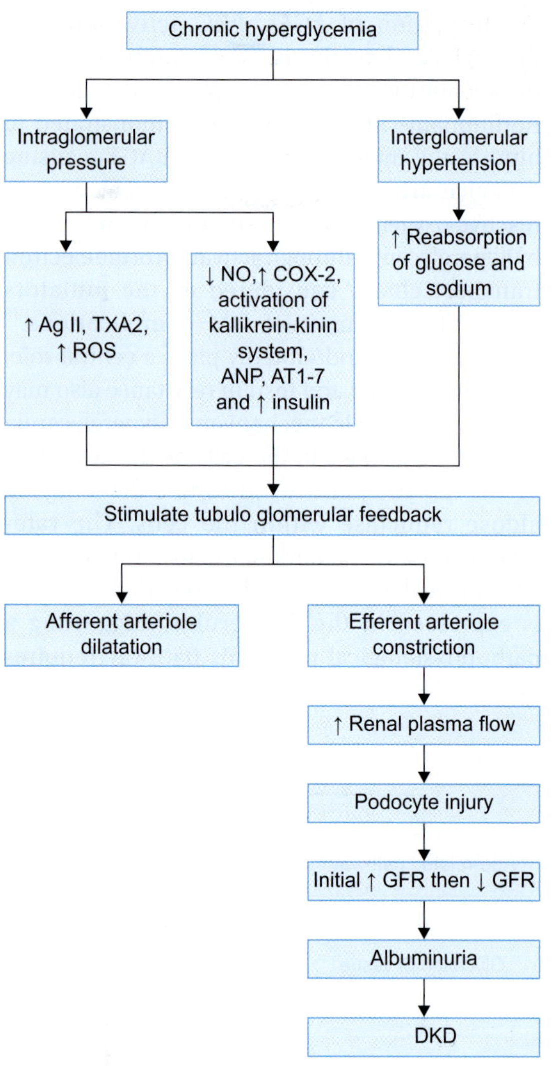

FLOWCHART 2: Biochemical cascade involved in the hemodynamic pathway of DKD.

(Ag II: angiotensin II; ANP: atrial natriuretic peptide; AT: angiotensin; COX-2: cyclooxygenase-2; DKD: diabetic kidney disease; GFR: glomerular filtration rate; NO: nitric oxide; ROS: reactive oxygen species; TXA2: thromboxane A2)

Likewise, angiopoietins can stimulate vascular growth and are thought to play a role in the development of DKD.[18] A strong association exists between the extent of macrophage infiltration and the later development of tubulointerstitial fibrosis, ultimately contributing to the progression of DKD.[19,20] ROS, angiotensin II, and activation of mineralocorticoid receptors (MRs) drive macrophages toward a proinflammatory M1 phenotype. These activated macrophages release profibrotic cytokines that enhance cellular proliferation, increase extracellular matrix accumulation, and promote fibrotic changes. At the molecular level, fibrosis is partly mediated through the activation of TGF-β1, which exerts two synergistic effects: Stimulation of connective tissue growth factor (CTGF) and suppression of matrix metalloproteinases (MMPs). Therefore, macrophages play a central role in the pathogenesis of DKD.[21]

In addition, these changes result in glomerular hyperfiltration, glomerular hypertension, renal hypertrophy, and altered glomerular composition, which is manifested clinically as albuminuria and hypertension.[11] Pathologically, the kidneys undergo several changes, including deposition of extracellular matrix, glomerular basement membrane thickening, proliferative changes, and tubular atrophy, ultimately resulting in interstitial fibrosis, and glomerulosclerosis (the final common pathway of many kidney diseases). Inflammation and fibrosis may also promote the progression of DKD and may result in acute kidney injury (AKI). Macrophage infiltration is common in AKI. AKI plays an important role in the progression of DKD. Frąk et al. outlined the new insights on the pathophysiology of DKD, which enhanced the understanding of molecular mechanisms of CKD. The latest information discussed was on oxidative stress, inflammation, neutrophil gelatinase-related lipocalin, MMPs, and uremic toxins.[22] Inflammation and the accumulation of uremic toxins may contribute to the risk of developing abnormalities in the skeletal muscle, such as sarcopenia.[23] The current understanding of obesity-related kidney disease pathogenesis includes nonpharmacological and pharmacological options such as sodium-glucose cotransporter-2 (SGLT2) inhibitors, nonsteroidal MR antagonists, and glucagon-like peptide 1 (GLP-1) analogs.[24] The inflammatory and fibrotic pathway involved in the pathophysiology of DKD is represented in **Flowchart 3**.

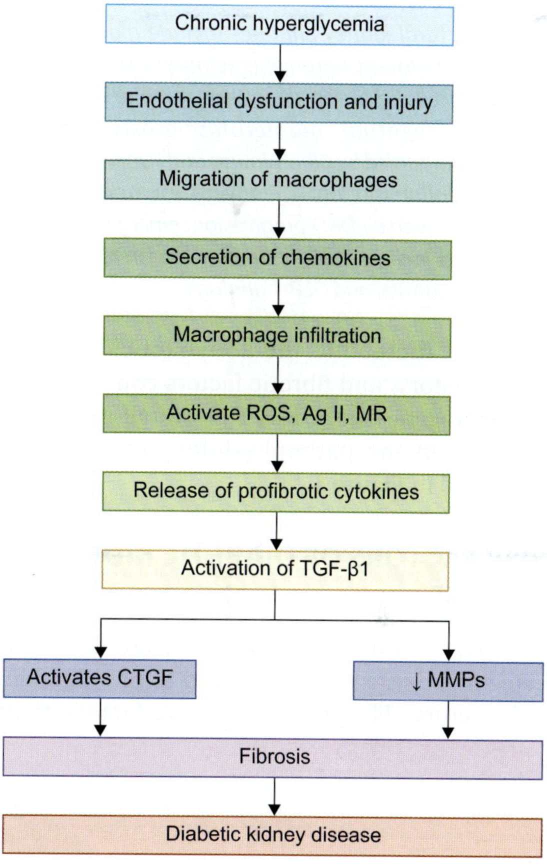

FLOWCHART 3: Schematic representation of inflammatory and fibrotic pathway of DKD.

(Ag: angiotensin; CTGF: connective tissue growth factor; MMPs: matrix metalloproteinases; MR: mineralocorticoid receptor; ROS: reactive oxygen species; TGF-β1: transforming growth factor beta 1)

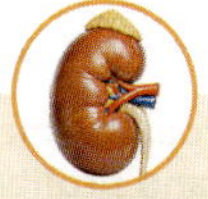

- *Early vascular mediators like VEGF and angiopoietins promote abnormal vascular growth, contributing to arteriosclerosis, hypertension, and DKD progression.*
- *Macrophage infiltration strongly correlates with tubulointerstitial fibrosis; ROS, angiotensin II, and MR activation push macrophages into a proinflammatory M1 phenotype that drives fibrosis via TGF-β1, CTGF, and decrease in MMPs.*

- *Structural kidney changes include glomerular hyperfiltration, basement membrane thickening, extracellular matrix deposition, tubular atrophy, and eventual glomerulosclerosis—often accompanied by albuminuria and hypertension.*
- *AKI, inflammation, oxidative stress, and uremic toxins worsen DKD progression; emerging treatments include SGLT2 inhibitors, nonsteroidal MR antagonists, and GLP-1 analogs.*

Thus, metabolic, hemodynamic, growth, inflammatory, and fibrotic factors contribute to the pathogenesis of DKD. The overall pathways involved in the pathophysiology of DKD are illustrated in **Figure 1**.

RISK FACTORS OF DIABETIC KIDNEY DISEASE

The risk factors of DKD can be broadly categorized into modifiable and nonmodifiable risk factors. The modifiable risk factors that contribute to the development and progression of DKD include uncontrolled DM, hypertension, obesity, proteinuria, dyslipidemia, dietary salt intake, and smoking whereas the nonmodifiable risk factors include age, sex, genetic factors, duration of DM and environmental factors such as pollution[25,26] are addressed in this chapter. The nonmodifiable and modifiable risk factors of DKD are diagrammatically represented in **Figure 2**.

NON-MODIFIABLE RISK FACTORS OF DIABETIC KIDNEY DISEASE

Age

Age is the most important nonmodifiable risk factor. With increasing age, several physiological and pathophysiological changes occur, including alterations in renal structure and function. A decline in renal mass, a reduced number of nephrons, and impaired renal blood flow are the common changes that can contribute to

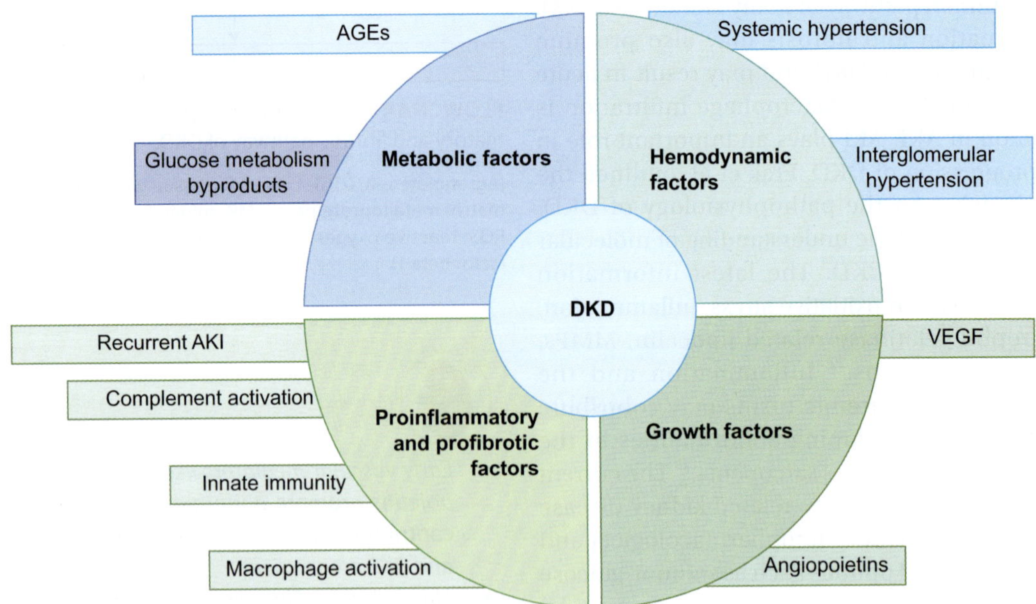

FIG. 1: Mechanistic overview of various pathways involved in the pathogenesis of DKD.

(AGE: advanced glycation end products; AKI: acute kidney injury; DKD: diabetic kidney disease; VEGF: vascular endothelial growth factor)

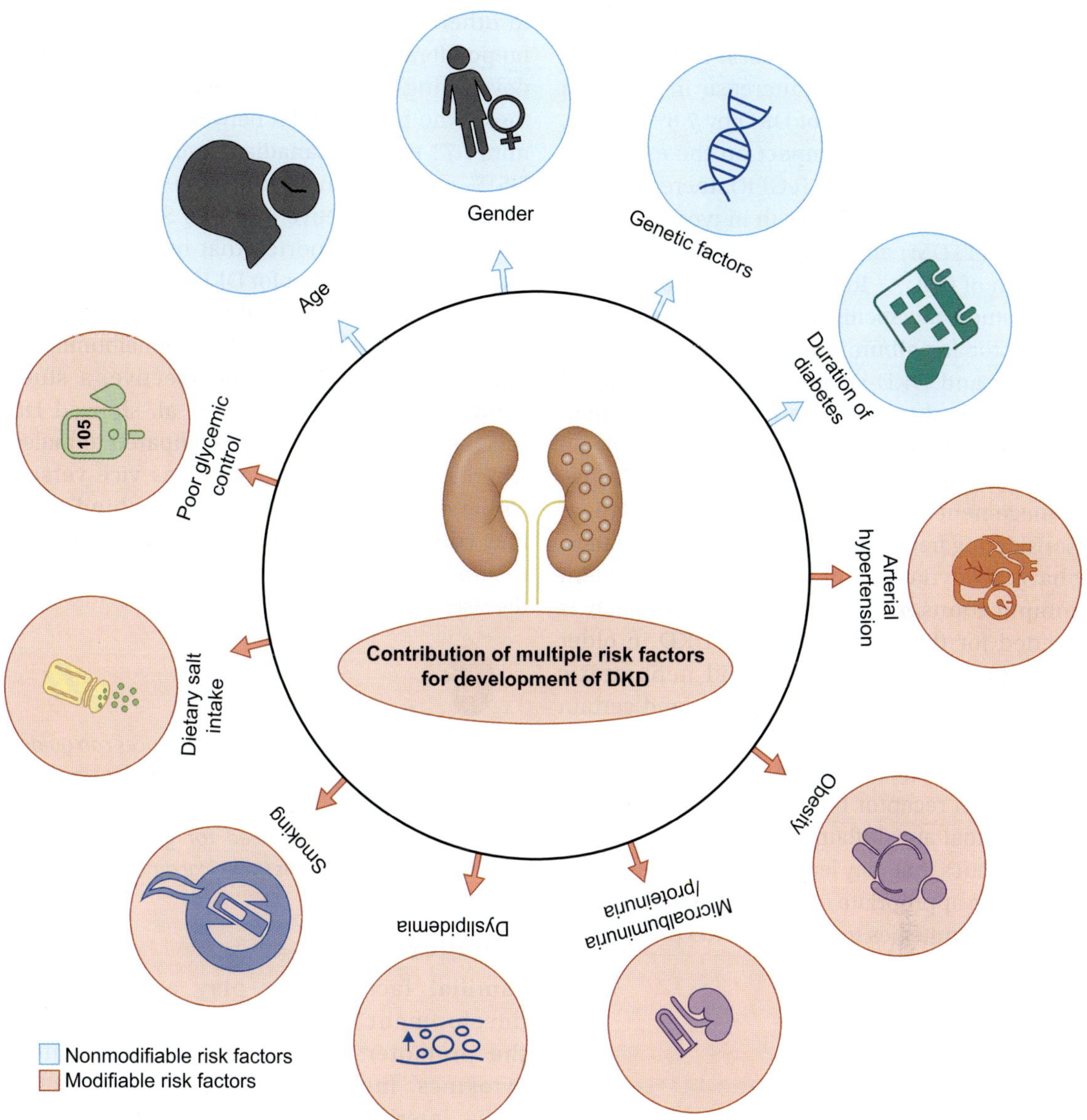

FIG. 2: Diagrammatic representation of nonmodifiable and modifiable risk factors of DKD.

the development and progression of DKD. Additionally, aging is associated with increased susceptibility to oxidative stress, inflammation, and fibrosis, all of which are implicated in the pathogenesis of DKD.[27] This, in turn, can cause increase in glomerular pressure, proteinuria, making it prone to increased risk of renal injury.

In the process of aging, cellular senescence has been implicated in the progression of DKD.[28] The accumulation of senescent cells releases proinflammatory cytokines, which can lead to tissue fibrosis. This senescence-associated secretory phenotype may exacerbate inflammation and promote the transformation of healthy tissue to fibrotic tissue. Thus, aging is often accompanied by several alterations in metabolic pathways. An increase in age by a year increased the odds of DKD by 7.8%.[29] Thus, advancing age has an impact on the estimated glomerular filtration rate (eGFR). Increasing age increases the risk of DKD both in type 1 diabetes mellitus (T1DM) and T2DM, irrespective of the duration of DM.[30,31] In an Australian population-based study, advancing age was an independent risk factor for albuminuria.[32] Both age-related changes and DKD-specific risk factors should be considered to optimize favorable treatment outcomes. There is limited evidence available on the guidelines and recommendations for effective management of DKD in the elderly population. Considering frailty, quality of life, life expectancy, pharmacodynamics of drugs, and treatment complications, a comprehensive approach is needed for the management of DKD in older individuals. It is better to avoid nephrotoxic antibiotics, radiocontrast exposure, and certain medication combinations, including angiotensin-converting enzyme inhibitors (ACEis) and angiotensin receptor blockers (ARBs), as well as nonsteroidal anti-inflammatory drugs (NSAIDs) and diuretics that may lead to AKI.[33] It is essential to develop appropriate interventions and specific treatment strategies to mitigate DKD progression in the aging population.

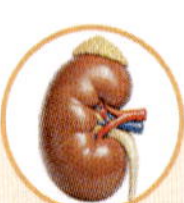

- *Aging is often accompanied by several alterations in metabolic pathways and advancing age is an independent risk factor for DKD.*
- *Appropriate interventions and specific treatment strategies are required to mitigate DKD progression in the aging population.*

Gender

Sex was reported as a risk factor for DKD, and it was found that men are more susceptible to DKD than women in T1DM and T2DM,[34] in contrast to other studies, which failed to show a male preponderance.[29] The lifetime risk of an individual developing ESRD was higher in men among those who had an eGFR between 44 and 59 mL/min/1.73 m^2 in a Canadian study. The risk was 7.51% in men compared to 3.21% in women.[35] In the UK Prospective Diabetes Study (UKPDS) 74 study, it was reported that male sex was an independent risk factor for DKD, as they follow an albuminuric pathway to a decline in eGFR, where females are more likely to follow a nonalbuminuric pathway.[36] In an Indian perspective, a study conducted by Viswanathan et al. showed DN was higher in females when compared to males, whereas the disease severity was vice versa.[37] Understanding the mechanisms behind these may contribute to personalized and sex-specific treatment for diabetic micro- and macrovascular diseases.

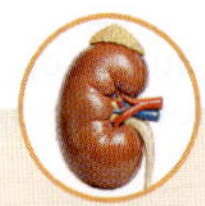

- *Understanding sex-specific differences can guide personalized treatment strategies for treating DKD.*
- *It emphasizes the need for gender-specific monitoring protocols in clinical practice.*

Genetic Factors

Familial factors may play a role in the development of DKD. Polymorphism in the promoter regions of the inflammatory cytokines, including tumor necrosis factor-alpha, interleukin 6, and interleukin-1β, along with changes in their production, has been linked to DKD susceptibility. Genes encoding the cytokines, ACE, proteins, and angiotensin II receptor participate in the metabolism. Evidence has suggested that polymorphism in the gene for the ACE contributes to either predisposing to nephropathy or accelerating its course. A South Indian study showed that a positive association exists between the D allele (ID and DD genotype) of the ACE polymorphism and proteinuria in people with T2DM.[38]

A familial aggregation study conducted in the South Indian population of T2DM with DN suggests that proteinuria was present in 50% and microalbuminuria in 26.7% of the diabetic siblings of probands with DN, in contrast to 0% and 3.3% among diabetic siblings of probands with normoalbuminuria, respectively.[39] It is clear that there are genetic factors involved in the risk of DKD. Many family-based linkage studies to identify a biological candidate gene for DKD have been performed.[40] Seaquist et al. showed that siblings of patients with T1DM who also had DM have a four-fold greater chance of developing DKD.[41] Freedman et al. have also shown that ESRD is five times higher in relatives of patients with T2DM with ESRD.[42] These observations alone do not prove a genetic contribution to DKD but may illustrate a socioeconomic/cultural clustering. However, several investigators employing molecular genetic techniques have performed linkage analyses to explain the vulnerability for DKD. In addition, genes associated with many modifiable factors may also play a promising role in the background of DKD predisposition. Parental history of hypertension, T2DM, cardiovascular disease (CVD), and insulin resistance appears to be a risk factor for DKD, suggesting that DKD may be linked by a complex interrelated genetic predisposition.[43,44]

Epigenetics

In recent times, epigenome-wide association studies have shown that specific deoxyribonucleic acid (DNA) methylation markers can predict the development and progression of DKD.[45] The epigenetic processes, such as histone changes, noncoding ribonucleic acid (RNA) and DNA methylation, might be crucial in the development of DKD. DKD can be attributed to epigenetic alterations caused by extrinsic and internal stimuli that can change the phenotype of the cell.[46] The DNA methylation mechanism of epigenetic regulation has been linked to DKD. The variations in DNA methylation act as biomarkers to predict the development and progression of DKD.[47] The

epigenetic modifications in histone methylation also lead to DKD. Epigenetic alterations, including aberrant DNA methylation of nuclear factor erythroid 2-related factor 2 (Nrf2) and alterations in histone modifications, are likely to play a major role in the progression of DN. A very recent South Indian expression study found that as the disease progresses, the expression of Nrf2, and its downstream targets is reduced gradually in individuals diagnosed with DKD. Epigenetic markers such as histone deacetylases and DNA methyltransferase are associated with Nrf2 regulation. This study provided evidence on the association between histone deacetylases and Nrf2 in the pathogenesis of DKD, shedding light on potential therapeutic targets.[48] Therefore, it is essential to elucidate the role of these epigenetic markers in DKD, paving the way to develop novel therapeutic strategies to combat DKD pathogenesis.

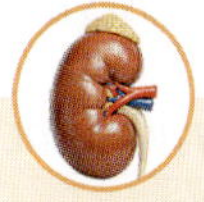

- *Familial factors may play a role in the development of DKD.*
- *DKD may be linked to a complex interrelated genetic predisposition.*
- *Epigenome-wide association studies have shown that specific DNA methylation markers can predict the development and progression of DKD.*

Duration of Diabetes Mellitus

The most important risk factor associated with DKD is having DM for a longer period. Individuals with DM for over 10 years are at significantly increased risk of developing DKD. In a 12-year observational study from India, it was reported that people with uncontrolled DM and an increase in blood pressure (BP) are at high risk of developing DN. Longer duration of DM emerged as a significant risk factor for the progression of DKD. Age, elevated BP, and presence of retinopathy are also associated with the progression of DN.[49] The Korean National Health and Nutrition Examination survey data reported that individuals with DM lasting >10 years or with glycated hemoglobin (HbA1c) of >8% had a higher risk of DKD. The adjusted odds ratio for DKD was 3.77 and 4.91 in people with DM lasting >20 years and HbA1c > 10%, respectively.[50] A cross-sectional study in T2DM patients reported that those with DM duration ≥15 years had 1.75-fold higher odds of being in a "high/very high" risk category for DKD progression,[51] whereas another observational study conducted among South Asian individuals with DM reported that 47.25% of them with a longer duration of DM were at an increased risk of DN.[52] Hence, a longer duration of DM is consistently associated with a higher risk of DKD.

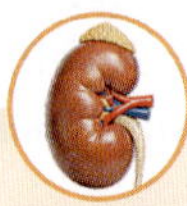

- *Longer duration of DM significantly increases the risk of developing DKD.*
- *Studies show prolonged DM is a strong predictor of nephropathy and DKD progression.*

MODIFIABLE RISK FACTORS OF DIABETIC KIDNEY DISEASE

Poor Glycemic Control

Poor glycemic control is a major and independent risk factor for the development and progression of DKD. The cellular mechanisms responsible for hyperglycemia-mediated renal damage include AGEs and activation of their receptor (RAGE). In addition, RAGE activation induces glomerular matrix production and increased oxidative stress. Also, there is a strong association between insulin resistance and DKD in the Indian population with T2DM.[51,53] Chronic hyperglycemia leads to glomerular hyperfiltration, thickening of the glomerular basement membrane, endothelial dysfunction, onset of albuminuria, progression to CKD, and eventually to ESRD.

Strict glucose control has been clearly shown to reduce the incidence of micro or macroalbuminuria and also slow GFR decline. Intensive glucose-lowering therapy in the DCCT trial significantly reduced the development of microalbuminuria by 36% and the EDIC (Epidemiology of Diabetes Intervention and Complication) study indicated that intensive DM therapy reduced the risk of impaired GFR by 50%.[54] Evidence also shows that glomerular hyperfiltration serves as an early predictor of microalbuminuria and overt proteinuria, both of which can be mitigated through improved glycemic regulation.[55] Another landmark trial (ADVANCE TRIAL)[56] showed that intensive glucose control can reduce the development of microalbuminuria and macroalbuminuria. Thus, maintaining stringent glycemic control, with an HbA1c target of <7.0% is recommended for adults with DM.[57] According to Kidney Disease: Improving Global Outcomes (KDIGO) recommendations, HbA1c targets for individuals with DKD who are not on dialysis should be personalized, typically within the range of <6.5–<8%, based on factors such as existing comorbidities, the stage of CKD, expected survival, and the risk of hypoglycemia.[58]

Therefore, maintaining the blood glucose levels within the target range can prevent or decrease disease progression. Intensified control of blood glucose is a cornerstone in the effort to delay the onset and progression of albuminuria and decreased eGFR.

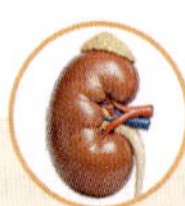

- *Poor glycemic control accelerates DKD through AGE–RAGE activation, oxidative stress, and insulin resistance.*
- *Tight glucose control significantly reduces microalbuminuria, proteinuria, and GFR decline in both T1DM and T2DM.*
- *Major trials have shown that intensive glycemic control lowers DKD risk.*

Arterial Hypertension

Uncontrolled BP can significantly increase the risk of DKD progressing to ESRD, CVD, and mortality.[59] The exact mechanism by which hypertension enhances the progression of DKD is not fully understood. However, it is widely accepted that management of hypertension is crucial to prevent or delay the progression of DKD. Many clinical trials in T1DM and T2DM have confirmed that reducing BP is associated with decreased progression to DKD. The Appropriate Blood Pressure Control in Diabetes (ABCD) trial[60] found a significant reduction in the development of microalbuminuria in normotensive but not in people with hypertensive T2DM, whereas the ADVANCE trial in T1DM highlighted that the systolic BP was found to be independently associated with the renal outcome.[61] In T2DM, lowering of BP was found to retard the onset and progression of DKD, independent of the antihypertensive agents used. Antihypertensive agents such as ACEi and ARBs are widely used for effectively lowering BP and for reducing proteinuria.[62] ACEis are considered the standard of care for delaying the progression of CKD.[63]

Several placebo-controlled trials have analyzed the risks and benefits of intense BP management in DM patients with diagnosed hypertension. Many studies have shown that intensive control of BP is associated with delayed albuminuria as well as decreased rates of serious extrarenal cardiac events.[64,65] Two landmark studies in people with T2DM—the UKPDS and the ABCD trial[66,67] demonstrated that intensive BP management offers clear advantages over less stringent control. Both studies showed that strict BP regulation significantly reduced the incidence of microalbuminuria in these patients. Nocturnal hypertension, defined as night-time BP above the goal, is another significant component of hypertension in CKD. The alterations in the circadian BP represent a stronger predictor of poor cardiorenal outcomes.[68] KDIGO guideline for patients with DKD suggests a target systolic BP of <120 mm Hg.[69] Hence, strict BP control is a key aspect of care to prevent DKD.

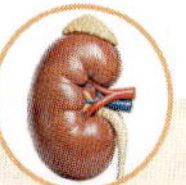

- *Uncontrolled BP accelerates the progression of DKD, CVD, and mortality.*
- *Intensive BP control lowers the risk of albuminuria and cardiovascular events and is crucial to delaying DKD progression.*
- *Nocturnal hypertension predicts poor cardiorenal outcomes.*
- *ACEis and ARBs lower BP, reduce proteinuria, and slow DKD progression.*

Obesity

Obesity is another important risk factor and there is documented evidence that obesity is associated with the development and progression of DKD and ESRD.[70] A strong association between DKD and obesity causes proteinuria, glomerular hypertrophy, and injury.[71] Two pathogenic mechanisms are involved in kidney injury in obesity. Direct mechanisms include hemodynamic and hormonal changes, which lead to glomerular hyperperfusion, i.e., increased renal plasma flow and glomerular hyperfiltration, which is evident from increased GFR. Increased glomerular capillary pressure subsequently leads to increased urinary albumin excretion, followed by proteinuria and declining GFR.[72] Increased body mass index (BMI) impairs kidney function through several mechanisms. Hemodynamic changes induced by obesity, cardiac output, and blood volume have an impact on the renal circulation. Obesity is commonly related to dyslipidemia; higher levels of triglyceride (TG) and low-density lipoprotein (LDL) cholesterol can also cause kidney damage as the accumulation of lipids damages the podocytes of tubular cells.[70] Ghrelin also plays a key role in renal pathology as it relates to obesity. The effect of ghrelin varies; it may act against oxidative stress, inflammation, renal fibrosis, or obstructive nephropathy, or it may stimulate glomerulosclerosis, interstitial fibrosis, podocyte damage, or increase angiotensin II-induced hypertension.[73] To prevent obesity-related DKD, weight reduction appears to be the most effective strategy.

A study conducted on a large and diverse population in the United States showed that the risk of DKD was directly proportional to the BMI; those who had severe obesity were found to have a seven times higher risk of DKD than the group of people with a normal BMI.[74] Similarly, Viswanathan et al., in a very recent study conducted among people with T2DM, found that increased BMI was independently associated with DKD. Those who were overweight and obese are four to five times at risk for DKD progression. It was suggested that lifestyle interventions and weight-lowering drugs may reduce the serious implications of obesity in individuals with T2DM and DKD.[75] In the Framingham Heart Study, it was observed that abdominal obesity is a more reliable predictor of CKD development than BMI.[76] Many observational studies have proved that weight loss is associated with a significant reduction in proteinuria and an improvement in eGFR. A systematic review and meta-analysis found that weight loss interventions, including dietary modification, physical activity, and bariatric surgery, were associated with significant improvements in the eGFR and proteinuria in people with DKD.[77]

Sodium-glucose cotransporter-2 inhibitors demonstrated renal protective effects, and GLP-1 receptor agonists target metabolic risk factors and improve renal outcomes. Drugs like SGLT2 inhibitors and GLP-1 receptor agonists (GLP-1 RAs), the new classes of glucose-lowering drugs, have shown benefits in reducing body weight and also in managing DKD and heart failure. Studies have shown that dapagliflozin, empagliflozin, and canagliflozin have consistent and biologically plausible class effects on cardiorenal outcomes in people with DM.[78] These agents are widely used to treat patients with DKD and CVDs. Thus, SGLT2 inhibitors reduce the progression of DKD and diminish the probability of heart failure and mortality in people with both DKD and T2DM. The Food and Drug Administration (FDA) approved GLP-1 RAs liraglutide and semaglutide for weight loss. The nephroprotective properties of subcutaneous once-weekly semaglutide in patients with advanced DKD were demonstrated in the FLOW trial.[79] Therefore, it is time to encourage the use of these drugs to improve cardiorenal outcomes and to prevent adverse complications. Weight loss was associated with significant improvement in the eGFR and proteinuria and weight loss should be gradual and sustainable.

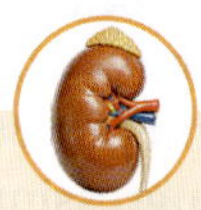

- *The central pathological event in DKD is chronic hyperglycemia, which initiates a cascade of molecular and cellular dysfunction.*
- *Progression of DKD involves inflammation, fibrosis, and altered glomerular dynamics (like hyperfiltration and hypertension), ultimately resulting in structural kidney changes such as glomerulosclerosis and interstitial fibrosis.*
- *Understanding of various pathological pathways of DKD will lead to the development of targeted therapies.*
- *Overweight and obese individuals are four to five times at risk for DKD progression.*
- *Targeted pharmacological therapies to treat DM in overweight and obese individuals provide better renal outcomes.*

Microalbuminuria/Proteinuria

Microalbuminuria is an important early indicator of DKD, as it reflects initial injury to the kidneys in people with DM. It serves as an early warning sign of worsening renal function and is strongly linked to the future development of overt proteinuria and ultimately, ESRD. Beyond signaling kidney involvement, microalbuminuria also represents systemic vascular damage, making it a significant predictor of CVD. Thus, its presence highlights both early glomerular injury and an elevated risk of broader vascular complications. Both KDIGO 2024 and the American Diabetes Association (ADA) 2025 Standards of Care emphasize the importance of classifying albuminuria and regularly monitoring kidney function for early detection of DKD. Albuminuria is categorized using the urine albumin–creatinine ratio (UACR): A1 (<30 mg/g) as normoalbuminuria, A2 (30–300 mg/g) as microalbuminuria, and A3 (>300 mg/g) as macroalbuminuria or proteinuria. KDIGO recommends assessing both albumin-creatinine ratio (ACR) and eGFR at least annually, with more frequent testing in patients at higher risk or those with worsening values. Similarly, the ADA recommends monitoring UACR and eGFR screening 1–4 times per year in T2DM, based on the severity and risk of progression. Both guidelines emphasize the need to confirm abnormal ACR results with repeat testing to ensure persistence of albuminuria before diagnosing DKD.

As DKD progresses, microalbuminuria often advances to proteinuria, a signature feature of more established kidney damage in DM and a potentially significant modifiable risk factor. Any glomerular injury that increases the permeability of the glomerular basement membrane will allow plasma proteins to escape into the urine, resulting in proteinuria. Some of these proteins are ingested by proximal tubular cells, initiating an inflammatory response that contributes to interstitial scarring. At the glomerulus level, hemodynamic effects and injury to the components of the glomerulus filtration barrier primarily lead to proteinuria. In addition, tubulointerstitial injury may diminish tubular protein reuptake. Proteinuria, along with other factors, may lead to progressive glomerulosclerosis and tubulointerstitial fibrosis, with a subsequent decline in GFR.[80] Proteinuria enhances the risk of rapid renal function decline as well as death.[81] Persistent proteinuria is a marker of kidney damage and the degree of proteinuria correlates with disease progression. Many studies[82,83] have considered proteinuria as a marker of significant renal

injury and persistent proteinuria may contribute to the progression of renal disease.[84] The 2024 KDIGO clinical practice guideline for evaluating and managing CKD includes proteinuria in the staging of CKD.[85] The recent post hoc analysis of the BRIGHTEN study demonstrated that the rate of eGFR loss in DKD was more rapid and resulted in increased proteinuria. Rapid decliners had a high level of proteinuria, but 30% of them with a urinary protein to creatinine ratio of ≥3.5 did not develop a rapid decline in kidney function, indicating that proteinuria alone does not predict rapid decline in kidney function.[86] Studies have demonstrated that ACEi or ARBs are considered first-line therapy for patients with hypertension and proteinuric CKD.[87,88] Another drug is finerenone, which reduces the risk of DKD. In the FIDELIO-DKD trial, treatment with finerenone lowered the risk of DKD progression and also cardiovascular events in patients with DKD and T2DM. Nonsteroidal MR antagonists such as finerenone add an antifibrotic mechanism of action. The patients should be closely monitored for hyperkalemia, especially those with eGFR <45 mL/min/1.73 m^2.[87] In clinical practice, the side effect profile should be monitored, especially in advanced DKD patients.

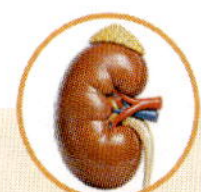

- *Proteinuria is a signature feature of DKD and serves as a marker for kidney damage.*
- *Persistent proteinuria correlates with progressive glomerulosclerosis and decline in GFR.*
- *High proteinuria increases the risk of rapid renal decline and mortality.*

Dyslipidemia

Dyslipidemia is another important risk factor for DKD. The dyslipidemia associated with DKD primarily comprises high TG levels and low high-density lipoprotein (HDL) cholesterol levels. Excess lipid accumulation causes damage to podocytes, tubular cells, and tubulointerstitial tissue by the production of ROS, lipid peroxidation, and mitochondrial damage, which leads to glomerular and tubular lesions.[89] The guidelines recommend statin therapy. The statin therapy advocates cardiovascular benefits in DKD, which demonstrated a reduction of major cardiovascular events by 23–28%.[90] According to findings from the Collaborative Atorvastatin Diabetes Study (CARDS) trial, the use of atorvastatin significantly lowered the incidence of cardiovascular events among people with DM with one or more coronary risk factors.[91] In parallel, a systematic review indicated that LDL cholesterol reduction effectively decreased total atherosclerotic events in both nondialysis CKD and kidney transplant populations.[92]

To conclude, effective treatment for hyperlipidemia in DKD patients is recommended due to its promising effects on CVD.

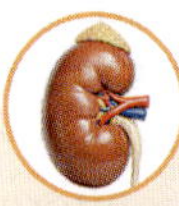

- *Dyslipidemia is an important risk factor for DKD, characterized by high TGs and low HDL cholesterol levels.*
- *Statin therapy is recommended as it reduces major cardiovascular events.*
- *Effective management of dyslipidemia in DKD improves both renal and cardiovascular outcomes.*

Dietary Salt Intake

Salt intake is an important modifiable risk factor. High salt intake can contribute to worsening DKD by volume expansion and glomerular hyperfiltration, leading to glomerular hypertension and ultimately to glomerulosclerosis.[93] High salt intake also promotes the inflammation of local tissues and endothelial dysfunction. Salt consumption of Indians was estimated to be higher than the recommended values, especially in the South Indian population.[94] A study conducted by Viswanathan et al. indicated the consumption of an alarmingly high amount

of dietary salt and an inappropriate proportion of macronutrients in people with DM and other comorbid conditions[95] and there is a high level of evidence for high dietary sodium intake to be associated with many adverse outcomes. A reduction in salt intake reduces systemic BP and thus minimizes hypertension, stress, and injury to the kidneys.[96] McMahon EJ et al. studied the effects of dietary sodium intake on BP, proteinuria, arterial rigidity, and extracellular volume in advanced stages of DKD patients and found that reducing salt intake significantly reduced 24-hour ambulatory BP, extracellular volume, albuminuria, and proteinuria.[97] The KDIGO guideline recommends lowering salt intake to <2 g/day of sodium (5 g of sodium chloride) to improve CV and other outcomes. Thus, sodium restriction is an important nonpharmacological intervention that can halt the progression of DKD. Practical suggestions would include less salt intake, less sodium, and less consumption of highly processed and packaged foods.

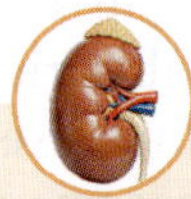

- *High salt intake worsens DKD via volume expansion, glomerular hyperfiltration, and glomerulosclerosis.*
- *Reducing salt lowers BP, proteinuria, and albuminuria.*
- *The KDIGO guideline recommends a sodium intake <2 g/day (<5 g of sodium chloride per day) to improve outcomes.*

Smoking

Smoking is an independent risk factor in the development and progression of DKD. The pathogenesis involved in smoking is multifactorial. Smoking can increase the risk of DKD through proinflammatory state, endothelial dysfunction, oxidative stress, glomerulosclerosis, and tubular atrophy. There is an increased risk of a decline in GFR for smokers when compared to their counterparts, provided the risk for progression to

ESRD was much increased in smokers.[98] The use of toxic chemicals and nicotine triggers the chronic vasoconstriction leading to kidney fibrosis[99] and also significantly increases the risk and severity of cardiovascular events in diabetic patients.[100] Hence, smoking cessation should be considered for renoprotection and prevention of DKD.

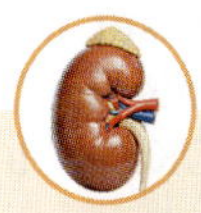

- *Smoking is an independent risk factor for the development and progression of DKD.*
- *Nicotine and toxic chemicals cause chronic vasoconstriction leading to kidney fibrosis.*
- *Smoking also increases the risk and severity of cardiovascular events in people with DM.*

ENVIRONMENTAL RISK FACTORS

Pollution: The latest research has identified pollution as an additional risk factor.[101] Exposure to environmental pollutants such as fine particulate matter and heavy metals can trigger or worsen DKD through mechanisms such as inflammation and oxidative stress. Air pollutants can damage blood vessels, causing vasoconstriction and endothelial dysfunction. Reduced blood flow, combined with high BP and air pollution exposure, can progress to DKD. Enhanced air quality monitoring and reducing intake of heavy metals through diet can help reduce the development and progression of DKD. To establish causal relationships between environmental pollution and DKD, detailed longitudinal studies with measurement of environmental exposures are required.

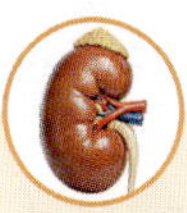

- *Pollution has been identified as a new risk factor for DKD.*
- *Fine particulate matter and heavy metals can trigger DKD.*
- *Improving air quality and reducing heavy metal intake can lower DKD risk.*

CHRONIC KIDNEY DISEASE OF UNKNOWN ETIOLOGY

Chronic kidney disease of unknown etiology (CKDu) is a phenomenon of developing CKD of unknown causes. The healthy population develops CKD without the presence of any of the above-mentioned risk factors. This was commonly found in agricultural farmers who work strenuously under intense heat. It was observed in a specific region, first in EL Salvador. CKDu was reported from other parts such as Srilanka and India.[102,103] The kidney injury arises from renal hypoperfusion caused by volume depletion.[104] The other risk factors studied include toxic elements used in agriculture and frequent self-use of NSAIDs. Evidence supporting a correlation between CKDu and the above-mentioned risk factors is yet to be documented.

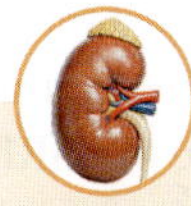

- *CKDu occurs in healthy individuals without traditional risk factors.*
- *It is common among agricultural workers exposed to heat stress and dehydration.*
- *Renal hypoperfusion from volume depletion is a major cause of CKDu.*

CONCLUSION

Understanding the above risk factors and the management of these risk factors can potentially slow the progression of DKD and ultimately improve patients' quality of life. Focusing nonmodifiable risk factors for the progression of CKD is crucial for improving patient outcomes, optimizing resource allocation, developing preventive measures, enhancing cost-efficiency, making a public health impact, and driving research and innovation in kidney disease management; whereas addressing modifiable risk factors, such as maintaining a healthy weight, controlling BP, reducing salt intake, and promoting a healthy lifestyle can play a crucial role in preventing or slowing the progression of DKD.

Thus, a comprehensive approach to managing these risk factors is essential in preventing and mitigating the impact of CKD on renal function. Currently, albuminuria, serum creatinine, and eGFR are the only available markers in clinical practice for the identification of DKD. So, there is a need for novel biomarkers for the early diagnosis of DKD. Emerging plasma and urinary biomarkers are showing promising results for the early diagnosis, which can be proven as a cost-effective tool to curtail the increasing prevalence rate, and to prevent the further development of DKD to its end stages. However, to translate these biomarkers into routine clinical practice and multicentric epidemiological studies is an urgent mission to validate their potential and applicability.

SUMMARY

Diabetes kidney disease is a major microvascular complication of DM and a leading cause of ESRD worldwide. Its pathogenesis is multifactorial, involving metabolic, hemodynamic, inflammatory, and hormonal pathways that cause glomerular and tubular injury through mechanisms such as oxidative stress, inflammation, and fibrosis. Both nonmodifiable factors, including age, gender, genetics, and duration of DM, and modifiable factors, like poor glycemic control, hypertension, obesity, proteinuria, dyslipidemia, high salt intake, and smoking, contribute to DKD onset and progression. Emerging evidence also highlights environmental pollution and CKDu as additional risk factors. Effective management requires early detection, strict control of blood glucose and BP, lifestyle modification, smoking cessation, and use of renoprotective drugs such as ACEis, ARBs, SGLT2 inhibitors, and statins. A comprehensive, multifactorial approach can significantly delay disease progression, reduce cardiovascular complications, and improve patient outcomes.

ACKNOWLEDGMENT

The author would like to thank Ms Rizwana Parveen for her assistance in the preparation of this chapter.

TAKE HOME MESSAGES

- ❑ Timely diagnosis, early detection, and appropriate interventions are the best approaches to deal with this catastrophic condition.
- ❑ Annual screening and identification of risk factors for the development of DKD are important for targeted prevention.
- ❑ Regular monitoring of eGFR and albuminuria guides disease staging and therapy adjustment.
- ❑ Physicians and policymakers should target modifiable risk factors to manage DKD and prevent its progression.

REFERENCES

1. International Diabetes Federation. IDF Diabetes Atlas, 11th edition, 2025. Brussels: International Diabetes Federation; 2025.

2. Alicic RZ, Rooney MT, Tuttle KR. Diabetic kidney disease. Clin J Am Soc Nephrol. 2017;12:2032-45.

3. Tuttle KR, Bakris GL, Bilous RW, Chiang JL, de Boer IH, Goldstein-Fuchs J, et al. Diabetic kidney disease: A report from an ADA consensus conference. Am J Kidney Dis. 2014;64(4):510-53.

4. Kovesdy CP. Epidemiology of chronic kidney disease: An update 2022. Kidney Int Suppl (2011). 2022;12(1):7-11.

5. Satyavani K, Kothandan H, Jayaraman M, Viswanathan V. Direct costs associated with chronic kidney disease among type 2 diabetic patients in India. Indian J Nephrol. 2014;24(3):141-7.

6. Nair N, Kalra R, Bhatt GC, Narang A, Kumar G, Raina R. The Effect and Prevalence of Comorbidities in

Adolescents with CKD and Obesity. Adv Chronic Kidney Dis. 2022;29:251-62.

7. Kofod DH, Carlson N, Ballegaard EF, Almdal TP, Torp-Pedersen C, Gislason G, et al. Cardiovascular mortality in patients with advanced chronic kidney disease with and without diabetes: A nationwide cohort study. Cardiovasc Diabetol. 2023;22:140.

8. Fineberg D, Jandeleit-Dahm KAM, Cooper ME. Diabetic nephropathy: Diagnosis and treatment. Nat Rev Endocrinol. 2013;9:713-23.

9. Usman MS, Khan MS, Butler J. The Interplay Between Diabetes, Cardiovascular Disease, and Kidney Disease. In: Chronic Kidney Disease and Type 2 Diabetes. Arlington: American Diabetes Association; 2021.

10. Zou H, Zhou B, Xu G. Correction to: SGLT2 inhibitors: A novel choice for the combination therapy in diabetic kidney disease. Cardiovasc Diabetol. 2018;17(1):38.

11. Toth-Manikowski S, Atta MG. Diabetic kidney disease: Pathophysiology and therapeutic targets. J. Diabetes Res. 2015;2015:697010.

12. Schena FP, Gesualdo L. Pathogenetic mechanisms of diabetic nephropathy. J Am Soc Nephrol. 2005;16:S30-3.

13. Vinod P. Pathophysiology of diabetic nephropathy. Clin Quer Nephrol. 2012;1:121-6.

14. Tonneijck L, Muskiet MH, Smits M, van Bommel EJ, Heerspink HJ, van Raalte DH, et al. Glomerular hyperfiltration in diabetes: mechanisms, clinical significance, and treatment. J Am Soc Nephrol. 2017;28:1023-39.

15. Vallon V, Komers R. Pathophysiology of the diabetic kidney. Compr Physiol. 2011;1:1175-232.

16. Helal I, Fick-Brosnahan GM, Reed-Gitomer B, Schrier RW. Glomerular Hyperfiltration: Definitions, Mechanisms and Clinical Implications. Nat Rev Nephrol. 2012;8:293-300.

17. Cooper ME, Vranes D, Youssef S, Stacker SA, Cox AJ, Rizkalla B, et al. Increased renal expression of vascular endothelial growth factor (VEGF) and its receptor VEGFR-2 in experimental diabetes. Diabetes; 1999;48:2229-39.

18. Gnudi L. Angiopoietins and diabetic nephropathy. Diabetologia. 2016;59:1616-20.

19. Nguyen D, Ping F, Mu W, Hill P, Atkins RC, Chadban SJ. Macrophage accumulation in human progressive diabetic nephropathy. Nephrology (Carlton). 2006;11:226-31.

20. Yonemoto S, Machiguchi T, Nomura K, Minakata T, Nanno M, Yoshida H. Correlations of tissue macrophages and cytoskeletal protein expression with renal fibrosis in patients with diabetes mellitus. Clin Exp Nephrol. 2006;10:186-92.

21. Tesch GH. Macrophages and diabetic nephropathy. Semin Nephrol. 2010;30:290-301.

22. Frąk W, Kućmierz J, Szlagor M, Młynarska E, Rysz J, Franczyk B. New Insights into Molecular Mechanisms of Chronic Kidney Disease. Biomedicines. 2022;10:2846.

23. Watanabe H, Enoki Y, Maruyama T. Sarcopenia in Chronic Kidney Disease: Factors, Mechanisms, and Therapeutic Interventions. Biol Pharm Bull. 2019;42:1437-45.

24. Kreiner FF, Schytz PA, Heerspink HJL, von Scholten BJ, Idorn T. Obesity-Related Kidney Disease: Current Understanding and Future Perspectives. Biomedicines. 2023;11:2498.

25. Kazancioğlu R. Risk factors for chronic kidney disease: An update. Kidney Int Suppl (2011). 2013;3(4):368-71.

26. Verma A, Popa C. The Interplay between Dietary Sodium Intake and Proteinuria in CKD. Kidney Int Rep. 2023;29:1133-6.

27. Leyane TS, Jere SW, Houreld NN. Oxidative Stress in Ageing and Chronic Degenerative Pathologies: Molecular Mechanisms Involved in Counteracting Oxidative Stress and Chronic Inflammation. Int J Mol Sci. 2022;23:7273.

28. Zhao JL, Qiao XH, Mao JH, Liu F, Fu HD. The interaction between cellular senescence and chronic kidney disease as a therapeutic opportunity. Front Pharmacol. 2022;13:974361.

29. Roy S, Schweiker-Kahn O, Jafry B, Masel-Miller R, Raju RS, O'Neill LMO, et al. Risk Factors and Comorbidities Associated with Diabetic Kidney Disease. J Prim Care Community Health. 2021;12:21501327211048556.

30. Harjutsalo V, Groop PH. Epidemiology and risk factors for diabetic kidney disease. Adv Chronic Kidney Dis. 2014;21(3):260-6.

31. Skupien J, Warram JH, Smiles AM, Niewczas MA, Gohda T, Pezzolesi MG, et al. The early decline in renal function in patients with type 1 diabetes and proteinuria predicts the risk of end-stage renal disease. Kidney Int. 2012;82(5):589-97.

32. Tapp RJ, Shaw JE, Zimmet PZ, Balkau B, Chadban SJ, Tonkin AM, et al. Albuminuria is evident in the early stages of diabetes onset: results from the Australian Diabetes, Obesity, and Lifestyle Study (AusDiab). Am J Kidney Dis. 2004;44(5):792-8.

33. Fassett RG. Current and emerging treatment options for the elderly patient with chronic kidney disease. Clin Interv Aging. 2014;9:191-9.

34. Maric C. Sex, diabetes and the kidney. Am J Physiol Renal Physiol. 2009;296(4):F680-8.

35. Turin TC, Tonelli M, Manns BJ, Ahmed SB, Ravani P, James M, et al. Lifetime risk of ESRD. J Am Soc Nephrol. 2012;23(9):1569-78.

36. Retnakaran R, Cull CA, Thorne KI, Adler AI, Holman RR; UKPDS Study Group. Risk factors for renal dysfunction intype 2 diabetes: U.K. Prospective Diabetes Study 74. Diabetes. 2006;55(6):1832-19.

37. Rani AA, Viswanathan V. Gender difference among T2DM patients with Diabetic nephropathy. Tamilnadu Association of physician of India. 2017;9(3).

38. Viswanathan V, Zhu Y, Bala K, Dunn S, Snehalatha C, Ramachandran A, et al. Association between ACE gene Polymorphism and diabetic nephropathy in South Indian patients. JOP. 2001;2(2):83-7.

39. Vijay V, Snehalatha C, Shina K, Lalitha S, Ramachandran A. Familial aggregation of diabetic kidney disease in Type 2 diabetes in South India. Diabetes Res Clin Pract. 1999;43:167-71.

40. Gu HF. Genetic and epigenetic studies in diabetic kidney disease. Front Genet. 2019;10:507.

41. Seaquist ER, Goetz FC, Rich S, Barbosa J. Familial clustering of diabetic kidney disease: Evidence for genetic susceptibility to diabetic nephropathy. N Engl J Med. 1989;320:1161-5.

42. Freedman BI, Spray BJ, Tuttle AB, Buckalew VM Jr. The familial risk of end-stage renal disease in African Americans. Am J Kidney Dis. 1993;21:387-93.

43. Earle K, Walker J, Hill C, Viberti G. Familial clustering of cardiovascular disease in patients with insulin-dependent diabetes and nephropathy. N Engl J Med. 1992;326(10):673-7.

44. Fagerudd JA, Pettersson-Fernholm KJ, Grönhagen-Riska C, Groop PH. The impact of a family history of type II (non-insulin-dependent) diabetes mellitus on the risk of diabetic nephropathyin patients with type I (insulin-dependent) diabetes mellitus. Diabetologia. 1999;42(5):519-26.

45. Sandholm N, Dahlstrom EH, Groop PH. Genetic and epigenetic background of diabetic kidney disease. Front Endocrinol. 2023;14:1163001.

46. Reddy MA, Natarajan R. Epigenetics in diabetic kidney disease. J Am Soc Nephrol. 2011;22(12):2182-5.

47. Bansal A, Pinney SE. DNA methylation and its role in the pathogenesis of diabetes. Pediatr Diabetes. 2017;18(3):167-77.

48. Harithpriya K, Juttada U, Jayasuriya R, Kumpatla S, Viswanathan V, Ramkumar KM. Comprehensive gene expression analysis of histone deacetylases and the transcription factor Nrf2 in the progression of diabetic nephropathy. Int J Diabetes Dev Ctries. 2025;45(2):462-71.

49. Viswanathan V, Tilak P, Kumpatla S. Risk factors associated with the development of overt nephropathy in type 2 diabetes patients: A 12 years observational study. Indian J Med Res. 2012;136(1):46-53.

50. Kim CS, Suh SH, Choi HS, Bae EH, Ma SK, Kim B, et al. Impact of diabetes duration and hyperglycemia on the progression of diabetic kidney disease: Insights from the KNHANES 2019-2021. World J Diabetes. 2025;16(5):102094.

51. Siddiqui K, George TP, Joy SS, Alfadda AA. Risk factors of chronic kidney disease among type 2 diabetic patients with longer duration of diabetes. Front Endocrinol (Lausanne). 2022;13:1079725.

52. Saha SK, Saifuddin MD, Moni TT, Kadir MR, Haque A, Mithila ST. Diabetic nephropathy and its risk factors among patients with diabetes mellitus-an observational study. Int J Res Med Sci. 2023;11(5):1439-43.

53. Viswanathan V, Tilak P, Meerza R, Kumpatla S. Insulin resistance at different stages of diabetic kidney disease in India. J Assoc Physicians India. 2010;58:612-5.

54. Writing Team for the Diabetes Control and Complications Trial/Epidemiology of Diabetes Interventions and Complications Research Group. Sustained effect of intensive treatment of type 1 diabetes mellitus on development and progression of diabetic nephropathy: The Epidemiology of Diabetes Interventions and Complications (EDIC) study. JAMA. 2023;290:2159-67.

55. Kalra OP. Preventive strategies for diabetic nephropathy. In: Singal RK (Ed). Medicine Update, volume 17. The Association of Physicians of India. New Delhi: Jaypee Brothers Medical Publishers; 2007. pp. 261-72.

56. Perkovic V, Heerspink HL, Chalmers J, Woodward M, Jun M, Li Q, et al. Intensive glucose control improves kidney outcomes in patients with type 2 diabetes. Kidney Int. 2013;83(3):517-23.

57. ElSayed NA, Aleppo G, Aroda VR, Bannuru RR, Brown FM, Bruemmer D, et al.; American Diabetes Association. 6. Glycemic targets: Standards of Care in Diabetes—2023. Diabetes Care. 2023;46(Suppl 1):S97-S110.

58. Kidney Disease: Improving Global Outcomes Diabetes Work Group. KDIGO 2020 clinical practice guideline for diabetes management in chronic kidney disease. Kidney Int. 2020;98(4S):S1-S115.

59. Georgianos PI, Agarwal R. Hypertension in chronic kidney disease-treatment standard 2023. Nephrol Dial Transplant. 2023;38:2694-703.

60. Hiatt W, Mehler P, Estacio R, Schrier R. Appropriate blood pressure control in hypertensive and normotensive type 2 diabetes mellitus: a summary of the ABCD trial. Nat Clin Pract Nephrol. 2007;3(8):428-38.

61. Wong TY, Shankar A, Klein R, Klein BE. Retinal vessel diameters and the incidence of gross proteinuria and renal insufficiency in people with type 1 diabetes. Diabetes. 2004;53:179-84.

62. Zhao M, Wang R, Yu Y, Chang M, Ma S, Zhang H, et al. Efficacy and Safety of Angiotensin-Converting Enzyme Inhibitor in Combination with Angiotensin-Receptor Blocker in Chronic Kidney Disease Based on

Dose: A Systematic Review and Meta-Analysis. Front Pharmacol. 2021;12:638611.

63. Ward F, Holian J, Murray PT. Drug therapies to delay the progression of chronic kidney disease. Clin Med (Lond). 2015;15(6):550-7.

64. ACCORD Study Group; Cushman WC, Evans GW, Byington RP, Goff DC Jr, Grimm RH Jr, Cutler JA, et al. Effects of intensive blood-pressure control in type 2 diabetes mellitus. N Engl J Med. 2010;362:1575-85.

65. Zac-Varghese S, Winocour P. Managing diabetic kidney disease. Br Med Bull. 2018;125:55-66.

66. UK Prospective Diabetes Study Group. Tight blood pressure control and risk of macrovascular and microvascular complications in type 2 diabetes: UKPDS 38. BMJ. 1998;317:703-13.

67. Estacio RO, Schrier RW. Antihypertensive therapy in type 2 diabetes: implications of the appropriate blood pressure control in diabetes (ABCD) trial. Am J Cardiol. 1998;82:9R-14R.

68. Park CH, Jhee JH, Chun KH, Seo J, Lee CJ, Park SH, et al. Nocturnal systolic blood pressure dipping and progression of chronic kidney disease. Hypertens Res. 2023;47:215-24.

69. Kidney Disease: Improving Global Outcomes (KDIGO) CKD Work Group. KDIGO 2024 Clinical Practice Guideline for the Evaluation and Management of Chronic Kidney Disease. Kidney Int. 2024;105(4S):S117-S314.

70. Lo R, Narasaki Y, Lei S, Rhee CM. Management of traditional risk factors for the development and progression of chronic kidney disease. Clin Kidney J. 2023;16:1737-50.

71. Wuerzner G, Pruijm M, Maillard M, Bovet P, Renaud C, Burnier M, et al. Marked Association Between Obesity and Glomerular Hyperfiltration: A Cross-sectional Study in an African Population. Am J Kidney Dis. 2010;56(2):303-12.

72. Kasiske BL, Crosson JT. Renal disease in patients with massive obesity. Arch Intern Med. 1986;146(6):1105-9.

73. Ibrahim M, Khalife L, Abdel-Latif R, Faour WH. Ghrelin hormone a new molecular modulator between obesity and glomerular damage. Mol Biol Rep. 2023;50(12):10525-33.

74. Hsu CY, McCulloch CE, Iribarren C, Darbinian J, Go AS. Body mass index and risk for end-stage renal disease. Ann Intern Med. 2006;144:21-8.

75. Viswanathan V, SelvaElavarasan S, Kumpatla S. Increased Body Mass Index is Independently Associated with Chronic Kidney Disease among People with Type 2 Diabetes. Indian J Nephrol. 2025;35:670-6.

76. Kwakernaak AJ, Zelle DM, Bakker SJ, Navis G. Central body fat distribution associates with unfavorable renal hemodynamics independent of body mass index. J Am Soc Nephrol. 2013;24:987-94.

77. Bolignano D, Zoccali C. Effects of weight loss on renal function in obese CKD patients: A systematic review. Nephrol Dial Transplant. 2013;28 (Suppl 4):iv82-98.

78. Kluger AY, Tecson KM, Lee AY, Lerma EV, Rangaswami J, Lepor NE, et al. Class effects of SGLT2 inhibitors on cardiorenal outcomes Cardiovasc Diabetol. 2019;18(1):99.

79. Perkovic V, Tuttle KR, Rossing P, Mahaffey KW, Mann JFE, Bakris G, et al.; FLOW Trial Committees and Investigators. Effects of Semaglutide on Chronic Kidney Disease in Patients with Type 2 Diabetes. N Engl J Med. 2024;391(2):109-21.

80. Jefferson JA, Shankland SJ, Pichler RH. Proteinuria in diabetic kidney disease: a mechanistic viewpoint. Kidney Int. 2008;74(1):22-36.

81. Haynes J, Haynes R. Proteinuria. BMJ. 2006; 332(7536):284.

82. Eddy AA. Interstitial nephritis induced by protein-overload proteinuria. Am J Pathol. 1998;135:719-33.

83. Remuzzi G, Bertani T. Is glomerulosclerosis a consequence of altered glomerular permeability to macromolecules? Kidney Int. 1990;38:384-94.

84. Nielsen R, Christensen EI. Proteinuria and events beyond the slit. Pediatr Nephrol. 2010;25(5):813-22.

85. Guideline Kidney Disease: Improving Global Outcomes (KDIGO) CKD Work Group. KDIGO 2024 Clinical Practice Guideline for the Evaluation and Management of Chronic Kidney Disease. Kidney Int. 2024;105(4S):S117-S314.

86. Gohda T, Murakoshi M, Suzuki Y, Kagimura T, Wada T, Narita I. Effect of proteinuria on the rapid kidney function decline in chronic kidney disease depends on the underlying disease: A post hoc analysis of the BRIGHTEN study. Diabetes Res Clin Pract. 2024;212:111682.

87. Kidney Disease: Improving Global Outcomes (KDIGO) Blood Pressure Work Group. KDIGO 2021 Clinical Practice Guideline for the Management of Blood Pressure in Chronic Kidney Disease. Kidney Int. 2021;99(3S):S1-S87.

88. Whelton PK, Carey RM, Aronow WS, Casey DE Jr, Collins KJ, Dennison Himmelfarb C, et al. 2017 ACC/AHA/AAPA/ABC/ACPM/AGS/APhA/ASH/ASPC/NMA/PCNA Guideline for the Prevention, Detection, Evaluation, and Management of High Blood Pressure in Adults: A Report of the American College of Cardiology/American Heart Association Task Force on Clinical Practice Guidelines. J Am Coll Cardiol. 2018;71(19):e127-e248.

89. Gai Z, Wang T, Visentin M, Kullak-Ublick GA, Fu X, Wang Z. Lipid Accumulation and Chronic Kidney Disease. Nutrients. 2019;11(4):722.

90. Heart Protection Study Collaborative Group. MRC/BHF Heart Protection Study of cholesterol lowering with simvastatin in 20,536 high-risk individuals: a randomised placebo-controlled trial. Lancet. 2002;360(9326):7-22.

91. Colhoun HM, Betteridge DJ, Durrington PN, Hitman GA, Neil HA, Livingstone SJ, et al. Primary prevention of cardiovascular disease with atorvastatin in type 2 diabetes in the Collaborative Atorvastatin Diabetes Study (CARDS): Multicentre randomised placebo-controlled trial. Lancet. 2004;364:685-96.

92. Ferro CJ, Mark PB, Kanbay M, Sarafidis P, Heine GH, Rossignol P, et al. Lipid management in patients with chronic kidney disease. Nat Rev Nephrol. 2018;14:727-49.

93. Shi H, Su X, Li C, Guo W, Wang L. Effect of a low-salt diet on chronic kidney disease outcomes: A systematic review and meta-analysis. BMJ Open. 2022;12:e050843.

94. Ravi S, Bermudez OI, Harivanzan V, Kenneth Chui KH, Vasudevan P, Must A, et al. Sodium Intake, Blood Pressure, and Dietary Sources of Sodium in an Adult South Indian Population. Ann Glob Health. 2016;82(2):234-42.

95. Smina TP, Kumpatla S, Viswanathan V. Higher dietary salt and inappropriate proportion of macronutrients consumption among people with diabetes and other co morbid conditions in South India: Estimation of salt intake with a formula. Diabetes Metab Syndr. 2019;13(5):2863-8.

96. Sulaiman MK. Diabetic nephropathy: Recent advances in pathophysiology and challenges in dietary management. Diabetol Metab Syndr. 2019;11:7.

97. McMahon EJ, Bauer JD, Hawley CM, Isbel NM, Stowasser M, Johnson DW, et al. A randomized trial of dietary sodium restriction in CKD. J Am Soc Nephrol. 2013;24:2096-103.

98. Orth SR, Stöckmann A, Conradt C, Ritz E, Ferro M, Kreusser W, et al. Smoking as a risk factor for end-stage renal failure in men with primary renal disease. Kidney Int. 1998;54:926-31.

99. Liao D, Ma L, Liu J, Fu P. Cigarette smoking as a risk factor for diabetic nephropathy: A systematic review and meta-analysis of prospective cohort studies. PLoS One. 2019;14:e0210213.

100. Onyenwenyi C, Ricardo AC. Impact of Lifestyle Modification on Diabetic Kidney Disease. Curr Diab Rep. 2015;15:60.

101. Tsai HJ, Wu PY, Huang JC, Chen SC. Environmental Pollution and Chronic Kidney Disease. Int J Med Sci. 2021;18:1121-9.

102. Wanigasuriya KP, Peiris-John RJ, Wickremasinghe R, Hittarage A. Chronic renal failure in North Central Province of Sri Lanka: an environmentally induced disease. Trans R Soc Trop Med Hyg. 2007;101(10):1013-7.

103. Ganguli A. Uddanam nephropathy/regional nephropathy in India: preliminary findings and a plea for further research. Am J Kidney Dis. 2016;68(3):344-8.

104. García-Trabanino R, Jarquín E, Wesseling C, Johnson RJ, González-Quiroz M, Weiss I, et al. Heat stress, dehydration, and kidney function in sugarcane cutters in El Salvador—A cross-shift study of workers at risk of Mesoamerican nephropathy. Environ Res. 2015;142:746-55.

Key Research Takeaway

Original Article

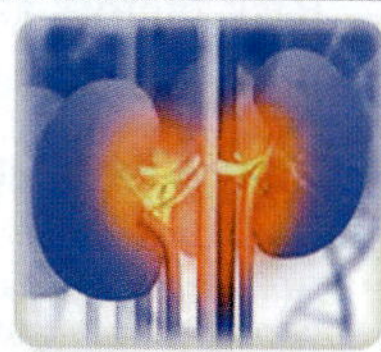

Increased Body Mass Index is Independently Associated with Chronic Kidney Disease among People with Type 2 Diabetes

Vijay Viswanathan[1], Sivashankari Selva Elavarasan[2], Satyavani Kumpatla[2]

[1]Department of Diabetology, [2]Diabetic Kidney Disease Research, M.V. Hospital for Diabetes and Prof. M. Viswanathan Diabetes Research Centre (IDF Centre for Excellence in Diabetes Care), Royapuram, Tamil Nadu, Chennai, India

Corresponding author: Vijay Viswanathan, Department of Diabetology, M.V. Hospital for Diabetes and Prof. M. Viswanathan Diabetes Research Centre (IDF Centre for Excellence in Diabetes Care), Royapuram, Chennai, Tamil Nadu, India.
E-mail: drvijay@mvdiabetes.com

Abstract

Background: The alarming increase in the prevalence of obesity has implications for chronic kidney disease (CKD) progression in type 2 diabetes (T2D). This study aimed to assess if increased body mass index (BMI) can be an independent risk factor for CKD and T2D in the Indian context. **Materials and Methods:** In this cross-sectional study, 602 (M:F = 378:224) participants were screened using Kidney Disease Improving Global Outcomes (KDIGO) from January to October 2023 in Chennai. Demographic, anthropometric, biochemical, clinical details, and comorbidities were recorded. T2D with CKD low risk was taken as control group, and CKD moderate and high risks were the study groups. BMI was classified based on the Asian criteria into normal (18.5–22.9), overweight (23–24.9), and obese (≥25 kg/m²). **Results:** Majority of participants in moderate and high risk categories were obese compared to the low risk category (60.5% and 66.4% vs. 39.1%; p < 0.001). A higher proportion of participants was on antihypertensive drugs in the high risk group and in the obese category (p < 0.001). Comorbidities and diabetic complications were higher in the high risk group (p < 0.001). Multivariate logistic regression revealed that age of ≥ 60 years [OR(95% CI); 6.3(2.2–18); p = 0.009]; increased BMI as overweight [3.6(2.1–6.3); p < 0.001] and obese [5.2(3.3–8.3); p < 0.001]; smoking [4.2(1.7–10.2); p = 0.002]; increased duration of diabetes of 5–15 years [2.3(1.2–4.5); p = 0.013], 16–25 years [4.8(2.2–10.4); p < 0.001], and >25 years [4.2(1.4–13); p = 0.011]; systolic blood pressure [1.01(1.0–1.03); p = 0.02]; and hemoglobin A1c [1.2(1.1–1.3); p < 0.001] were independent risk factors for the progression of CKD. **Conclusion:** Increased BMI was independently associated with CKD in T2D. Overweight and obese individuals are four to five times at risk for CKD progression. Early identification, lifestyle intervention, and weight-lowering drugs may reduce the complications of obesity in T2D and CKD.

DOI: 10.25259/IJN_319_2024

Indian J Med Res 136, July 2012, pp 46-53

Risk factors associated with the development of overt nephropathy in type 2 diabetes patients: A 12 years observational study

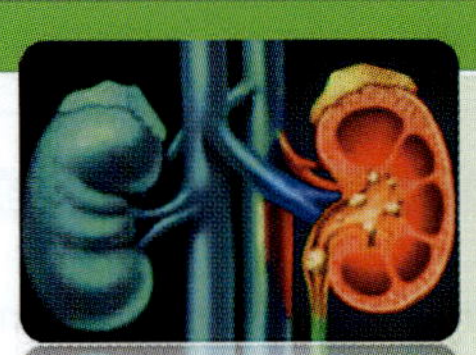

Vijay Viswanathan, Priyanka Tilak & Satyavani Kumpatla

M.V. Hospital for Diabetes & Prof. M. Viswanathan Diabetes Research Centre, WHO Collaborating Centre for Research, Education & Training in Diabetes, Chennai, India

Received August 27, 2010

Background & objectives: Diabetic nephropathy (DN) is the leading cause of chronic kidney disease and end-stage renal disease in developing countries. Early detection and risk reduction measures can prevent DN. The aim of the study was to determine the risk factors for the development of proteinuria over a period of 12 years of follow up in normoalbuminuric type 2 diabetes patients attending a specialized centre.

Methods: Of the 2630 type 2 diabetes subjects newly registered in 1996, 152 (M:F;92:60) normoalbuminuric subjects had baseline and subsequent measurements of anthropometric, haemodynamic and biochemical details spanning 12 years. The subjects were divided into 2 groups based on the renal status during follow up visits. Group 1 (non-progressors) had persistent normoalbuminuria and group 2 (progressors) had persistent proteinuria. Presence of other diabetic complications during follow up and details on antidiabetic and antihypertensive agents were noted.

Results: During median follow up of 11 years in subjects with normal renal function at baseline, 44.1 per cent developed proteinuria at follow up. Glucose levels, HbA$_1$c, systolic blood pressure (SBP), triglycerides, and urea levels were significantly higher at baseline among progressors than non-progressors. Progressors had a longer duration of diabetes and significant fall in estimated glomerular filtration rate (eGFR) levels at follow up. In Cox's regression analysis, baseline age, duration of diabetes, baseline HbA$_1$c and mean values of HbA$_1$c, triglycerides, SBP and presence of retinopathy showed significant association with the development of macroalbuminuria.

Interpretation & conclusions: Type 2 diabetes patients with uncontrolled diabetes and increase in blood pressure are at high risk of developing nephropathy. Age, long duration of diabetes, elevated BP, poor glycaemic control and presence of retinopathy were significantly associated with the progression of diabetic nephropathy.

3

Estimation of Glomerular Filtration Rate, Albuminuria, and KDIGO Guidelines

Sivashankari Selva Elavarasan, Vijay Viswanathan

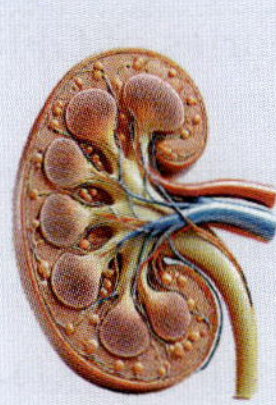

- ➢ Criteria for the diagnosis of chronic kidney disease (CKD)
- ➢ Evaluation of the cause of CKD
- ➢ Additional tests for the evaluation of CKD
- ➢ History of evolution of estimated glomerular filtration rate (eGFR)
- ➢ Gold standard method of calculating GFR
- ➢ Assessment of albuminuria
- ➢ Dipstick versus micral
- ➢ Albumin excretion rate and albumin-creatinine ratio
- ➢ Proteinuria
- ➢ Kidney failure risk equation
- ➢ What do the recent guidelines say?
- ➢ Need for referral to a nephrologist

Abstract

Diabetic kidney disease (DKD) is one of the most important, chronic, and common complications that develops among people with type 2 diabetes. The evaluation of chronic kidney disease (CKD) is based on two important criteria, namely estimated glomerular filtration rate (eGFR) and albuminuria, and we have to assess the prognosis of the patients based on the risk stratification system given by Kidney Disease: Improving Global Outcomes (KDIGO). Most recently, a kidney failure risk equation was advocated by KDIGO to evaluate the risk of renal failure. The etiology of CKD has to be identified and the patient must be periodically evaluated and assessed. Regular screening, at least annual evaluation of CKD and adherence to the prescribed treatment remain the cornerstones of management of DKD. The adaptation of recommended guidelines to adhere to the needs of the community based on the resources available, without compromising on the basic evaluation of the patient to prevent the onset of complications, remains the principle of appropriate intervention for people with DKD. A referral to a nephrologist should always be considered when difficulties are encountered in identifying the etiology or any sudden or drastic change observed in the evaluation of eGFR and albuminuria. A multipronged approach, comprehensive intervention, and individualized targeted therapy are required to diagnose the condition early, decrease the progression of the disease, and thereby prevent complications like end-stage renal disease.

Keywords: Diabetic kidney disease, Kidney Disease: Improving Global Outcomes, estimated glomerular filtration rate, albuminuria, screening.

INTRODUCTION

Diabetic kidney disease (DKD) is recognized as one of the slow-onset complications of diabetes, which eventually develops over time. Chronic kidney disease (CKD) is sometimes diagnosed at the time of diagnosis of diabetes for people with type 2 diabetes because type 2 diabetes remains undiagnosed for years. At times, the onset of complications makes the diagnosis apparent. A comprehensive intervention and targeted therapy are required to diagnose the condition early, decrease the progression of the disease, and thereby prevent complications like end-stage renal disease (ESRD). Thus, periodic screening of DKD is required to make a prompt diagnosis and current guidelines recommend at least annual screening for DKD for people living with diabetes. Estimating the glomerular filtration rate using serum creatinine and measuring albuminuria remain the key principles for an early diagnosis of DKD.

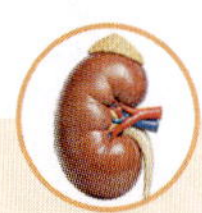

Regular screening of people with diabetes is essential to make an early diagnosis of DKD. eGFR calculated using serum creatinine and albuminuria measurement are the cornerstones for making an early diagnosis of DKD.

CRITERIA FOR DIAGNOSIS OF CHRONIC KIDNEY DISEASE

Chronic kidney disease is defined as any abnormalities in the structure and function of the kidney, which have been present for a minimum of 3 months. The latest Kidney Disease: Improving Global Outcomes (KDIGO) guidelines suggest classification of CKD based on cause, glomerular filtration rate category (GFR), and albuminuria categories. There are numerous reasons for CKD, some of which can be congenital or genetic and others can be systemic or primary. The criteria for diagnosis of CKD are as follows.

A decline in GFR < 60 mL/min for > 3 months, presence of either one or more of the following markers of kidney damage such as persistent hematuria, abnormal presence of urine sediments, albuminuria ($\geq$30 mg/g), any histological abnormalities detected in the biopsy or any structural abnormalities detected by imaging, or history of renal transplantation are recognized as the criteria for diagnosis for CKD.

The KDIGO 2024 guidelines suggest the classification of CKD based on cause, GFR, and albuminuria. There are four risk categories based on the KDIGO heatmap namely: CKD low risk, CKD moderately increased risk, CKD high risk, and CKD very high risk categories **(Fig. 1)**. These categories are based on the categories of eGFR and albuminuria. The various categories of GFR are enlisted in **Table 1**.

There are three stages of albuminuria namely: (1) normoalbuminuria, (2) microalbuminuria, and (3) macroalbuminuria **(Fig. 2)**.

The CKD epidemiology collaboration (CKD-EPI) formula, based on serum creatinine, is used for estimating GFR in resource-constrained settings like India.

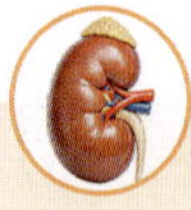

Any abnormalities in the structure and function of kidney for more than 3 months is called CKD. The classification of CKD is based on cause, GFR and albuminuria (CGA) according to the latest KDIGO guidelines. The CKD-EPI formula, based on serum creatinine, is used for estimating GFR in resource-constrained settings like India. The three categories of albuminuria are normoalbuminuria, microalbuminuria, and macroalbuminuria.

EVALUATION OF CAUSE OF CHRONIC KIDNEY DISEASE

Healthcare providers should establish the cause of CKD based on physical examination of the patient, social and environmental history, medical and family history, signs and symptoms

KDIGO: Prognosis of CKD by GFR and albuminuria categories				Persistent albuminuria categories — Description and range		
				A1 Normal to mildly increased <30 mg/g <3 mg/mmol	**A2** Moderately increased 30–300 mg/g 3–30 mg/mmol	**A3** Severely increased >300 mg/g >30 mg/mmol
GFR categories (mL/min/1.73 m²) — Description and range	G1	Normal or high	≥90			
	G2	Mildly decreased	60–89			
	G3a	Mildly to moderately decreased	45–59			
	G3b	Moderately to severely decreased	30–44			
	G4	Severely decreased	15–29			
	G5	Kidney failure	<15			

Green: Low risk (if no other markers of kidney disease, no CKD); Yellow: Moderately increased risk; Orange: High risk; Red: Very high risk. GFR, glomerular filtration rate

FIG. 1: The prognosis of chronic kidney disease (CKD) based on glomerular filtration rate (GFR) and albuminuria as defined by Kidney Disease: Improving Global Outcomes (KDIGO) and the various colors in the heat map describe the risk categories.[1]

TABLE 1: The different categories of glomerular filtration rate (GFR) in Kidney Disease: Improving Global Outcomes (KDIGO) based on eGFR values.

Category of GFR	eGFR (mL/min/1.73 m²)
G1	≥ 90
G2	60–89
G3a	45–59
G3b	30–44
G4	15–29
G5	< 15

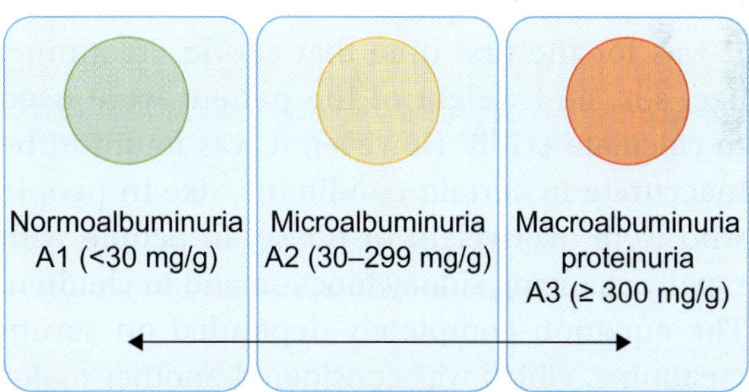

FIG. 2: The three categories of albuminuria (A1, A2, A3).

of urinary tract infections or systemic diseases, nephrotoxic medications and with the use of laboratory investigation techniques. Laboratory investigations like analysis of the urine for sediments and albumin-creatinine ratio (ACR), serological and genetic tests, ultrasound imaging and renal biopsy can be used for the evaluation of a person with CKD based on the resources available.

ADDITIONAL TESTS FOR EVALUATION OF CHRONIC KIDNEY DISEASE

The use of imaging techniques such as ultrasound, magnetic resonance imaging (MRI), or computed tomography (CT) can be considered to detect the structural abnormalities in the kidney shape, size, and symmetry. Biopsy of the kidney is a safe and acceptable method for evaluation of CKD in clinically appropriate situations. The use of genetic testing is evolving as a new technique to establish a diagnosis of CKD even in cases without a positive family history of CKD. However, it is important to make use of these tests based on the resources available.

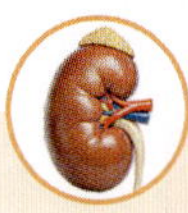

It is mandatory to establish the cause of CKD based on the physical examination, history, signs and symptoms, as well as laboratory investigations. The use of techniques like USG, biopsy, or genetic testing should be used in clinically appropriate situations based on the resources available.

HISTORY OF EVOLUTION OF ESTIMATED GLOMERULAR FILTRATION RATE

In 1957, the first formula to calculate creatinine clearance was given by Effersøe. Later in 1976, the Cockrofft–Gault equation came into existence. It was for the first time that serum creatinine, age, sex, and weight of the patient were used to calculate eGFR. However, it was found to be inaccurate in certain conditions, like in people who were overweight or obese, in people with rapidly changing kidney function and in children. The equation completely depended on serum creatinine, which was considered another major limitation. In 1994, Löfberg and Grubb identified cystatin C, which is filtered by the kidneys and not secreted and can be used for the calculation of eGFR. Cystatin C was a relatively new marker in 1994 and a lack of adequate research, its limited availability, lack of accountability, and standardization, as well as the higher cost were the primary reasons for the limited clinical and practical utility of cystatin C. A study compared the use of cystatin C and serum creatinine for the

assessment of kidney function. It stated that the high cost of creatinine acted as a huge barrier to adopting the use of cystatin C for routine clinical settings.[2]

In 1999, the modification of diet in renal disease equation (MDRD) was introduced to calculate eGFR. This equation initially had six variables and was later modified with four variables: Age, gender, ethnicity, and serum creatinine. However, the MDRD equation was found to be inaccurate among certain populations, such as the elderly and people with normal or high eGFR and people with fluctuating creatinine levels. This was the primary reason for the overestimation of GFR and was soon superseded by the new equations that evolved.

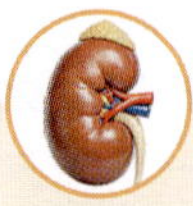

The Cockcroft–Gault equation used serum creatinine, age, sex, and weight of the patient to calculate eGFR. But, it was found to be inaccurate among people who were overweight or obese, in people with rapidly changing kidney function and in children. Cystatin C was not used due to its high cost and lack of standardization. The MDRD equation was used to calculate eGFR. This was later modified with four variables, namely age, gender, ethnicity, and serum creatinine, and was found to be inaccurate among the elderly, people with high eGFR or fluctuating creatinine levels.

In 2009, Levey and his colleagues developed the CKD-EPI equation. This new equation had higher accuracy when compared to MDRD and especially at higher GFR levels. In 2012, the CKD-EPI equation was updated and modified to include cystatin C to yield more accurate results. Kumpatla et al. compared the accuracy and the bias of MDRD with the CKD-EPI equation, including both serum creatinine (Scr) and cystatin C. The overall mean absolute bias and precision were lowest when MDRD and CKD-EPI were compared, which suggested that there was good and consistent agreement between the two equations.[3] Hence, CKD-EPI (Scr) can be used widely among clinicians to assess the eGFR in routine practice. The eGFR that is calculated using serum creatinine is cost-effective and hence found wide acceptance and usage among clinicians in their clinical practice.[4]

In 2021, the race variable was removed from the equation and a new race-free CKD-EPI equation was developed to remove health inequities in treatment. The CKD-EPI (Scr) 2021 equation overestimated the GFR when compared to CKD-EPI (Scr) 2009 and this decreased the kidney disease burden among people with type 2 diabetes in India. This was the first study in which the CKD-EPI (Scr) 2021 equation was validated in the Indian population among people with type 2 diabetes and it was observed that the CKD-EPI (Scr) 2021 equation classified 85.9% of the participants accurately and the renal function was overestimated in 14% of the population studied. A considerable proportion of the participants (28%), whose eGFR was < 60 mL/min, were reclassified to higher GFR categories and this reclassification can have a potential impact on the early referral and management of people living with CKD and type 2 diabetes.[5] The evolution of the history of eGFR can be illustrated in a **Flowchart 1**.

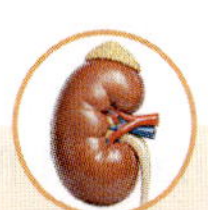

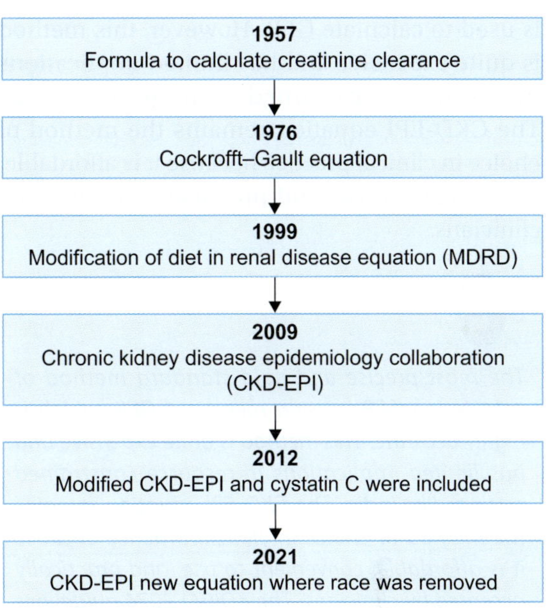

FLOWCHART 1: The evolution of estimated glomerular filtration rate (eGFR) formula to calculate GFR.

The CKD-EPI equation had higher accuracy when compared to MDRD and especially at higher GFR levels. CKD-EPI (Scr) can be used widely among clinicians to assess the eGFR in routine practice. In 2021, the race variable was removed from the equation and a new race-free CKD-EPI equation was developed to remove health inequities in treatment. The CKD-EPI (Scr) 2021 equation overestimated the GFR when compared to CKD-EPI (Scr) 2009 and this decreased the kidney disease burden among people with type 2 diabetes in India.

In 2024, the KDIGO guidelines suggest the use of a combination of eGFR cr-cys for the accurate estimation of eGFR, if available, because creatinine is directly related to muscle mass. Sometimes, the use of a creatinine-based equation can be misleading, especially in cases of spinal cord injury or sarcopenia. Similarly, cancer or thyroid disturbances, or the use of steroids, can impact the levels of cystatin and, therefore, both creatinine and cystatin are not perfect markers in assessing the GFR. But KDIGO recommends the combination of cystatin and creatinine-based equation to calculate eGFR accurately. The best or the gold standard method is always the direct measurement of GFR.

GOLD STANDARD METHOD OF CALCULATING GLOMERULAR FILTRATION RATE

The most precise and gold standard method of calculating GFR is using measured GFR. This method has a higher level of accuracy, and it utilizes the concept of clearance of exogenous markers, such as inulin, iohexol, iothalamate, or radioisotopes such as technetium and chromium, because a direct measurement of kidney function is used to calculate GFR. However, this method is quite expensive and has limited implications in resource-constrained settings like India. The CKD-EPI equation remains the method of choice in clinical practice because it is affordable, convenient to use, and practically accepted by clinicians.

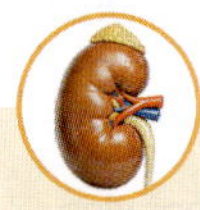

The most precise and gold standard method of calculating GFR is using measured GFR, which is highly accurate. This method is quite expensive and has limited implications in resource-constrained settings like India. The CKD-EPI equation remains the method of choice in clinical practice because it is affordable, convenient to use, and practically accepted by clinicians. The KDIGO 2024 guidelines recommend the use of a combination of eGFR cr-cys for the accurate estimation of eGFR.

There are several online calculators available to calculate eGFR using the three variables, namely, age, sex, and serum creatinine. The KDIGO 2024 guidelines recommend the use of the eGFR cr-cys equation to calculate eGFR in cases where eGFR (Scr) is less accurate and also affects the clinical decision-making for referral and management. The CKD-EPI (Scr) 2021 equation is widely used in cases where there are resource constraints and cystatin C is not available for GFR calculation.

ASSESSMENT OF ALBUMINURIA

Dipstick versus Micral

Albumin is a protein that is normally present in the blood, and the kidneys prevent it from leaking into the urine. When the kidneys are damaged, they start passing into the urine and it is called albuminuria. The presence of albuminuria poses an increased risk for cardiovascular disease. Incipient diabetic nephropathy can be detected by using a stick. A chemically treated strip is dipped into urine to check for protein. A color change is noted with the increase in the concentration of protein and a darker color indicates a higher concentration of protein. But, this test may not be sensitive to detect microalbuminuria. A micral test can be done to evaluate for microalbuminuria using an immunological reaction. This test is also reported using the change in color in the strips and is considered sensitive to detect even small amounts of albumin in the urine. The micral test is more expensive than the urine dipstick. Both the dipstick method and micral tests are semiquantitative tests used for screening and detection of albumin in the urine in routine clinical settings and community settings in a simple and cost-effective manner. A study by Vijay et al. concluded that urine dipstick can be an inexpensive method to diagnose incipient diabetic nephropathy, especially among people with diabetes. This method was fairly sensitive and highly specific to detect microalbuminuria.[6]

Albumin Excretion Rate and Albumin–Creatinine Ratio

The total amount of albumin that is excreted in 24 hours is calculated using albumin excretion rate (AER). A complete and accurate collection of 24-hour urine is required to calculate AER. This process is quite cumbersome and time-consuming and is also considered the gold standard method to diagnose albuminuria accurately. However, this method is prone to errors if all the urine over 24 hours is not collected.

A single spot urine can be used to measure ACR using an early morning sample. This method is more convenient for the patients and is also the most preferred method used for screening. A result of 30 mg/g is considered positive for microalbuminuria. In a study by Vijay et al., the urine albumin-creatinine ratio (UACR) was determined using both random and early morning samples of urine. Similarly, AER was also measured for all the participants and it was observed that AER can be estimated from ACR in the early morning sample and the measured AER had good sensitivity and specificity. Hence, the ACR, which was calculated in the early morning sample from AER, can be used as a simple and reliable method to determine albuminuria in routine clinical settings.[7]

PROTEINURIA (MACROALBUMINURIA)

Estimated protein excretion (EPE) is used to evaluate proteinuria or protein-creatinine ratio (PCR) using a single random sample of urine. This method is more convenient and less cumbersome than the 24-hour collection method. In a 6-year follow-up study by Vijay et al., it was found that the EPE was a reliable method to assess proteinuria and renal function in developing countries regularly.[8] The PCR can be estimated using the spot urine and the normal value is estimated to be < 0.2 mg. A 24-hour urine collection can also be done, which is considered the gold standard method of calculating proteinuria, but it is less convenient and time-consuming. Nayak et al. studied the accuracy of estimating the PCR from spot urine by comparing it with the 24-hour urine collection method. He found that spot urine PCR predicted 24-hour urine protein and a correction factor was adapted in a subgroup of patients with nephrotic range proteinuria, especially among people with stage 3 and 4 CKD in the Asian Indian population.[9] Both the KDIGO 2024 and American Diabetes Association (ADA) 2025 guidelines recommend the use of angiotensin converting enzyme inhibitors (ACEi)/angiotensin receptor blockers (ARB) for the management of people with proteinuria.[1,10] Diuretics can also help reduce the fluid overload and help treat patients with moderate-to-severe proteinuria. It is always mandatory to address underlying conditions such as diabetes and hypertension, along with dietary salt restriction, to manage proteinuria among people with DKD.

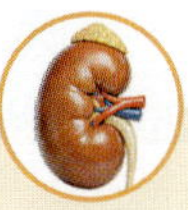

The dipstick method and micral tests are semiquantitative tests used for screening and detection of albumin in the urine in routine clinical settings and community settings in a simple and cost-effective manner. The total amount of albumin that is excreted in 24 hours is calculated using AER. A complete and accurate collection of 24-hour urine is required to calculate AER. This process is quite cumbersome and time-consuming and is also considered the gold standard method to diagnose albuminuria accurately. A single spot urine can be used to measure ACR using an early morning sample. This method is more convenient for the patients and is also the most preferred method used for screening. A result of 30 mg/g is considered positive for microalbuminuria. Estimated protein excretion is used to evaluate proteinuria or PCR using a single random sample of urine.

KIDNEY FAILURE RISK EQUATION

An externally validated risk equation like kidney failure risk equation (KFRE) can be used to estimate the 2-year and 5-year risk of people with CKD to reach end-stage renal failure (ESRD), especially for people in CKD stage 3a to 5. This equation can use either the four variables or the eight variables to assess the baseline risk of ESRD. The eight-variable equation provides a comprehensive risk assessment using variables such as age, sex, UACR, eGFR, serum albumin, serum calcium, serum phosphate, and serum bicarbonate. An improved accuracy and a comprehensive assessment are possible with the use of an eight-variable equation. However, in resource-limited settings, the four-variable KFRE is simple, convenient, practically applicable, and also comparable to the eight-variable KFRE. KFRE is validated in multiple international cohorts and is also recommended for use by the KDIGO **(Table 2)**.

TABLE 2: The various risk categories based on kidney failure risk equation (KFRE).

Risk category	Time period	Interpretation
3–5%	Over 5 years	Referral to nephrologist
10%	Over 2 years	Need for a comprehensive team base care
20–40%	Over 2 years	Plan for future procedures like renal replacement therapy (RRT)

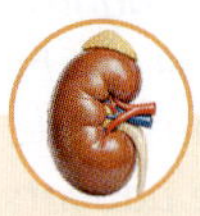

An externally validated risk equation like KFRE is used to estimate the 2-year and 5-year risk of people with CKD to reach ESRD, especially for people in CKD stage 3a to 5. The four variable KFRE is simple, convenient, practically applicable, and also comparable to the eight variable KFRE and is validated in multiple international cohorts.

WHAT DO THE RECENT GUIDELINES SAY?

The KDIGO 2025 guidelines suggest the following important recommendations **(Fig. 3)**.[11]

- *Evaluation of CKD*:
  - The use of the serum creatinine-based GFR equation and the cystatin-based equation when both methods are available. If cystatin C is unavailable, CKD-EPI (Scr) can be used for the estimation of eGFR.
  - UACR has to be measured either using laboratory methods or point-of-care testing.
- *Risk assessment:* The use of validated KFRE can be used to estimate the two-year and five-year risk of developing ESRD for people in CKD stages 3–5.
- *Interventions to curb the progression of CKD and mitigate complications:* KDIGO 2025 recommends the use of sodium-glucose cotransporter-2 inhibitors (SGLT2i) for people with CKD with eGFR >20 mg/mL to delay the

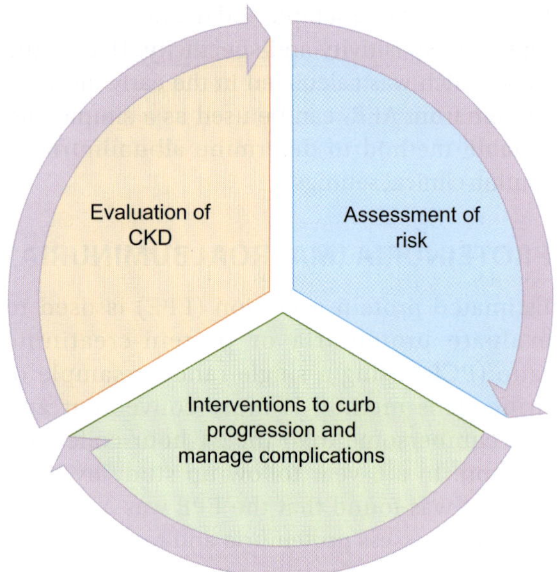

FIG. 3: The important recommendations given by Kidney Disease: Improving Global Outcomes (KDIGO) 2025.

(CKD: chronic kidney disease)

progression and the use of statins to prevent the occurrence of any adverse coronary events.

The KDIGO 2024 guidelines suggest the use of four pillars of therapy, such as the use of renin–angiotensin–aldosterone system (RAAS) blockers (ACEi or ARB) as the first line of therapy. SGLT2i is recommended as the second line of therapy for people with eGFR ≥ 20 mL/min. Nonsteroidal mineralocorticoid receptor antagonists like Finerenone are recommended for microalbuminuria and long-term cardiovascular benefits. However, the serum levels of potassium have to be constantly monitored due to the potential risk for hyperkalemia. Glucagon-like peptide-1 receptor agonists (GLP1-RA) is also recommended as the fourth pillar of therapy among people who are unable to meet the individualized glycemic control despite the use of metformin and SGLT2i.[1]

Lifestyle interventions, like including physical activity for 150 minutes per week and reducing the intake of salt to < 5 g/day are also recommended. Optimizing glycemic and blood pressure control is an essential part and parcel of all the guidelines.

ADA 2025 guidelines recommend maintaining HbA1c of < 7% for people living with CKD and diabetes. The KDIGO recommends maintaining a systolic blood pressure of < 120 mm Hg, whereas the ADA 2025 suggests maintaining a blood pressure (BP) of < 130/80 mm Hg.

The ADA 2025 guidelines also suggest screening for complications through various laboratory investigations **(Fig. 4)**.[10]

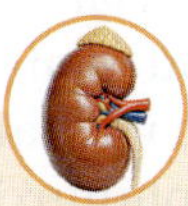

The KDIGO 2025 guidelines suggest the evaluation of CKD, assessment of risk, and interventions to curb the progression of CKD and manage the potential associated complications. KDIGO 2024 guidelines suggest the use of four pillars of therapy, such as the use of RAAS blockers, SGLT2i, Finerenone, and GLP1-RA. ADA 2025 guidelines recommend maintaining HbA1c of < 7% for people living with CKD and diabetes. The KDIGO recommends maintaining a systolic blood pressure of < 120 mm Hg, whereas the ADA 2025 suggests maintaining a BP of < 130/80 mm Hg. ADA 2025 guidelines recommend screening for complications such as high blood pressure, volume overload, metabolic acidosis, anemia, or metabolic bone diseases.

NEED FOR REFERRAL TO NEPHROLOGIST

Diabetologists and general physicians should consider referring the patients to nephrologists when there is a rapid decline in eGFR or when there is a persistent increase in albuminuria or when the etiology of CKD is unknown. Recently, CKD of unknown etiology (CKDu) has been identified in rural populations across the world after eliminating conditions such as diabetes and hypertension. These cases are common in tropical climates and agricultural regions due to factors such as dehydration, heat stress, and exposure to pesticides, and are now recognized as a global noncommunicable disease. The referral to a nephrologist depends upon the stage at which the healthcare professional identifies the patient. Appropriate and timely referral to a nephrologist can delay the progression to ESRD. There are different conditions in which people with CKD and diabetes have to be referred to a nephrologist **(Fig. 5)**.

When there is a decline in eGFR by > 30% or when the eGFR declines by > 5 mL/min in 6 months or if ACR doubles in subsequent visits, referral to a nephrologist has to be considered.

The prevalence and severity of the symptoms among people with CKD and diabetes have to

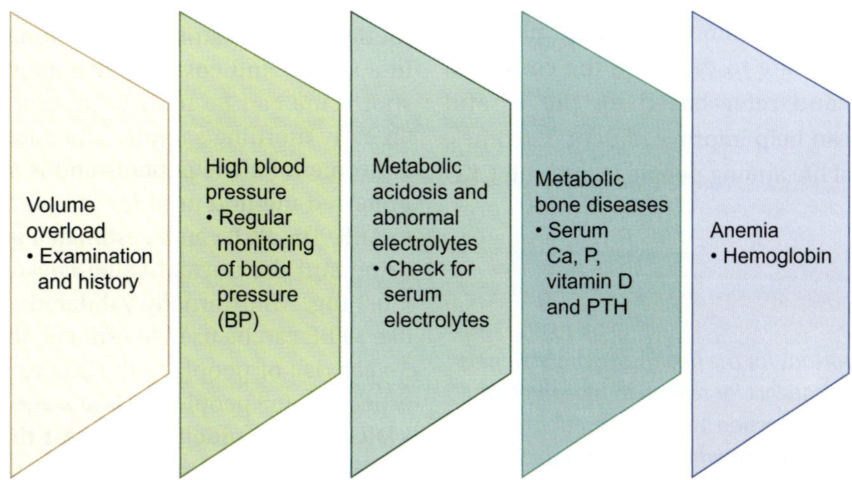

FIG. 4: The American Diabetes Association (ADA) 2025 guidelines for screening for complications.

(PTH: parathyroid hormone)

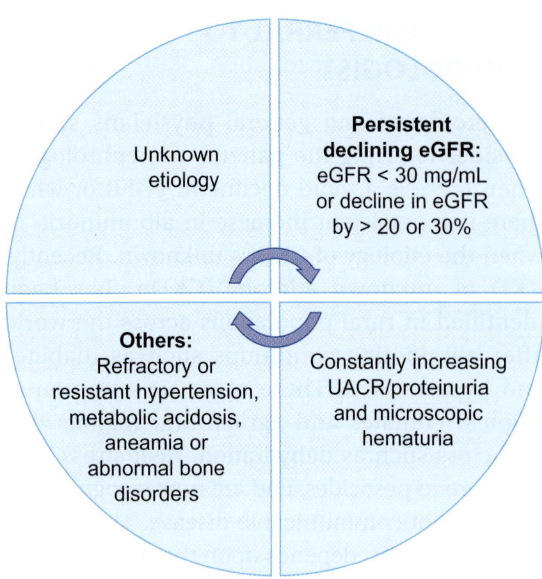

FIG. 5: The different conditions in which referral to a nephrologist is recommended for people with diabetes and chronic kidney disease (CKD).

(eGFR: estimated glomerular filtration rate; UACR: urine albumin-creatinine ratio)

be assessed to establish an early diagnosis. The healthcare professionals must be educated about the treatment of some of the common symptoms of people with CKD. A multidisciplinary approach to stratify patients and also treat them appropriately remain the need of the hour. Systematic planning and integrated care to diagnose the condition early, treat and refer based on the careful assessment can help improve patient outcomes, and quality of life among people living with CKD and diabetes.

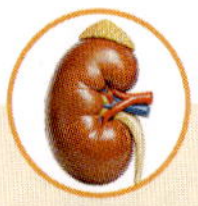

It is very important for the healthcare professionals to identify the patients for referral to a nephrologist, to delay the progression to ESRD. A referral to a nephrologist is required when there is a decline in eGFR by 5 mL/min in 6 months or if the ACR doubles in subsequent visits.

SUMMARY

Diabetic kidney disease remains one of the most important, chronic, and common complications among people with type 2 diabetes. Estimating the GFR using serum creatinine and measuring albuminuria remain the key principles for an early diagnosis of DKD. Healthcare providers should establish the cause of CKD based on physical examination of the patient, social and environmental history, medical and family history, signs and symptoms of urinary tract infections or systemic diseases, nephrotoxic medications and with the use of laboratory investigation techniques. The use of imaging techniques such as ultrasound, MRI, or CT can be considered to detect the structural abnormalities in the kidney shape, size, and symmetry. Biopsy and genetic testing can be done based on the resources available and when the need arises. The most precise and gold standard method of calculating GFR is using measured GFR. However, this method is quite expensive and has limited implications in resource-constrained settings like India and the CKD-EPI equation remains the method of choice in clinical practice because it is affordable, convenient to use, and practically accepted by the clinicians. The dipstick method and micral tests are semiquantitative tests used for screening and detection of albumin in the urine in routine clinical settings and community settings in a simple and cost-effective manner. A single spot urine can be used to measure ACR using an early morning sample. This method is more convenient for the patients and is also the most preferred method used for screening compared to AER. The PCR can be estimated using the spot urine and the normal value is estimated to be < 0.2 mg. An externally validated risk equation like KFRE can be used to estimate the 2-year and 5-year risk of people with CKD to reach ESRD, especially for people in CKD stage 3a to 5. The KDIGO 2025 guidelines suggest the evaluation of CKD, assessment of risk and interventions to curb the progression of CKD, and manage the potential associated complications. KDIGO

2024 guidelines suggest the use of four pillars of therapy, such as the use of RAAS blockers, SGLT2i, Finerenone, and GLP1-RA. ADA 2025 guidelines recommend screening for complications such as high blood pressure, volume overload, metabolic acidosis, anemia, or metabolic bone diseases. Diabetologists and general physicians should consider referring the patients to nephrologists when there is a rapid decline in eGFR or when there is a persistent increase in albuminuria or when the etiology of CKD is unknown. The referral to a nephrologist depends upon the stage at which the healthcare professional identifies the patient. Appropriate and timely referral to a nephrologist can delay the progression to ESRD.

CONCLUSION

Early diagnosis of DKD involves the assessment of eGFR and albuminuria using KDIGO guidelines. While eGFR can be calculated using a serum-based creatinine equation like CKD-EPI to assess kidney function, albuminuria can be assessed using semiquantitative methods like dipstick or micral, or quantitative methods like ACR or PCR to evaluate endothelial or glomerular injury. The assessment of both these diagnostic parameters helps clinicians to identify people at an increased risk of developing CKD. Optimizing blood pressure and glycemic control remains the mainstay of management of people with CKD. The KDIGO recommends using the four pillars of therapy for management of people with DKD, namely: RAAS blockers, SGLT2i, Finerenone, and GLP1-RA. Identifying patients early, stratifying them based on risk and tailoring targeted intervention therapy are the cornerstones of prevention and management of DKD. Early diagnosis and management of DKD can improve the quality of life of patients, reduce the financial burden, and also prevent the progression of the disease and the onset of complications like ESRD.

TAKE HOME MESSAGES

- Early screening and diagnosis of people with DKD is important because of the absence of symptoms of CKD in its early stages.
- We recommend estimation of eGFR using the serum creatinine-based equation (CKD-EPI) and assessment of ACR or PCR simultaneously, and evaluating the CKD staging based on the KDIGO heat map.
- Adherence to these guidelines can improve the accuracy of diagnosis of CKD, decrease the progression, and prevent adverse treatment outcomes.
- Screening for DKD should be included as a part of routine clinic visits to enable early diagnosis and management of DKD.

REFERENCES

1. Kidney Disease: Improving Global Outcomes (KDIGO), CKD Work Group. KDIGO 2024 Clinical Practice Guideline for the Evaluation and Management of Chronic Kidney Disease. Kidney Int. 2024;105(4S):S117-314.
2. Viswanathan V, Snehalatha C, Nair MB, Ramachandran A. Comparative assessment of cystatin c and creatinine for determining renal function. Indian J Nephrol. 2005;15(3):91-4.
3. Kumpatla S, Soni A, Viswanathan V. Comparison of Two Creatinine Based Equations for Routine Estimation of GFR in a Speciality Clinic for Diabetes. J Assoc Physicians India. 2017;65(8):38-41.
4. Rani AA, Viswanathan V. Estimated Glomerular Filtration Rate Using Creatinine-Based Chronic Kidney Disease Epidemiology Collaboration Equation. Indian J Nephrol. 2018;28(6):492-3.
5. Selva Elavarasan S, Kumpatla S, Viswanathan V. Comparison of estimated Glomerular Filtration Rate using the CKD-EPI (Scr) 2009 and CKD-EPI (Scr) 2021 (race-free) equations among people with type 2 diabetes in a tertiary care setting in India. Int J Diabet Developing Countries. 2025:1-8.
6. Viswanathan V, Nair MB, Suresh S, Chamukuttan S, Ambady R; An Inexpensive Method to Diagnose

Incipient Diabetic Nephropathy in Developing Countries. Diabetes Care. 2005;28(5):1259-60.

7. Viswanathan V, Snehalatha C, Nair BM, Ramachandran A. Validation of a method to determine albumin excretion rate in type 2 diabetes mellitus. Indian J Nephrol. 2003;13(3):85.

8. Viswanathan V, Chamukuttan S, Kuniyil S, Ambady R. Evaluation of a simple, random urine test for prospective analysis of proteinuria in Type 2 diabetes: a six year follow-up study. Diabetes Res Clin Pract. 2000;49(2-3):143-7.

9. Nayak R, Annigeri RA, Vadamalai V, Seshadri R, Balasubramanian S, Rao BS, et al. Accuracy of spot urine protein creatinine ratio in measuring proteinuria in chronic kidney disease stage 3 and 4. Indian J Nephrol. 2013;23(6):428-33.

10. American Diabetes Association Professional Practice Committee; Chronic Kidney Disease and Risk Management: Standards of Care in Diabetes—2025. Diabetes Care. 2025;48(Supplement_1):S239-51.

11. Madero M, Levin A, Ahmed SB, Carrero JJ, Foster B, Francis A, et al. Evaluation and management of chronic kidney disease: Synopsis of the kidney disease: Improving Global Outcomes 2024 clinical practice guideline. Ann Intern Med. 2025;178(5):01926.

Key Research Takeaway

Indian J Nephrol 2005;15: 91-94

Comparative assessment of cystatin c and creatinine for determining renal function

ARTICLE

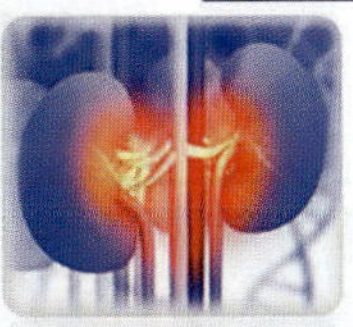

V Viswanathan, C Snehalatha, MB Nair, A Ramachandran

Diabetes Research Centre, 4, Main Road, Royapuram, Chennai

Abstract

Aims: To determine whether plasma cystatin C was a better marker of glomerular filtration rate (GFR) when compared with plasma creatinine in South Indian type 2 diabetic subjects with moderately elevated plasma creatinine.

Materials and methods: Among the 60 study subjects, 40 were type 2 diabetic patients and the other 20 subjects were non-diabetic subjects (NGT). Diabetic subjects were categorized into 2 groups, those with normoalbuminuria and without any complications (n=20,NAU) and those with diabetic nephropathy and retinopathy (n=20,PROT). Plasma cystatin C was measured by particle enhanced turbidimetric (PET) assay (DAKO A/S, Denmark). GFR was determined using the Cockroft-Gault equation.

Results: As expected, PROT group had significantly ($p < 0.05$) higher levels of plasma creatinine (1.1 ± 0.4 mg / dl) when compared with the NGT group (0.8 ± 0.1 mg/dl) and the NAU subjects (0.8 ± 0.1 mg /dl). However no difference in creatinine levels was noted between NGT and NAU groups. NAU (1.4 ± 0.6 mg /dl) and PROT (1.1 ± 0.6 mg /dl) groups had significantly higher levels of cystatin C when compared with NGT group (0.7 ± 0.3 mg/dl). The cystatin C levels did not differ significantly ($p = 0.4$) between the NAU and the PROT groups.

In the total group, a significant correlation was observed between both cystatin C and creatinine ($r=0.50$; $p<0.0001$).

Conclusion: Cystatin C was a better marker of moderately impaired renal function when compared with creatinine. Cystatin C had a good correlation with creatinine.

ORIGINAL ARTICLE

Comparison of Two Creatinine Based Equations for Routine Estimation of GFR in a Speciality Clinic for Diabetes

Satyavani Kumpatla[1], Anju Soni[2], Vijay Viswanathan[3]

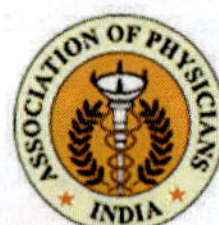

Abstract

Objectives: To compare the bias, absolute bias, precision and accuracies between the equations, viz., CKD-EPI (Scr), CKD-EPI (Scys) and MDRD in Indian patients with type 2 diabetes.

Methods: 198 patients who underwent 24 h urinary collection for assessing kidney function between November 2014-January 2015 were included. Cohen's κ coefficient, Bland-Altman plot were calculated between estimated kidney function equations, and bias, precision, accuracies was calculated between the formulae.

Results: The mean eGFR based on MDRD, CKD-EPI (Scr) and CKD-EPI (Scys) equations were 64.5±21.9, 70.2±25.1 and 74.7±31.0 ml/min/ $1.73m_2$ respectively. The overall mean absolute bias was smallest for MDRD vs CKD EPI (Scr). The precision was also least for MDRD vs CKD EPI (Scr) indicating that the agreement between these equations is consistent for the range of values. MDRD vs CKD EPI (Scr) had the highest accuracy in comparison to other compared formula. The performance between MDRD versus CKD EPI (Scys) was different. There was a good agreement between MDRD and CKD EPI (Scr).in both stage 3 and stage 4 CKD. The MDRD vs CKD EPI (Scr) classified 72.2% of the patients correctly.

Conclusion: In conclusion, there was a good agreement between CKD-EPI (Scr) and MDRD equations. CKD-EPI equation based on creatinine estimation is widely accepted method and clinicians may use this equation in routine clinical practice to assess kidney function among patients with type 2 diabetes.

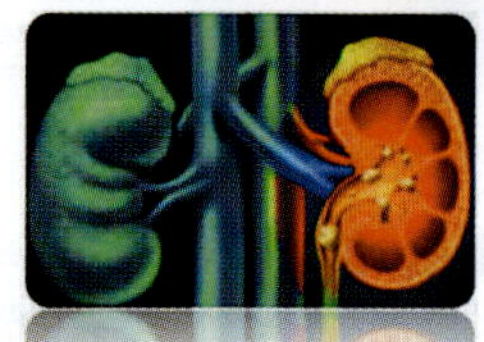

1Lab Director, 2Research Associate, 3Head and Chief Diabetologist, M.V. Hospital for Diabetes and Prof. M. Viswanathan Diabetes Research Centre, Royapuram, Chennai, Tamil Nadu

Received: 04.01.2016; Accepted: 28.04.2017

Editorial Viewpoint

- There are various methodsto measure GFR with variable accuracy.
- This study concludes a good agreement between CKD-EPI (Scr) and MDRD equations.

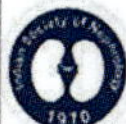

Estimated Glomerular Filtration Rate Using Creatinine-Based Chronic Kidney Disease Epidemiology Collaboration Equation

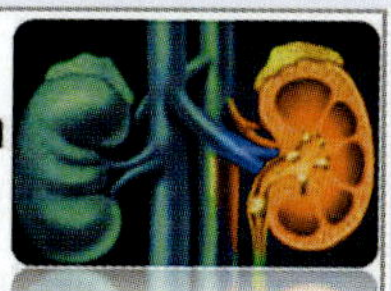

A. A. Rani, V. Viswanathan

Department for Diabetic Kidney Disease, Prof. M. Viswanathan Diabetes Research Centre
M.V. Hospital for Diabetes, Chennai, Tamil Nadu, India

Indian Journal of Nephrology | Volume 28 | Issue 6 | November-December 2018

Sir,

Recently, we have been reading articles on estimating glomerular filtration rate (eGFR) in Indian population with great interest. With the understanding that there is a rising epidemic of type 2 diabetes mellitus and the subsequent increase in its associated complications, it poses a nationwide threat. Diabetic nephropathy is the significant cause of chronic kidney disease (CKD). An Indian study showed that patients with CKD spend more toward their hospital admission than those without diabetic complications.[1] Hence, glomerular filtration rate (GFR) assessment is important for the clinicians to assess the kidney function, detect and estimate the progression of CKD. eGFR using CKD epidemiology collaboration (CKD-EPI) equation[2] is a major indicator of kidney function, and it plays an important role in detecting, evaluating, and also in managing CKD. Serum creatinine (Scr) or serum cystatin (Scys) is used to estimate GFR. A population-based Indian study emphasized that Cystatin C identifies more patients in early CKD and also in patients with normoalbuminuric CKD when compared to creatinine.[3] This study focused on the creatinine-based equations, such as Cockcroft-Gault and modification of diet in renal disease (MDRD), by comparing it with CKD-EPI equation using Cystatin C. An earlier study by Viswanathan *et al.*[4] suggested that Cystatin C was a better marker for moderately impaired renal function when compared to creatinine using Cockcroft-Gault. In developing countries like India, use of Cystatin C in clinical practice is limited due to its cost.

At present, Cystatin C has an advantage in detecting theearly CKD, but it is not a cost-effective test and cannotbe recommended for routine clinical practice.To overcome this limitation, creatinine can be used for eGFR. A recent study in 2017 compared the estimation of GFR using gamma camera-based Gates protocol and Scr-based predicting equations with GFR measured by plasma clearance of Tc-99m DTPA in North Indian population. The finding highlighted that CKD-EPI correlated with Tc-99m DTPA and showed least bias and highest precision when compared to GFR estimate using Cockroft-Gault, MDRD, and Gates protocol. Kumpatla *et al.*[5] compared MDRD equation versus CKD-EPI using Scr and MDRD equation versus CKD-EPI using Scys to estimate eGFR in a clinical setting in South Indian population. The mean bias, mean absolute bias and precision were lesser in MDRD versus CKD-EPI using Scr when compared to that of MDRD versus CKD-EPI using Scys. Likewise, Scr showed highest accuracy when compared with Scys. This showed that creatinine-based CKD-EPI can identify CKD at an early stage. Thus, for an Indian population, CKD-EPI equation using creatinine predicts GFR best than other equations. This underlines the importance of standardization of eGFR calculation among Indian population. Further research is needed in large sample to determine the best methods by comparing eGFR equations with the gold standard methods. In conclusion, CKD-EPI equation using Scr was found to be superior in terms of estimating kidney function and is cost-effective; hence, it can be implemented in the routine clinicalpractice.

Comparison of estimated Glomerular Filtration Rate using the CKD-EPI (Scr) 2009 and CKD-EPI (Scr) 2021 (race-free) equations among people with type 2 diabetes in a tertiary care setting in India

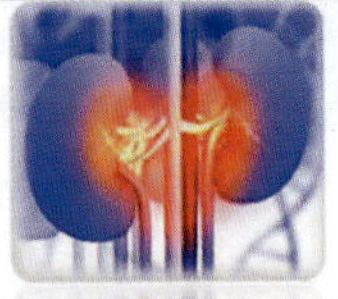

Sivashankari Selva Elavarasan · Satyavani Kumpatla · Vijay Viswanathan

ORIGINAL ARTICLE

Abstract

Background: Limited studies are available to assess transition effect in eGFR using the CKD-EPI (Scr) 2021 among Indians with type 2 diabetes (T2DM) using KDIGO.

Objective: The aim was to compare eGFR using CKD-EPI 2009 (Scr) versus 2021, assess changes in eGFR, reclassification across KDIGO categories and agreement between the two equations.

Methods: A total of 2059 participants were screened from April-June 2024 for this cross sectional study. Demographic, anthropometric, clinical and biochemical details were recorded. eGFR was calculated for the participants using both the equations and were classified based on KDIGO.

Results: Overall median eGFR was higher with CKD-EPI (Scr) 2021 versus 2009 (73 vs 69; $p < 0.001$). Median eGFR deviation was 4 ml/min/1.73m^2 among those aged above 45 years. Highest difference in median eGFR was seen in moderately increased risk category [CKD-EPI 2021 vs 2009] (71 vs 66; $p < 0.001$) followed by low risk (79 vs 76; $p < 0.001$) and high risk categories (59 vs 57;$p = 0.098$). CKD-EPI 2021 classified 85.9% of the participants accurately, in 14.1% of them kidney function was overestimated (kappa $\kappa = 0.76$). Around 28% of participants, whose eGFR was less than 60 ml/min/1.73m^2 reclassified to an improved GFR category when the new equation was employed.

Conclusion: The new race-free CKD-EPI (Scr) 2021 equation provided higher eGFR values than 2009 equation. One in every seven person has the possibility of being classified to higher eGFR category based on KDIGO and this reclassification may have implications on early referral and management among people with T2DM and CKD.

International Journal of Diabetes in Developing Countries   https://doi.org/10.1007/s13410-025-01556-0

Indian J Nephrol 2003;13: 85–88

8 5

ARTICLE

Validation of a method to determine albumin excretion rate in type 2 diabetes mellitus

V Viswanathan, C Snehalatha, B M Nair, A Ramachandran

Diabetes Research Centre, Chennai, India

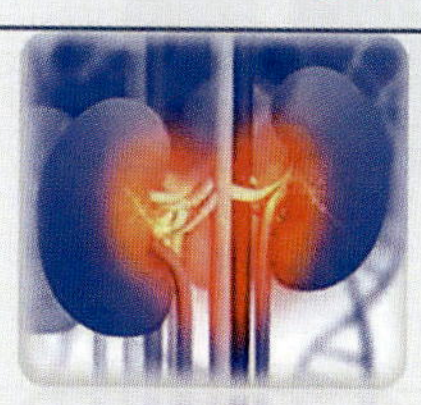

Background & Objective: Determination of albuminuria is important in identifying early renal disorders. A simple and reliable method for determination of albuminuria needs to be validated for routine clinical purpose. The present study was done to determine the sensitivity and specificity of albumin / creatinine ratio (ACR) estimated from a random and early morning urine sample to identify microalbuminuria (MAU) and to determine the validity of derivation of albumin excretion rate (AER) from albumin / creatinine ratio (ACR) in type 2 diabetics. As ACR can be determined in random urine sample it may be possible to calculate AER from ACR. This will avoid the cumbersome 24-hour urine collection.

Methods: Random ACR (RACR, n = 84) and early morning ACR (EACR, n = 60) were determined on the same day by estimating the urine albumin to creatinine ratio in type 2 diabetic subjects. 24-hour AER was also determined in all the patients. The correlation between the RACR, EACR and the 24-hour AER was determined using Pearson's Linear Correlation method. The regression equation for deriving AER from RACR and EACR was calculated. The specificity and sensitivity of AER calculated from RACR and EACR was also determined.

Results: The correlation between EACR and 24-hour AER was stronger when compared with RACR. AER calculated from EACR had 100% sensitivity and 100% specificity to identify microalbuminuria. While the AER calculated from RACR had 58% sensitivity and 92% specificity.

Interpretation & Conclusion: AER can be calculated in type 2 diabetic patients from ACR determined in an early morning urine sample. The calculated AER has good sensitivity, specificity. This calculation would be helpful to determine AER in outpatients and may obviate the cumbersome 24-hour urine collection.

4

Biomarkers for the Early Detection of Diabetic Kidney Diseases

Udyama Juttada, Vijay Viswanathan

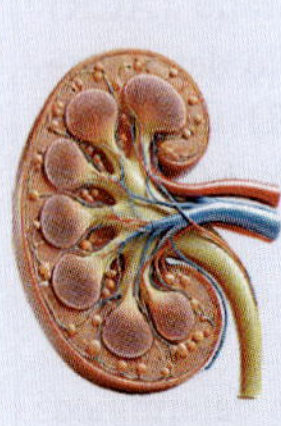

- ➢ Classification of DKD biomarkers
- ➢ Clinical biomarkers for DKD
  - ◆ Diagnostic biomarkers
  - ◆ Novel biomarkers
- ➢ Genetics biomarkers of DKD
  - ◆ Common genetic variants associated with DKD
  - ◆ Epigenetics

Abstract

Diabetic kidney disease (DKD) remains one of the major microvascular complications that lead to reduced lifespan in diabetes individuals. The importance of both prognostic and endpoint biomarkers for the diagnosis of advanced DKD and end-stage renal disease (ESRD) has received significant advancements and interest in recent years. Although the regularly practiced markers of DKD, albuminuria, and estimated glomerular filtration rate (eGFR) have shown positive feedback in established DKD, their limitations in sensitivity and specificity have led to the identification of novel biomarkers that could improve risk stratification. Considering the complex pathophysiology of DKD which involves several mechanisms such as hyperglycemia-induced inflammation, oxidative stress, and tubular damage, eventually leading to kidney damage and fibrosis, many novel biomarkers have captured one specific mechanism of the disease and are helpful in early diagnosis. We also reviewed in the chapter the current information from genetic and epigenetic studies of DKD and ESRD in patients with diabetes, including the approaches of genome-wide association study (GWAS) or epigenome-wide association study (EWAS) and candidate gene association analyses which are challenging for taking studies using candidate approaches through to actual clinical biomarker.

Keywords: Biomarkers, diabetic kidney disease (DKD), diagnosis, epigenetics.

INTRODUCTION

Diabetic kidney disease (DKD), previously called diabetic nephropathy, DKD is a chronic microvascular complication of diabetes and progresses gradually among 30–40% of individuals with increasing history of diabetes.[1]

DKD is a major cause of chronic kidney disease (CKD) worldwide and one of the reasons for end-stage-renal disease (ESRD) leading to dialysis or transplantation. The prevalence of CKD is a concerning reason for the mortality rate among people with diabetes[2] which makes it very important for the early diagnosis and prevention of ESRD. Along with some well-known risk factors, there are some diagnostic tests to confirm the presence of DKD, but only after the onset of the disease or when the disease has progressed to ESRD, due to this, there is increasing interest in the development of prognostic or predictive biomarkers to allow for risk stratification into clinical trials, as well as eventually for targeting preventive therapy. There is a substantial focus on the development of biomarkers of drug response that were implemented for DKD treatment. Therefore, the therapeutic goal of any biomarker should be to prevent the disease at earlier stages, not just ESRD.

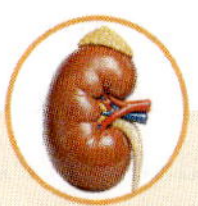

There is an increasing interest in the development of prognostic or predictive biomarkers for risk stratification in clinical trials, as well as for targeting preventive therapy.

CLASSIFICATION OF DIABETIC KIDNEY DISEASE BIOMARKERS

Biomarkers were classified based on the disease pathophysiology and the stage at which they are expressed **(Flowchart 1)**. These biomarkers should have few attempts to build and validate predictive equations using the available clinical data which would form the basis for evaluating the *marginal* improvement in prediction with biomarkers.

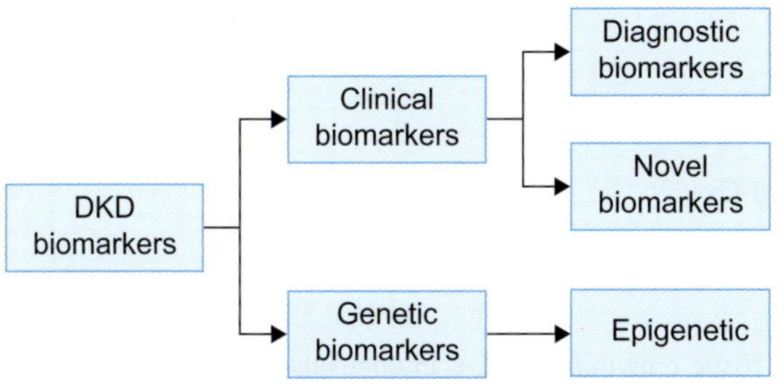

FLOWCHART 1: Classification of biomarkers related to diabetic kidney disease (DKD).

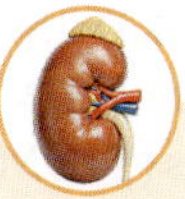

Classification of clinical biomarkers for diabetes kidney diseases.

Diagnostic Biomarkers

Common diagnostic markers for identifying DKD are estimated glomerular filtration rate (eGFR) and albuminuria. eGFR is a calculation based on serum creatinine level, age, and gender. Albuminuria is the amount of albumin excreted in urine, and it strongly predicts the progression of DKD. However, it lacks specificity and sensitivity for ESRD and progressive decline in eGFR. It has been shown that the coexistence of albuminuria among diabetes individuals makes DKD more prominent rather than non-diabetic CKD in people with type 2 diabetes mellitus (T2DM).[3] Identifying DKD at early stages will promote better outcomes in therapeutic intervention. One of the better ways to achieve this is through the development of prognostic or predictive biomarkers for risk stratification DKD is a multifactorial pathogenic progressive disease that includes glomerular, tubular, and inflammatory factors which results in the prognosis of renal fibrosis.[4] Uncontrolled blood sugar, smoking, dyslipidemia, hypertension, and obesity are the major risk factors associated with DKD.[5] The physiology of DKD involves nearly every nephron structure in our body: glomerular endothelia and epithelia, podocytes, mesangial matrix, as well as renal tubular epithelia.[6] Thus, biomarkers beyond proteinuria, based on the pathophysiology of DKD are important in the treatment algorithm of DKD patients.

Albuminuria is also a strong predictive diagnostic marker for the progression of DKD, but it lacks specificity and sensitivity for ESRD and progressive decline in eGFR. Many people with T2DM cases show a large proportion of normoalbuminuria with progression renal disease.[7,8] There is also evidence that the coexistence of albuminuria makes DKD than non-diabetic CKD among people with T2DM.[9] However, even in type 1 diabetes mellitus (T1DM), where non-diabetic CKD is much less common, albuminuria was reported to have a poor positive predictive value for DKD as only about one-third of those with microalbuminuria will have progressive renal function decline Albumin excretion also had low sensitivity, as only about half of those with progressive renal function decline were albuminuria.[10] Many cohort studies from all over the world have highlighted that the eGFR slope, albumin to creatinine ratio (ACR) and HbA1c had a C statistic (not cross-validated) for ESRD within the range of 0.67–0.80.[11-13]

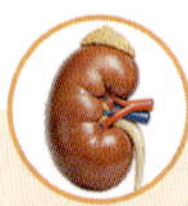

Estimated glomerular filtration rate and albuminuria are the strong predictive diagnostic markers for progression of DKD as suggested by updated KDIGO 2025 guidelines for people living with CKD.

Novel Biomarkers

Along with the traditional biomarkers, many alternative biomarkers are also validated in order to enable nephrologists to focus on DKD patients with poor prognoses. These novel markers are better biomarkers that help in earlier detection of the disease. Serum creatinine, eGFR, and proteinuria are insensitive and depending on these might result in extensive time-lapse where successful interventions could be tested and applied. Numerous biomarkers were identified for this purpose, and initial findings from many studies are enlightening. These novel biomarkers can be classified according to the pathological effects on renal structure and its response. Detailed classification has been tabulated in **Table 1**.

Along with the traditional biomarkers for the diagnosis of DKD some specific novel biomarkers such as kidney injury molecule 1 (KIM-1), N-Acetyl-β-O-glucosaminidase, liver-type fatty acid-binding protein (L-FABP), tenascin and tissue inhibitor of metalloproteinases 1, glomerular injury: urinary nephrin, podocin, and podocalyxin are more prominently in practice which was represented in **Figure 1**.

In one of our previous studies, we identified high levels of urinary liver-type fatty acid binding protein (u-LFABP) in association with declining renal function in T2DM. Macroalbuminuric study subjects showed higher levels of u-LFABP as compared to normoalbuminuric and

TABLE 1: Shows classification of novel biomarkers.[17]			
Glomerular biomarkers	*Tubular biomarkers*	*Biomarkers of oxidative stress*	*Biomarkers of inflammation*
Type IV collagen	NGAL 8oxodG	Uric acid	Tumor necrotic factor-α
• Fibronectin • Serum cystatin C • Transferrin • L-PGDS • Glycosaminoglycans (GAGs)	Urinary cystatin C	Pentosidine	• Tumor necrotic factor-α receptors • IL-6
Laminin	KIM-1	8oxodG 8-Oxo	MCP-1
Immunoglobulin G	RBP4		TGF-β
Ceruloplasmin	L-FABP		CTGF

(8oxodG: 8-Oxo-7,8-dihydro-2-deoxyguanosine; CTGF: connective tissue growth factor; IL-6: interleukins-6; KIM-1: kidney injury molecule-1; L-FABP: liver-type fatty acid-binding protein; L-PGDS: lipocalin-type prostaglandin D synthase; MCP-1: monocyte chemoattractant protein; NGAL: neutrophil gelatinase-associated lipocalin; RBP4: retinol-binding protein 4; TGF-β transforming growth factor-beta)

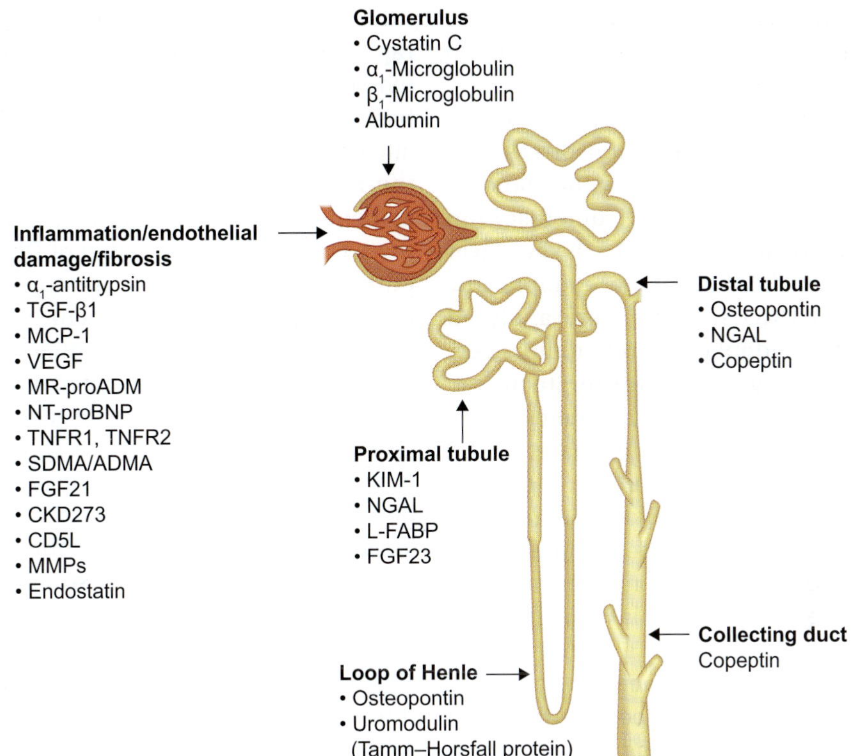

FIG. 1: Shows the diagrammatic representation of the novel biomarkers identified for the diabetic kidney disease (DKD) progression at various parts of kidney.[18]

microalbuminuric subjects. The results suggest the importance of tubular damage in the development of renal dysfunction among DKD individuals and its correlation with other clinical parameters[14] also the study showed u-LFABP levels were elevated in patients with reduced eGFR and showed a positive correlation with systolic blood pressure and protein to creatinine ratio in the total study subjects.

In another study from MV research team demonstrated that urinary monocyte chemoattractant protein-1 (uMCP-1) which is a strong chemotactic factor for monocytes, and its role in upregulated in diabetic nephropathy was analyzed as a great significance in the diagnosis and intervention of early diabetic nephropathy. This study has shown a positive association among the levels of uMCP-1 which increased gradually in type 2 diabetic subjects with deteriorating renal function. It was also significantly associated with the other risk factors of diabetic nephropathy.[15]

The identification of novel biomarkers based on the pathogenesis of DKD involving various renal structures is a prominent approach to identifying renal damage earlier. The potential 22 novel biomarkers mentioned in the table concerning the pathogenesis of DKD development are very promising. Each biomarker has its role in either identifying DKD early or predicting the progression of DKD over and above clinical history and standardized markers such as albuminuria and creatinine. Some biomarkers are useful for predicting other micro and macrovascular complications such as retinopathy and cardiovascular disease. This panel of biomarkers now warrants further validation in large-scale longitudinal studies involving people with T1DM and T2DM before their transition to clinical routine practice.

In another study by Victor et al., the crosstalk between endoplasmic reticulum stress and oxidative stress is highlighted by understanding the role of protein disulfide isomerase and endoplasmic reticulum oxidase 1α, a key player in redox protein folding in the endoplasmic reticulum.[16] 90 DKD subjects were analyzed and found that endoplasmic reticulum stress markers, activating transcription factor 6, inositol-requiring enzyme 1α, protein kinase RNA-like endoplasmic reticulum kinase, C/EBP homologous protein, and glucose-regulated protein-78; oxidative stress markers, thioredoxin-interacting protein and cytochrome b-245 light chain; and the crosstalk markers, protein disulfide isomerase and endoplasmic reticulum oxidase-1α, were progressively elevated in DKD subjects. The association between the crosstalk markers showed a positive correlation with endoplasmic reticulum stress and oxidative stress markers. Further, phosphorylation of eIF2α in high glucose-exposed cells was studied using western blot. In conclusion, our results shed light on the crosstalk between endoplasmic reticulum stress and oxidative stress and significantly contribute toward the onset and progression of diabetic nephropathy and also represent the major therapeutic targets for alleviating micro- and macrovascular complications associated with this metabolic disturbance.

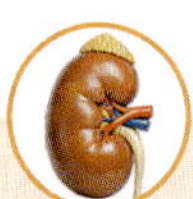

Novel biomarkers are more accurate and sensitive and significantly contribute to the diagnosis even before the onset of DKD.

GENETICS BIOMARKERS OF DIABETIC KIDNEY DISEASE

It is widely acknowledged that the greater the genetic susceptibility to T2DM in an individual, the earlier the disease manifestation and more rapid progression. Along with diagnostic biomarkers it is established that DKD has a genetic basis and prominence in certain ethnic groups and families among T2DM individuals suggesting the role of genetic factors. Both clinical and epidemiological studies have demonstrated that there is a familial aggregation of DKD in various ethnic groups, indicating that genetic factors contribute to the development of the disease. Scientific approaches for identifying genes that predispose to DKD are being mainly performed using linkage scans, candidate gene analysis and GWAS. Various studies have shown evidence of genetic determinants that may influence the development of kidney disease in patients with T2DM. GWAS has enlightened the knowledge of DKD heritability. The major advantage of genetic studies in DKD diagnosis is that it would permit the identification of individuals at risk of DKD shortly after diagnosis of diabetes rather than much later when microalbuminuria advances. There is substantial evidence of renal injury. This would also permit clinicians to target therapeutic interventions aimed at primary prevention rather than secondary treatment of established DKD. Secondly, and perhaps more importantly, if the susceptibility variants are located in genes that have not previously been implicated in DKD, this may lead to a clear understanding of its pathophysiology and the development of novel treatments.

Single nucleotide polymorphisms (SNPs) are the common mode to understand DNA variation. The updated dbSNP database in GWAS has >500 million reference SNPs (rs) with allele frequency data that has provided fundamental information for genetic studies of complex diseases including, DKD.[19] Estimated genetic variants were as high as 59% when adjusted for sex, diabetes duration and age at diabetes diagnosis, and with a tendency to higher heritability estimates for the more severe definitions.[20] Similar analyses in individuals with T2DM suggested only 8–25% heritability for DKD, potentially reflecting more heterogeneous mechanisms leading to DKD in T2DM in addition to a more important contribution of environmental factors.[21,22] Scientific evidence suggests higher rates of diabetic kidney disease are seen in Indo-Asians in the UK, in African-Americans,[23] in Nauruans[24] and Pima Indians.[25] The reason scientists predict genetic susceptibility for these interracial differences is the incidence of DKD.

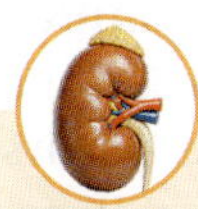

Genetics studies will enlighten the knowledge on DKD heritability and identification of individuals at risk of DKD shortly after diagnosis of diabetes.

COMMON GENETIC VARIANTS ASSOCIATED WITH DIABETIC KIDNEY DISEASE

In a study by Viswanathan et al., was among the first to report about the familial aggregation of *ACE* gene polymorphism among DKD in T2DM individuals. In this study, siblings of people with diabetes with the proband history of DKD were studied and those without proband DKD history were considered as controls and their genetic profiles were visualized. The results showed that there was strong familial clustering of DKD in south Indians with T2DM which was further independent of the familial clustering of diabetes. This study further laid the path of genetic studies on DKD, and they also noticed that the prevalence of other vascular complications was also higher among individuals with DKD siblings.[26] In another study by Viswanathan et al., also found that there was a strong association of the D allele of the *ACE* gene with diabetic nephropathy. DD genotype conferred the maximum risk, whereas the ACE II genotype seemed to confer a protective role against the development of diabetic and nondiabetic CKD.[27] Further, the ID and DD genotypes of the *ACE* gene conferred a greater role in genetic variations underlying the high-risk stage of DKD especially in women.[28]

The crucial role of tumor necrosis factor-α (TNF-α) on renal function in patients with diabetic nephropathy and further genetic association of TNF-α [-308G/A, (rs1800629)] SNP on the susceptibility to DKD individuals were also studied. The correlation between the plasma levels of TNF-α along with circulatory TNF-α receptor superfamily cytokines was also analyzed (sTNFR-1 and sTNFR-2).

Results of the study showed a remarkable stepwise increase in the levels of circulatory biomarkers such as TNF-α, sTNF-R1, and sTNF-R2 from normoalbuminuria to macroalbuminuria. In established DKD subjects, the TNF-α levels were higher in individuals who had mutant AA, than the wild GG genotype of *TNF*-α gene. Our results conclude that rs1800629 polymorphism in the *TNF*-α gene was associated with renal complications in T2DM subjects.[29]

Studies by OP Kalra have also highlighted the SNP's found in the oxidative stress (OS) pathology which plays a significant role in the development of DKD and that glutathione S-transferase theta-1 and/or glutathione S-transferase Mu-1 null genotypes are associated with higher OS in patients with DN.[30] In addition, Kalra et al. found that increased levels of inflammatory mediators, i.e., TNF-α, high-sensitivity C-reactive protein (hsCRP) and uMCP-1 play a significant role in contributing to oxidative stress.[31] Genetic polymorphism of the *NF-κB* gene and *TNF*-α gene play a pivotal role in determining the serum levels of various inflammatory markers and oxidant stress parameters. A significant association of -429T/C and Gly82Ser receptors for advanced glycation end-products (RAGE) polymorphisms were found to be associated with the development of macrovascular and microvascular complications, respectively in T2DM subjects.

Another Indian study on[19] inflammatory cytokine genes *TGFB1*: T869C (Leu10Pro) and Tyr81His; *CCL2*: A-2518G and insertion/deletion (I/D); *CCR5*: insertion/deletion (I/D) and G59029A; *IL8*: T-251Λ; *MMP9*: Arg279Gln

(G>A) have shown effect on risk of DN and a combination of risk alleles confer a substantial increased risk of DKD.

A recent meta-analysis also highlighted the genetic variants associated with DKD, such as angiotensin-converting enzyme 1, ApoE, and nitric oxide synthase.[32] In another study, an association of DKD with hemicentin 1 (HMCN1) polymorphism was identified among the Mexican-American population with renal disease.[33]

Some of this evidence paved the way for predicting and developing potential genetic risk scores (GRS) for DKD progression in patients with T2DM and major cardiovascular events (MCVE) and all-cause mortality (ACM) as secondary outcomes.

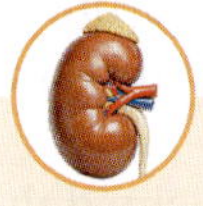

Angiotensin-converting enzyme (ACE) gene shows a strong association with DKD and confers a greater role in genetic variations underlying the high-risk stage of DKD.

EPIGENETICS

Epigenetics is denoted as any changes in gene expression that occur without alternating the underlying DNA sequence, its variation mainly includes DNA methylation, histone modification and changes in the noncoding RNA expression profile, which is an integrated part of DKD-related inflammation, oxidative stress, hemodynamics, and the activation of abnormal signaling pathways. MicroRNA (miRNAs) are an important element of epigenetics. These are short non-coding RNAs that influence gene expression through post-transcriptional processes carried by exosome/microvesicle. In recent years, evidence shows that microRNA is involved in the DKD progression via inflammation, hypertrophy, autophagy, endoplasmic reticulum (ER) stress, oxidative stress, insulin resistance, and podocyte injury and positive correlation

of miRNA expression is observed for TGF-β stimulator with albuminuria and reported good diagnostic efficiency.[34] Epigenetic studies secured the evidence for a pathogenic role of noncoding RNAs, such as miRNAs (miRs) in DKD.[35] miRs are a family of endogenous short, 21-nucleotide long, noncoding RNAs that recognize target mRNAs through partial complementary elements in the 3′-UTR of the mRNAs and inhibit their expression by translational repression or destabilization. Kato et al. first identified miR-192 as a regulator of collagen synthesis in DKD.[36]

A significant decrease was observed in the gene expression of nuclear factor erythroid-2-related factor 2 (Nrf2) in the DKD group compared to healthy controls. The transcription factor of Nrf2 is useful in maintaining cellular homeostasis. The regulation of Nrf2 expression is also an established target for treating DKD, and this regulation has been reported to be influenced by epigenetics. A parallel and significant downregulation of HDAC3/7/8/9/10/11 and SIRT1/2/3/4/7 was observed in DKD subjects compared to T2DM.[37] Our study findings provide compelling evidence of the association between HDACs and Nrf2 in the pathogenesis of DKD, shedding light on potential therapeutic avenues for this condition.

With ongoing rapid advancements in genome technologies including microarrays and next-generation sequencing, it is imperative to initiate the Human Epigenome Project.[38] It is possible to quantify genome-wide DNA methylation and histone PTMs, which will play a key chromatin marks among various clinical cohorts and assess their role in epigenetic modulation of a wide range of kidney diseases. These efforts will soon lead to the development of essential novel therapies for DKD. Lastly, combining genetic, epigenetic, and phenotypic studies will generate information to understand new pathogenic pathways and to search for new biomarkers for early diagnosis and prediction as part of prevention programs in DKD.

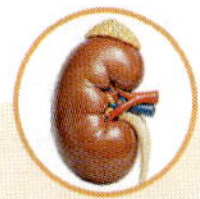

Epigenetic studies secured the evidence for a pathogenic role of noncoding RNAs, such as miRNAs in DKD.

SUMMARY

Clinical therapeutic strategies and the existing diagnostic biomarkers only partially slow the progression of DKD and roughly predict disease progression. Therefore, novel therapeutic methods, targets, and novel biomarkers are urgently needed to meet clinical requirements. Various genome-wide meta-analyses like[39] SUMMIT study for DKD had analyzed several different renal phenotypes among people with T1DM and T2DM. There is an urgent need for biomarker identification for early diagnosis of DKD. Drugs or biomarkers designed for a single target are probably not accurate, and the joint use of multiple epigenetic drugs targeting different epigenetic variations should be considered in future DKD treatment. To summarize biomarkers are one of the reliable ways to predict the DKD progression even without the presence of any risk factors.

CONCLUSION

Advancements in proteomics technologies, sample conditioning, and analysis methods have greatly influenced the productivity and efficiency of biomarker discovery, many clinical trials have influenced biomarker verification and validation making it a routine practice in the diagnosis process of DKD and it remains a significant, costly, and high-risk undertaking in the commercial development and deployment of novel biomarkers for DKD. Researchers have also made major efforts to undertake well-powered genetic and epigenetic studies in DKD to help understand its pathogenesis and further risk stratification of the disease.

TAKE HOME MESSAGES

- Diagnosis of DKD early or even before the onset of the disease is possible through novel and genetic markers biomarkers.
- Clinical implications and validation of these biomarkers are required on a larger scale to implement them in routine clinical practice.

REFERENCES

1. Harjutsalo V, Groop PH. Epidemiology and risk factors for diabetic kidney disease. Adv Chronic Kidney Dis. 2014;21(3):260-6.
2. Dousdampanis P, Trigka K, Mouzaki A. Tregs and kidney: From diabetic nephropathy to renal transplantation. World J Transplant. 2016 Sep 24;6(3):556-63.
3. Skupien J, Warram JH, Smiles AM, Stanton RC, Krolewski AS. Patterns of estimated glomerular filtration rate decline leading to end-stage renal disease in type 1 diabetes. Diabetes Care. 2016;39:2262-9.
4. Schlondorff DO. Overview of factors contributing to the pathophysiology of progressive renal disease. Kidney Int. 2008;74(7):860-6.
5. Hussain S, Jamali MC, Habib A, Hussain MS, Akhtar M, Najmi AK. Diabetic kidney disease: an overview of prevalence, risk factors, and biomarkers. Clin Epidemiol Glob Health. 2021;9:2-6.
6. Ilyas Z, Chaiban JT, Krikorian A. Novel insights into the pathophysiology and clinical aspects of diabetic nephropathy. Rev Endocr Metab Disord. 2017;18(1):21-8.
7. Macisaac RJ, Ekinci EI, Jerums G. Markers of and risk factors for the development and progression of diabetic kidney disease. Am J Kidney Dis. 2014;63(2 Suppl 2):S39-62.

8. Retnakaran R, Cull CA, Thorne KI, Adler AI, Holman RR. Risk factors for renal dysfunction in type 2 diabetes: U.K. Prospective Diabetes Study 74. Diabetes. 2006;55:1832-9.

9. Ekinci EI, Jerums G, Skene A, Crammer P, Power D, Cheong KY, et al. Renal structure in normoalbuminuric and albuminuric patients with type 2 diabetes and impaired renal function. Diabetes Care. 2013;36:3620-6.

10. Krolewski AS. Progressive renal decline: the new paradigm of diabetic nephropathy in type 1 diabetes. Diabetes Care. 2015;38:954-62.

11. Rosolowsky ET, Skupien J, Smiles AM, Niewczas M, Roshan B, Stanton R, et al. Risk for ESRD in type 1 diabetes remains high despite renoprotection. J Am Soc Nephrol. 2011;22:545-53.

12. Skupien J, Warram JH, Smiles AM, Niewczas MA, Gohda T, Pezzolesi MG, et al. The early decline in renal function in patients with type 1 diabetes and proteinuria predicts the risk of end stage renal disease. Kidney Int. 2012;82:589-97.

13. Forsblom C, Harjutsalo V, Groop PH. Kuka sairastuu diabeettiseen nefropatiaan? [Who will develop diabetic nephropathy?]. Duodecim. 2014;130(12):1253-9.

14. Viswanathan V, Sivakumar S, Sekar V, Umapathy D, Kumpatla S. Clinical significance of urinary liver-type fatty acid binding protein at various stages of nephropathy. Indian J Nephrol. 2015;25(5):269-73.

15. Tilak P, Khashim Z, Kumpatla S, Babu M, Viswanathan V. Clinical significance of urinary Monocyte Chemoattractant Protein-1 (uMCP-1) in Indian type 2 diabetic patients at different stages of diabetic nephropathy. Intern J Diabetes Mellitus. 2010;2:15-9.

16. Victor P, Umapathy D, George L, Juttada U, Ganesh GV, Amin KN, et al. Crosstalk between endoplasmic reticulum stress and oxidative stress in the progression of diabetic nephropathy. Cell Stress Chaperones. 2021;26(2):311-21.

17. Swaminathan SM, Rao IR, Shenoy SV, Prabhu AR, Basthi P, Rangaswamy MD, et al. Novel biomarkers for prognosticating diabetic kidney disease progression. Intern Urol Nephrol. 2023;55:913-28.

18. Colhoun HM, Marcovecchio ML. Biomarkers of diabetic kidney disease. Diabetologia. 2018;61(5):996-1011.

19. Ahluwalia TS, Khullar M, Ahuja M, Kohli HS, Bhansali A, Mohan V, et al. Common variants of inflammatory cytokine genes are associated with risk of nephropathy in type 2 diabetes among Asian Indians. PLoS One. 2009;4(4):e5168.

20. Sandholm N, Van Zuydam N, Ahlqvist E, Juliusdottir T, Deshmukh HA, Rayner NW, et al. The genetic landscape of renal complications in type 1 diabetes. J Am Soc Nephrol. 2017;28:557-74.

21. van Zuydam NR, Ahlqvist E, Sandholm N, Deshmukh H, Rayner NW, Abdalla M, et al. A genome-wide association study of diabetic kidney disease in subjects with type 2 diabetes. Diabetes. 2018;67:1414-27.

22. Kim J, Jensen A, Ko S, Raghavan S, Phillips LS, Hung A, et al. Systematic heritability and heritability enrichment analysis for diabetes complications in UK biobank and ACCORD studies. Diabetes. 2022;71:1137-48.

23. Cowie CC, Port FK, Wolfe RA, Savage PJ, Moll PP, Hawthorne VM. Disparities in incidence of diabetic end-stage renal disease according to race and type of diabetes. N Engl J Med. 1989;321:1074-9.

24. Collins VR, Dowse GK, Finch CF, Zimmet PZ, Linnanae AW. Prevalence and risk factors for micro- and macroalbuminuria in diabetic subjects and entire population of Nauru. Diabetes. 1989;38:1602-10.

25. Pettitt DJ, Saad MF, Bennett PH, Nelson RG, Knowler WC. Familial predisposition to renal disease in two generations of Pima Indians with type 2 (non-insulin-dependent) diabetes mellitus. Diabetologia. 1990;33:438-43.

26. Vijay V, Snehalatha C, Shina K, Lalitha S, Ramachandran A. Familial aggregation of diabetic kidney disease in Type 2 diabetes in south India. Diabetes Res Clin Pract. 1999;43:167-71.

27. Viswanathan V, Zhu Y, Bala K, Dunn S, Snehalatha C, Ramachandran A, et al. Association between ACE gene polymorphism and diabetic nephropathy in South Indian patients. JOP. 2001;2(2):83-7.

28. Viswanathan V, Krishnamoorthy E, Kumpatla S. Higher prevalence of deletion allele in angiotensin converting enzyme Gene among type 2 diabetic subjects with lower estimated glomerular. Intern J Curr Res. 2018;10(6):70930-6.

29. Umapathy D, Krishnamoorthy E, Mariappanadar V, Viswanathan V, Ramkumar KM. Increased levels of circulating (TNF-α) are associated with (-308G/A) promoter polymorphism of TNF-α gene in Diabetic Nephropathy. Int J Biol Macromol. 2018;107 (Pt B):2113-21.

30. Gautam A, Kalra OP, Agarwal S, Gambhir JK, Gupta S, Mehndiratta M. Association of nuclear factor kappa B1gene polymorphism in relation to the risk of developing nephropathy in type 2 diabetes mellitus. Proc Annu Conf Indian Soc. Nephrol. 2012;6-9:28-9.

31. Gupta S, Mehndiratta M, Kalra S, Kalra OP, Shukla R, Gambhir JK. Association of tumor necrosis factor (TNF) promoter polymorphisms with plasma TNF-α levels and susceptibility to diabetic nephropathy in North Indian population. J Diab Compl. 2015;29: 338-42.

32. Mooyaart AL, Valk EJ, van Es LA, Bruijn JA, de Heer E, Freedman BI, et al. Genetic associations in diabetic nephropathy: a meta-analysis. Diabetologia. 2011; 54(3):544-53.

33. Kim S, Abboud HE, Pahl MV, Tayek J, Snyder S, Tamkin J, et al. Examination of association with candidate genes for diabetic nephropathy in a Mexican American population. Clin J Am Soc Nephrol. 2010;5(6): 1072-8.

34. Cao Q, Chen XM, Huang C, Pollock CA. MicroRNA as novel biomarkers and therapeutic targets in diabetic kidney disease: an update. FASEB Bio Adv. 2019;1(6):375-88.

35. Kato M, Zhang J, Wang M, Lanting L, Yuan H, Rossi JJ, et al. MicroRNA-192 in diabetic kidney glomeruli and its function in TGF-beta-induced collagen expression via inhibition of E-box repressors. Proc Natl Acad Sci USA. 2007;104(9):3432-7.

36. Kato M, Park JT, Natarajan R. MicroRNAs and the glomerulus. Exp Cell Res. 2012;318(9):993-1000.

37. Harithpriya K, Juttada U, Jayasuriya R, Kumpatla S, Viswanathan V, Ramkumar KM. Comprehensive gene expression analysis of histone deacetylases and the transcription factor Nrf2 in the progression of diabetic nephropathy. Int J Diabetes Dev Ctries. 2025;45:462-71.

38. Reddy MA, Natarajan R. Epigenetics in diabetic kidney disease. J Am Soc Nephrol. 2011;22(12):2182-5.

39. Looker HC, Colombo M, Hess S, Brosnan MJ, Farran B, Dalton RN, et al. Biomarkers of rapid chronic kidney disease progression in type 2 diabetes. Kidney Int. 2015;88(4):888-96.

Key Research Takeaway

Familial aggregation of diabetic kidney disease in Type 2 diabetes in south India

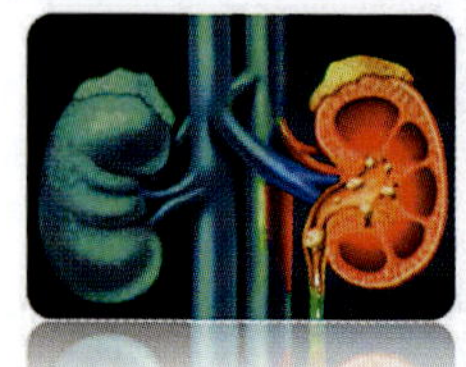

V. Vijay *, C. Snehalatha, K. Shina, S. Lalitha, A. Ramachandran

Diabetes Research Centre, No. 4, Main Road, Royapuram, Madras 600 013, India

Received 7 October 1998; received in revised form 20 October 1998; accepted 5 January 1999

Abstract

The study was done to assess whether there was a familial aggregation of diabetic kidney disease (DKD) in Type 2 diabetic subjects. The profile of associated complications was also studied. Two groups of diabetic siblings of Type 2 diabetic patients, matched for age, body mass index (BMI) and duration of diabetes mellitus were studied. The siblings also had Type 2 diabetes. Group A comprised of siblings of probands with diabetic nephropathy and retinopathy ($n = 30$, M:F = 20:10) and Group B were siblings of probands without diabetic nephropathy or microalbuminuria (MAU) ($n = 30$, M:F = 14:16). Anthropometry, measurement of blood pressure and tests for proteinuria, MAU and retinopathy and ECG and biothesiometry were carried out for all study subjects. Persistent proteinuria was present in 15 (50%) siblings in group A and none in group B. MAU was detected in 26.7% ($n = 7$) in Group A and 3.3% ($n = 1$) in Group B ($P = 0.057$). Thus a total of 22 out of 30 cases in Group A had albuminuria. In Group A, seven (23.3%) had proteinuria and hypertension. Hypertension was present in nine (30.0%) in group A, and in five (16.7%) in group B (NS). Occurrence of retinopathy was found to be significantly higher in group A than in group B (33.3 vs 6.7%, $\chi^2 = 5.1$, $P = 0.023$). Abnormal ECG changes were present in 10% and 6.7% in Group A and Group B, respectively. In Group A, one patient had peripheral vascular disease (PVD) while in Group B none had PVD. A comparison of sib pairs, matched for age, duration of diabetes and the level of metabolic control showed that there was strong familial clustering of diabetic kidney disease in south Indians with Type 2 diabetes. This was independent of the familial clustering of diabetes. Prevalence of other vascular complications were also higher in Group A. © 1999 Elsevier Science Ireland Ltd. All rights reserved.

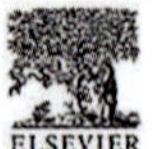

Diabetes Research and Clinical Practice 43 (1999) 167–171

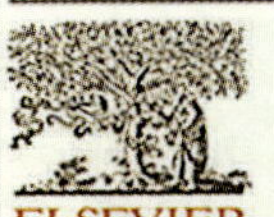

Contents lists available at ScienceDirect

International Journal of Diabetes Mellitus

journal homepage: ees.elsevier.com/locate/ijdm

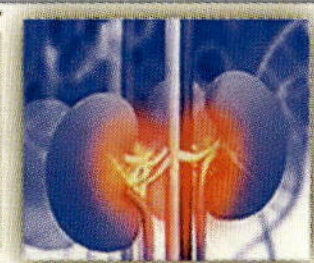

Original Article

Clinical significance of urinary Monocyte Chemoattractant Protein-1 (uMCP-1) in Indian type 2 diabetic patients at different stages of diabetic nephropathy

Priyanka Tilak, Zenith Khashim, Satyavani Kumpatla, Mary Babu, Vijay Viswanathan *

M.V. Hospital for Diabetes and Diabetes Research Centre, No. 5, Main Road, Royapuram, Chennai 600 013, India

ARTICLE INFO

Article history:
Received 20 July 2009
Accepted 13 October 2009

Keywords:
Urinary MCP-1
Diabetic nephropathy
Type 2 diabetes
India

ABSTRACT

Objective: Monocyte Chemoattractant Protein-1 (MCP-1) is the strongest known chemotactic factor for monocytes and is upregulated in diabetic nephropathy. So measuring urinary MCP-1 is of great significance in the diagnosis and intervention of early diabetic nephropathy. This study aims at determining the levels of urinary MCP-1 (uMCP-1) at different stages of diabetic nephropathy and to see its correlation with other parameters in Indian type2 diabetic subjects.

Materials and methods: A total of 64 (M:F; 40:24) type 2 diabetic subjects were divided into three groups based on their renal function and were compared with non-diabetic controls (Group 1) $n = 20$ (M:F; 13:7). The study groups were Group 2 (normoalbuminuria) $n = 16$, Group 3 (microalbuminuria) $n = 23$ and Group 4 (macroalbuminuria) $n = 25$. Demographic, anthropometric and biochemical details were recorded for all the subjects. Urinary MCP-1 levels were measured by using solid phase ELISA method.

Results: Mean levels of uMCP-1 in subjects with type 2 diabetes were significantly higher than in controls ($p < 0.05$). The levels of uMCP-1 in type 2 diabetic subjects increased gradually with deteriorating renal function ($p = 0.006$). There was a significant difference in urinary MCP-1 levels between Group 2 and Group 1 ($p < 0.001$). Levels of uMCP-1 were significantly higher in subjects with eGFR <60 ml/min compared to eGFR >60 ml/min ($p = 0.008$). uMCP-1 levels correlated positively with uACR or uPCR ($r = 0.551$, $p < 0.0001$), urea ($r = 0.43$, $p < 0.0001$) and creatinine ($r = 0.478$, $p < 0.0001$). A negative correlation between uMCP-1 and eGFR ($r = -0.338$, $p = 0.006$) was noted.

Conclusion: Our study demonstrated that urinary MCP-1 levels increased gradually in type 2 diabetic subjects with deteriorating renal function. It is significantly associated with the other risk factors of diabetic nephropathy.

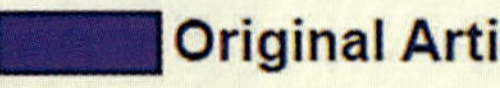 **Original Article**

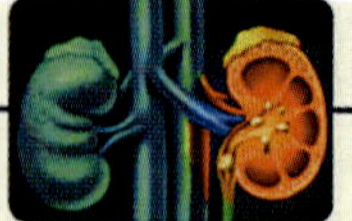

Clinical significance of urinary liver-type fatty acid binding protein at various stages of nephropathy

V. Viswanathan, S. Sivakumar[1], V. Sekar[1], D. Umapathy[1], S. Kumpatla[1]

Departments of Diabetology, [1]Biochemistry and Molecular Genetics, M.V. Hospital for Diabetes and Prof. M. Viswanathan Diabetes Research Center (WHO Collaborating Center for Research Education and Training in Diabetes), Royapuram, Chennai, Tamil Nadu, India

ABSTRACT

This cross-sectional study was to evaluate the levels of urinary liver-type fatty acid binding protein (u-LFABP pg/mg urine creatinine ratio) at different stages of diabetic nephropathy and to see its correlation with other clinical parameters in South Indian patients with type 2 diabetes mellitus (T2DM). A total of 65 (M: F; 42:23) T2DM subjects were divided into three groups, and were compared with 13 (M: F; 3:10) nondiabetic controls. The study groups were as follows: normoalbuminuric ($n = 22$), microalbuminuric ($n = 22$) and macroalbuminuric ($n = 21$). Estimated glomerular filtration rate (eGFR) was calculated using Cockcroft and Gault formula. u-LFABP levels in spot urine samples were measured with a solid phase enzyme linked immunosorbent assay. This study showed that u-LFABP levels were undetectable in healthy controls and was very low in the normoalbuminuric subjects. Elevated levels of u-LFABP are evident from the microalbuminuric stage indicating tubular damage. The levels of u-LFABP increased gradually with declining renal function. Geometric mean (95% confidence interval) for normoalbuminuria was 0.65 (0.47–0.97), microalbuminuria was 0.99 (0.55–1.97) and macroalbuminuria was 5.16 (1.8–14.5), ($P = 0.005$). In conclusion, u-LFABP levels were elevated in patients with reduced eGFR and showed a positive correlation with systolic blood pressure and protein to creatinine ratio in the total study subjects.

JOP. J. Pancreas (Online) 2001; 2(2):83-87.

Association between ACE Gene Polymorphism and Diabetic Nephropathy in South Indian Patients

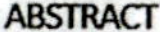

Vijay Viswanathan1, Yanqing Zhu2, Karthik Bala2, Stephen Dunn2 , Chamukuttan Snehalatha1, Ambady Ramachandran1, Muthu Jayaraman1, Kumar Sharma2

1Diabetes Research Centre. Madras, India. 2Division of Nephrology, Dorrance Hamilton Research Laboratories, Department of Medicine, Thomas Jefferson University. Philadelphia, USA

ABSTRACT

Objective To study the association of ACEgene polymorphism and diabetic nephropathyin South Indian subjects.

Setting Outpatient clinic of a specialized hospital.

Patients The study included 109 South Indiantype 2 diabetic patients (72 males and 37females; age 56.7±9.0 years, mean±SD). Thepatients were subdivided into two groups:nephropathic (n=86) and normoalbuminuricpatients (n=23).

Interventions Genomic DNA was isolated from the peripheral blood leukocytes. To determine the ACE genotype, genomic DNA was amplified by PCR initially using a flanking primer pair and, subsequently when necessary, with a primer pair that recognizes the insertion specific sequence for confirmation of the specificity of the amplification reactions.

Main outcome measures ACE genotype distribution in the two study groups.

Results In the nephropathic patients, ID and DD genotypes were present in 52.3% and 27.9% of the patients, respectively as compared to 34.8% and 21.7% respectively in those with normoalbuminuria. The D allele was present in 80.2% of the nephropathic patients and 56.5% of the normoalbuminuric patients (c2=4.28, P=0.039; odds ratio 3.12). Therefore, the higher percentage of II genotype in the normoalbuminuric group was 43.5% as compared to the 19.8% in nephropathic patients.

Conclusions This study showed a positive association between the D allele (ID and DD genotype) of the ACE polymorphism and diabetic proteinuria in South Indian type 2 diabetic patients. Our findings are in keeping with several earlier studies showing a strong association of the D allele of the ACE gene with diabetic nephropathy.

INTRODUCTION South Asian type 2 diabetic patients have been shown to have a higher prevalence of nephropathy when compared to Europeans [1,2]. ACE polymorphism appears to have a significant impact on the progression of diabetic nephropathy [3]. Several Japanese studies have found the D allele to be an independent risk factor for diabetic nephropathy [4]. It is important to look for the gene association in the Asian Indian population, in view of the high prevalence of diabetic nephropathy and to see whether the associationdiffers from other populations. To our knowledge, there have been no studies on ACE

5

Beyond Diagnosis: Psychological Dimensions of Diabetic Kidney Disease

Vaishnavi Vijay, Manjula Arunraj

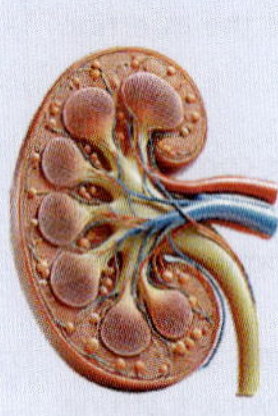

- ➤ The mind-body loop
- ➤ Cognitive decline in diabetic kidney disease
- ➤ The 3-way link (HbA1c—depression/anxiety—kidney function)
- ➤ The brain–kidney axis
- ➤ Psychologically driven physical symptoms
- ➤ Misinterpretations in diabetic kidney disease
- ➤ The evolving role of psychologists
- ➤ Real—world experiences from MV Hospital
- ➤ Breaking stigma within the medical community about interventions
- ➤ Opportunities for screening, early interventions, and collaborative care

Abstract

Chronic illnesses like chronic kidney disease (CKD) among people with type 2 diabetes (T2D) demand a holistic approach that goes beyond physical treatment. This chapter examines the integration of psychological care into CKD treatment, starting with the mind-body loop and the influence of emotional health on physical outcomes. It highlights emerging evidence of cognitive decline in patients with diabetic kidney disease (DKD), as well as the significant three-way relationship between glycemic control (HbA1c), depression/anxiety, and kidney function. It also examines the brain-kidney axis and the role of stress hormones in mediating both renal and neuropsychological decline. Psychologists are increasingly becoming core members of multidisciplinary teams, contributing to bedside assessments, emotional regulation strategies, and discharge planning. The challenges posed by psychosomatic symptoms and misinterpretations further underline the need for integrated psychological care. The integration of psychology in renal and endocrine care is not just beneficial—it is essential. Through early detection, collaborative care models, and innovative therapeutic tools, this chapter advocates for a paradigm shift in how DKD is understood and managed.

Keywords: Mind and body, stress hormones, psychosomatic symptoms, diabetic kidney disease.

INTRODUCTION

Diabetic kidney disease (DKD) is more than a physical condition it is a complex interplay between biological, psychological, and behavioral factors. As kidney function declines, patients often face not only increasing physical symptoms but also cognitive impairment and emotional distress. These mental and emotional challenges, in turn, can influence self-care behaviors and treatment adherence, creating a cycle that may accelerate disease progression. In the evolving landscape of chronic illness care, psychologists are becoming integral members of inpatient teams, particularly in addressing the mental health challenges associated with DKD. This chapter explores the vital connection between the mind and body in DKD, highlighting how cognitive decline develops across disease stages and how psychological health profoundly shapes clinical outcomes and also how a psychologist's role and psychological interventions improve outcomes, reduce stigma, and enable early, collaborative mental healthcare in renal and endocrine settings.

PSYCHO NEPHROLOGY: EXPLORING INTERPLAY OF MENTAL HEALTH AND KIDNEY DISEASE

Mind-body Loop

The interconnectedness between an individual's physical and mental state is called the mind and body loop. The thoughts and emotions of a person impact the physical body and both can influence one another. The reciprocal association between kidney function and mental health is known as the "mind-body loop" in renal illness. A single factor might negatively impact both poor mental health and kidney function. For instance, chronic renal disease can cause fatigue, sadness, and cognitive impairment, while stress and worry can exacerbate the advancement of kidney disease **(Flowchart 1)**.

The kidney and the brain interact in a strong and complicated way, often leading to abnormal cognitive function for patients with CKD.[1] Cognitive dysfunction, or abnormal cognitive performance, is considered a serious complication of CKD among people with type 2 diabetes (T2D) as well as end-stage renal disease (ESRD). It impacts memory, processing speed, executive function, and attention, all of which are essential for day-to-day functioning and treatment compliance.

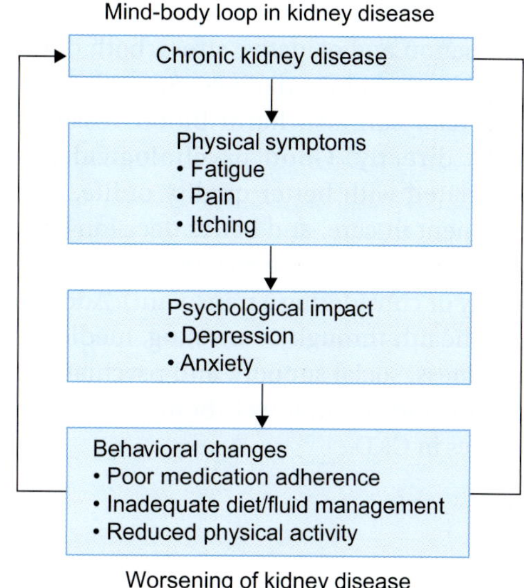

FLOWCHART 1: The interconnection between physiological and psychological factors.

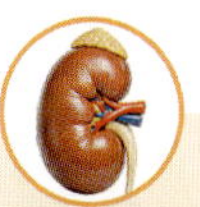

There is a reciprocal relationship between mental health, kidney function, and diabetic kidney disease which can lead to cognitive and emotional challenges, while psychological stress and poor mental health can worsen kidney outcomes.

PSYCHOLOGICAL HEALTH AND KIDNEY DISEASE OUTCOMES

Patients with diabetes and CKD often experience depression, anxiety, and cognitive decline. Depression rates among people with CKD are significantly greater than in the general population, often reaching 20–30% depending on the disease stage. Poor mental health is linked to faster disease progression, higher rates of hospitalization, and increased mortality. Depression can reduce adherence to medications, dialysis schedules, diet, and fluid restrictions, which worsens kidney outcomes. Psychological stress increases systemic inflammation and oxidative stress, both of which can accelerate kidney damage. Stress hormones like cortisol can also harm blood vessels and kidneys directly. Good psychological health is associated with better quality of life, greater engagement in care, and better decision-making about treatments (like choosing the best dialysis modality or considering a transplant). Addressing mental health through counseling, medications, mindfulness, social support, and psychiatric care improves both mental well-being and physical outcomes in CKD.

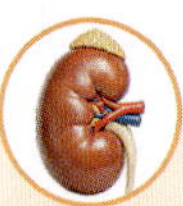

Addressing mental health through interventions like counseling, medication, and support improves the quality of life of people living with diabetes and can significantly slow DKD progression and improve treatment adherence.

COGNITIVE DECLINE IN DIABETIC KIDNEY DISEASE

Cognitive decline is increasingly recognized as a serious and underappreciated complication of DKD, resulting from the complex interplay between chronic hyperglycemia, vascular damage, inflammation, and uremic toxicity. Patients with DKD, particularly in advanced stages, frequently exhibit impairments in attention, executive function, memory, and processing speed **(Flowchart 2)**. The mechanisms involve microvascular damage to the brain, similar to diabetic retinopathy or nephropathy, and chronic inflammation. The progression of kidney disease leads to systemic inflammation, oxidative stress, anemia, and endothelial dysfunction, which further compromise cerebral perfusion and contribute to neurodegeneration.

These cognitive impairments can hinder medication adherence, dietary compliance, and decision-making, creating a vicious cycle

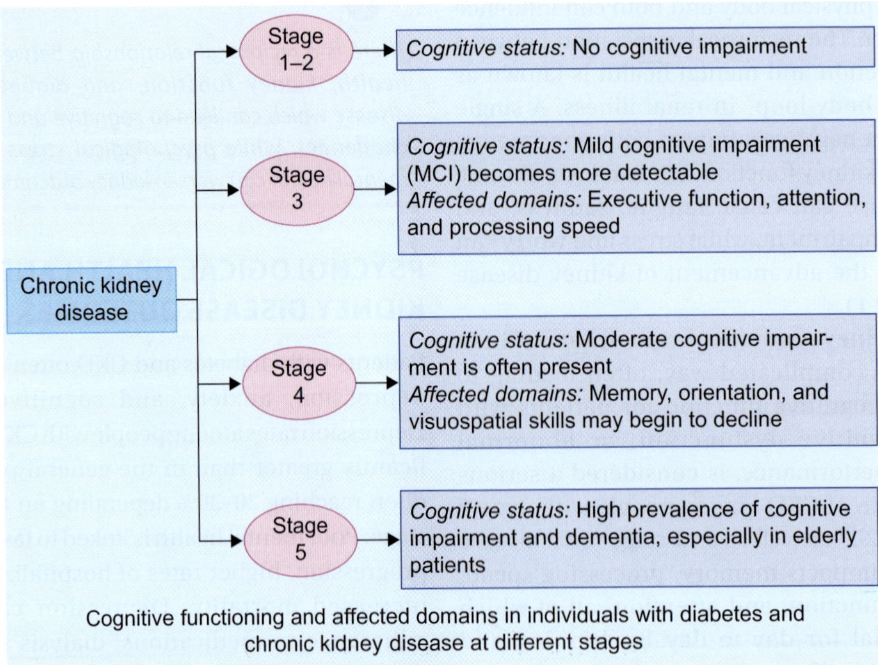

FLOWCHART 2: The stagewise cognitive status of chronic kidney disease in patients living with diabetes.

that worsens both kidney and brain outcomes. Therefore, early cognitive screening, personalized education, mental health support, and optimal control of metabolic and vascular risk factors are essential components of care in patients with DKD to preserve cognitive function and enhance long-term outcomes. Cognitive impairment is a significant and often underrecognized complication of CKD, with its prevalence and severity increasing as kidney function declines. While cognitive impairment is less studied in early CKD stages, some research suggests that cognitive decline can begin early and parallels kidney function decline.[2]

The severity of cognitive decline correlates with the progression of kidney disease, becoming more pronounced as the estimated glomerular filtration rate (eGFR) falls below 45 mL/min/1.73 m².[3] Hemodialysis patients may experience "dialysis-related cognitive decline" due to hemodynamic instability or "brain stunning." Peritoneal dialysis may be associated with better cognitive outcomes compared to hemodialysis. Commonly used cognitive screening instruments include the trail making test (Trial A/B), the Montreal cognitive assessment (MoCA), and the mini-mental status examination (MMSE). Additionally, several neuroimaging techniques can be used to detect lesions in the white matter.

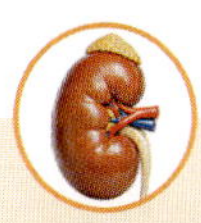

Cognitive impairment affects attention, memory, and executive function. It is a significant but often underrecognized complication of diabetic and CKD, exacerbated by systemic inflammation, vascular damage, and uremic toxins.

Management Strategies

- *Control comorbidities:* Effective management of comorbid conditions such as hypertension, diabetes mellitus, and dyslipidemia is critical in slowing both renal and cognitive decline. Strict glycemic control in diabetic patients has also been shown to reduce the risk of

microvascular complications that impact the brain. Regular monitoring and comprehensive cardiovascular risk reduction are essential components of preserving cognitive function.

- *Optimize dialysis:* Avoid intradialytic hypotension and consider dialysis modality adjustments. Dialysis adequacy and modality selection can significantly influence cognitive outcomes. Individualized dialysis prescriptions based on patient tolerance and cognitive status are recommended.
- *Cognitive rehabilitation:* Therapy and structured activities may help preserve function. The integration of such interventions into nephrology care including referrals to occupational or neuropsychologists can enhance quality of life and independence.
- *Medication review:* Avoid drugs with anticholinergic effects or sedatives that may worsen cognition. Making medication schedules simpler and educating patients and caregivers about the cognitive risks of certain drugs are also key steps.

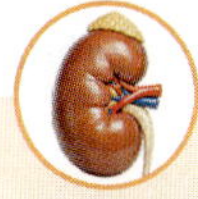

Early cognitive screening, personalized treatment plans, optimized dialysis, and targeted control of comorbidities (such as diabetes and hypertension) are critical strategies to preserve brain function and improve long-term outcomes in DKD patients.

3-WAY LINK (HbA1c—DEPRESSION/ANXIETY—KIDNEY FUNCTION)

Glycated hemoglobin (HbA1c) is a blood test that indicates the mean blood glucose levels during the preceding 2–3 months. It is mainly used to diagnose and monitor diabetes. An increased risk of anxiety and depression is associated with a higher HbA1c. Depression and anxiety can result from improper blood sugar control. Chronic elevated glucose levels may have an effect on neurotransmitters such as serotonin and dopamine. People with poorly controlled diabetes often report more symptoms of depression and anxiety compared to those with better control.

Higher HbA1c levels (indicating poor blood glucose control) are strongly associated with an increased risk of CKD. Long-term hyperglycemia damages the glomeruli in the kidneys.[4] Poorer glucose management can contribute to anxiety and depression. Patients with depression often show higher HbA1c levels, possibly due to lower medication adherence, unhealthy behaviors, and biological factors (like increased cortisol levels).[5] Moreover, kidney disease itself can lead to depression through a toxic build-up of chemicals that influence the brain. Depression and anxiety also make it more difficult to manage diabetes (people may skip medications, eat worse, etc.), which worsens HbA1c and accelerates kidney damage **(Fig. 1)**.

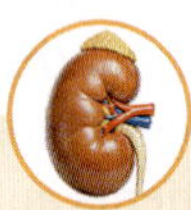

Poor glycemic control (high HbA1c) is linked to increased depression and anxiety, which in turn worsen diabetes management and accelerate kidney damage which creates a self-reinforcing cycle that affects both mental and physical health.

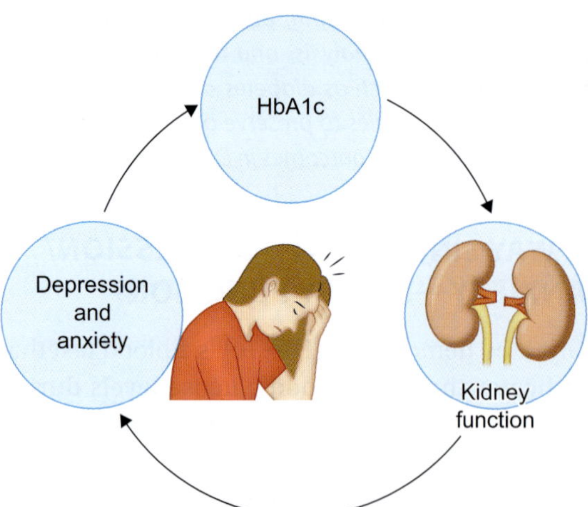

FIG. 1: A vicious loop in which a high glycated hemoglobin (HbA1c) can decrease our mood and cause poor diabetes control, which, in turn, can lead to a decrease in kidney function and an even worse mood.

Management Strategies

Effective management includes optimizing glycemic control with medications such as sodium-glucose cotransporter-2 (SGLT2) inhibitors and glucagon-like peptide-1 (GLP-1) receptor agonists, which also protect kidney function, alongside blood pressure control (target < 130/80 mm Hg) using angiotensin-converting enzyme (ACE) inhibitors or angiotensin II receptor blockers (ARBs) to slow CKD progression. Mental health should be addressed through regular screening (e.g., PHQ-9, GAD-7), cognitive behavioral therapy (CBT), and antidepressants like selective serotonin reuptake inhibitors (SSRIs) (adjusted for renal function), as treating depression can improve glycemic outcomes. A multidisciplinary team including endocrinologists, nephrologists, mental health professionals, dietitians, and primary care providers should collaborate to deliver patient-centered care that also includes lifestyle education, self-management support, and digital tools for monitoring and adherence. This integrated approach, supported by guidelines such as Kidney Disease: Improving Global Outcomes (KDIGO) 2022, American Diabetes Association (ADA) 2024, and NICE CG91, can significantly improve outcomes and quality of life for patients managing these interrelated conditions.

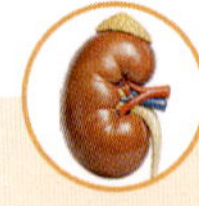

Combining optimized blood sugar and blood pressure control with regular mental health screening and support from a coordinated care team significantly improves clinical outcomes and quality of life for patients with diabetes, kidney disease, and mood disorders.

BRAIN–KIDNEY AXIS AND ROLE OF STRESS HORMONES

The brain-kidney axis represents a dynamic bi-directional relationship in which neural, hormonal, and inflammatory processes connect brain and kidney health, with cortisol—a key stress hormone—playing a central role. Chronic psychological stress activates the hypothalamic–pituitary–adrenal (HPA) axis, increasing cortisol levels, which in turn elevates blood pressure, blood glucose, and systemic inflammation—all of which contribute to renal injury and CKD progression. High cortisol levels also decrease hippocampus function and mood regulation, encouraging feelings of depression and anxiety, all of which are common in CKD, and exacerbating HPA axis dysfunction in an endless cycle.[6]

Damaged kidneys can cause neuroinflammation, cognitive impairment, and psychiatric symptoms by releasing proinflammatory cytokines such as interleukin (IL)-6 and tumor necrosis factor alpha (TNF-α) and failing to remove neurotoxic uremic solutes such as indoxyl sulfate, which can penetrate the blood–brain barrier. Furthermore, increased sympathetic nervous system activity—which occurs in both stress and CKD—causes vasoconstriction and sodium retention, worsening hypertension and renal injury. This brain–kidney–stress loop emphasizes the necessity for holistic management of both physiological and psychological health in individuals with diabetic kidney disease.

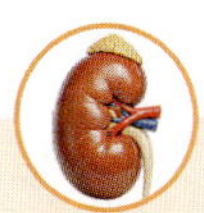

Chronic stress elevates cortisol, which worsens blood pressure, glucose control, and inflammation contributing to a decrease in kidney function. Impaired kidneys release neurotoxin substances that further damage brain function and mood, perpetuating the cycle.

Management Strategies

Management of brain–kidney axis dysfunction, particularly in patients with CKD and elevated stress hormones like cortisol, requires a multidisciplinary and integrative approach that targets both physiological and psychological domains.

- Medical strategies include optimizing kidney function through strict blood pressure control with ACE inhibitors or ARBs, managing diabetes with SGLT2 inhibitors or GLP-1 receptor agonists, correcting metabolic derangements, and reducing systemic inflammation. Cortisol modulation involves avoiding unnecessary corticosteroids, screening for adrenal dysfunction, and cautiously treating hypercortisolism if present.
- Psychological care is critical and includes routine screening for depression, anxiety, and cognitive impairment using tools such as PHQ-9, GAD-7, and MoCA, along with mental health interventions such as training for stress management, cognitive behavioral therapy (CBT), and mindfulness-based stress reduction (MBSR).
- Pharmacologic support may include renal-adjusted doses of SSRIs, avoiding benzodiazepines due to central nervous system (CNS) sensitivity.
- Lifestyle modifications such as a renal-friendly diet, moderate physical activity, and sleep hygiene further support both brain and kidney health.
- Collaborative care models involving nephrologists, endocrinologists, mental health professionals, and dietitians enhance outcomes while emerging strategies like hair cortisol monitoring, gut microbiota modulation, and neuroprotective therapies offer additional promise.

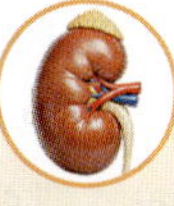

Holistic, patient-centered management improves both clinical outcomes and quality of life in individuals affected by the brain–kidney–stress interplay.

PSYCHOLOGICALLY DRIVEN PHYSICAL SYMPTOMS AND MISINTERPRETATIONS IN DIABETIC KIDNEY DISEASE

Psychosomatic symptoms are physical symptoms that stem from psychological or emotional factors rather than direct organic pathology, and they are highly prevalent in patients with diabetic kidney disease (DKD). These patients often report fatigue, sleep disturbances, gastrointestinal discomfort, pain, and cognitive impairment, which are commonly misattributed to nonspecific or unrelated causes. For instance, fatigue is frequently seen as a result of "just high blood sugar" or overwork, while gastrointestinal issues may be blamed on diet rather than uremia or medication side effects. Similarly, mood changes, cognitive decline, or irritability are often dismissed as normal aging or stress, masking underlying depression, anxiety, or neuroinflammatory effects of CKD **(Table 1)**. These misattributions delay the recognition of mental health issues and interfere with effective symptom management. Studies have shown that such symptoms often correlate with elevated levels of proinflammatory cytokines, HPA axis dysregulation, and uremic toxin accumulation, which impact both peripheral and central nervous systems. Psychological distress in chronic renal disease was significantly predicted by patients' views of their condition, underscoring the importance of cognitive variables in symptom interpretation.[7] The increased rate of depression among those with CKD is associated with adverse outcomes, including poor quality of life and increased mortality.[8] It is important to use integrated care techniques that address both the physical and psychological elements of DKD in order to ensure comprehensive management and better patient outcomes.

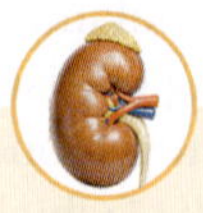

Psychosomatic symptoms in DKD are common but often misinterpreted, delaying mental health diagnosis and effective care. Integrated care improves recognition and management of both physical and psychological symptoms, leading to better outcomes.

PSYCHOLOGISTS IN WARD: REDEFINING ROLES IN RENAL AND ENDOCRINE CARE

Evolving Role of Psychologists

Traditionally, psychological services in hospitals were viewed as incidental. However, the modern care model is transforming this view, especially in chronic conditions like diabetic kidney disease (DKD), where mental health significantly affects disease management and quality of life.

Psychologists now work alongside endocrinologists and nephrologists to support patients through:

- Adjustment to diagnosis
- Treatment adherence

TABLE 1: The possible misattributions among people living with diabetes and chronic kidney disease (CKD).	
Psychosomatic symptom	*Possible misattribution by patient*
Fatigue and low energy	"It is just my blood sugar" or "I am just tired from work"
Sleep disturbances (insomnia or hypersomnia)	"I cannot sleep because of stress" or "Maybe it is my pain meds"
Gastrointestinal discomfort (nausea, bloating)	"It is something I ate" or "Maybe it is just gas"
Muscle cramps and joint pain	"I am just aging" or "It is arthritis"
Cognitive issues (poor concentration, memory)	"I must be getting old" or "It is just stress from family/work"
Breathlessness or pain in the chest	An attack related to anxiety or "I am feeling unwell"
Palpitations or dizziness	"Panic attacks" or "I need more sugar"
Loss of appetite or weight loss	"I am just not hungry" or "It is my depression meds"
Tingling or numbness (neuropathy)	"I must have slept wrong" or "Circulation problem"
Emotional lability (irritability, sadness)	"I am just moody" or "This is normal stress"

- Managing their emotions and diabetes distress

A 2022 review indicated that up to 30% of patients with diabetes experience depression, and up to 40% report diabetes distress, which significantly impairs treatment adherence and glycemic control.[9]

In renal care, psychological distress is even more prevalent. Patients undergoing dialysis often face:

- Social isolation
- Sleep disturbances
- Cognitive challenges
- Grief related to lifestyle changes

Psychologists can help by providing brief cognitive-behavioral interventions, psychoeducation, and supportive counseling during admissions **(Flowchart 3)**. Their roles have expanded from postdischarge care to proactive involvement at the bedside, conducting early risk assessments, and contributing to multidisciplinary discussions.[10]

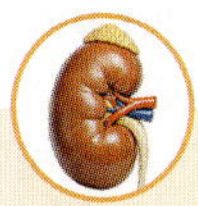

Psychologists play a vital role in the multidisciplinary care of diabetic kidney disease, addressing emotional, cognitive, and behavioral challenges that impact treatment adherence and quality of life—shifting from incidental support to integrated, proactive care.

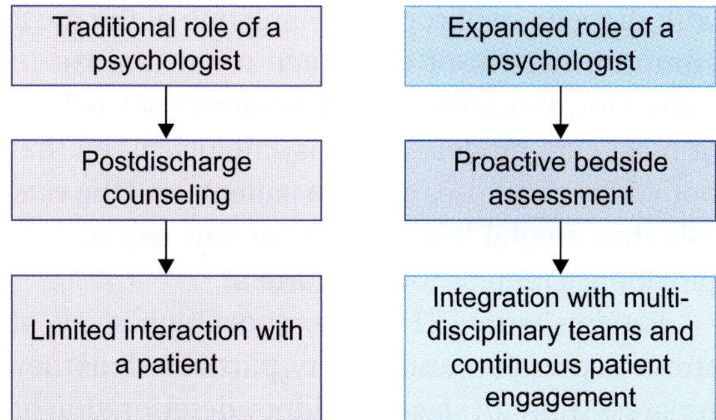

FLOWCHART 3: Displays psychologists' traditional and expanding roles in providing psychological care for individuals with diabetic kidney disease (DKD).

REAL WORLD EXPERIENCES FROM THE "MIND-WELLNESS CLINIC" OF MV HOSPITAL

A study conducted at MV Hospital titled "Assessment of Diabetes-Related Distress Among Subjects with Type 2 Diabetes in South India"[11] underscored the substantial psychological burden experienced by people living with T2D. The study employed a structured distress assessment framework among outpatients attending the hospital's diabetes clinic and found that a significant proportion of about 77.5% of individuals experienced moderate-to-high levels of diabetes-related distress (DRD). These findings are especially salient in the context of CKD, where psychological distress can act as both a consequence and a contributing factor. The study clearly emphasized that unmanaged emotional distress could lead to poor adherence to medication, unhealthy coping behaviors and disengagement from self-care routines each of which increases the likelihood of renal complications. Therefore, routine assessment and management of psychological distress in individuals with diabetes is not merely a supportive measure but a preventive one, particularly when aiming to delay or mitigate the onset of diabetic nephropathy. By identifying and addressing distress early through the support of trained psychologists, hospitals can empower patients to better adhere to their medical regimens and make lifestyle modifications that preserve renal function over time. This study served as a catalyst for MV Hospital's continued focus on psychological screening and intervention as part of routine diabetes and kidney health monitoring.

Another significant contribution from MV Hospital's mental health integration efforts is demonstrated in the study titled "A Study on the Positive Impact of Intensive Psychological Counselling on Psychological Well-being of Type 2 Diabetic Patients Undergoing Amputation".[12] The study focused on patients who underwent an amputation due to diabetes-related complications whose prognosis often includes the potential for

CKD due to years of uncontrolled diabetes and associated vascular deterioration. These patients were provided with intensive psychological counseling before and after surgery. Such sessions usually include providing emotional support, cognitive restructuring, psychoeducation, and techniques to build resilience and body acceptance. The outcomes were promising, patients who received intensive counseling showed better psychological outcomes on the quality of life questionnaire compared to a regular counseling session. Although the study's primary objective was psychological well-being post-amputation, its implications extend directly to patients with or at risk of developing CKD. First, the findings reinforce the importance of psychological resilience in managing the consequences of long-term diabetes complications. Second, they demonstrate that intensive psychological intervention can serve as a stabilizing force during major health crises something commonly experienced by patients facing CKD diagnosis. Emotional trauma, denial and fear are common reactions to the progression of kidney disease; this study highlights that well-timed psychological support can reduce long-term mental health complications and improve patient engagement with ongoing care.

The intervention model used short-term but intensive therapy delivered within a medical setting and serves as a blueprint for integrating psychologists within units. As CKD patients often undergo multiple hospitalizations, psychological care during these periods of vulnerability could significantly improve both shorthand long-term outcomes.

The third study, "The Effect of Progressive Muscle Relaxation Therapy on Diabetes Distress and Anxiety among Patients with Type 2 Diabetes"[13] explored a different kind of intervention one that was non-invasive, easy to implement and scalable. Participants were taught progressive muscle relaxation (PMR) techniques during outpatient visits and were encouraged to practice them regularly through regular follow-ups on WhatsApp as well. The study observed measurable reductions in both DRD and generalized anxiety symptoms following the intervention period. PMR, a technique that involves systematically tensing and relaxing muscle groups, not only supports psychological well-being but also impacts physiological parameters by reducing stress hormones, stabilizing blood pressure and promoting parasympathetic nervous system activity. These effects are particularly beneficial for individuals with CKD or at risk of CKD, as elevated stress levels are known to accelerate kidney function decline through pathways involving hypertension, inflammation, and poor metabolic control. Importantly, this study presents a practical, low-barrier intervention that can be incorporated into standard diabetes and CKD care. Unlike more resource-intensive therapies, PMR requires minimal time, no specialized equipment, and can be taught by trained psychologists. Its inclusion in patient education programs, especially for those managing multiple comorbidities, represents a cost-effective, evidence-based strategy to support both mental and physical health.

Taken together, these three studies reflect MV Hospital's commitment to understanding and addressing the psychological dimensions of chronic illness. They also provide critical evidence for how psychological interventions can influence medical outcomes and patient well-being, particularly in the context of kidney health. The overlap between diabetes and CKD is clinically well established, with diabetic nephropathy being one of the most common causes of end-stage renal disease in India. However, what remains underacknowledged in most care models is the psychological toll that both these diagnoses exert on patients and the vital role that mental health professionals can play in providing a remedy for this burden.

Patients with CKD often report high levels of stress, depression, and anxiety, particularly as they progress through stages of kidney deterioration or initiate dialysis. These mental health challenges can reduce treatment adherence, impair decision-making about transplant options, and increase hospitalization rates. The success of MV Hospital's psychological interventions in the context of diabetes therefore provides a roadmap for replicating similar strategies within renal care settings. Each of these approaches requires institutional commitment and interdisciplinary collaboration. Psychologists must be seen not as secondary staff, but as core members of chronic disease management teams. Their expertise in navigating emotional complexity, building coping strategies, and fostering resilience directly complements the medical goals of the doctors.

By integrating mental health professionals within medical teams and drawing on the evidence from our institution, we can pave the way for a more humane, responsive, and effective model of chronic disease management. This is a proven reality and holds promise for replication and scaling across the broader healthcare landscape in India and beyond.

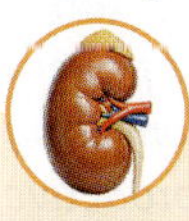

The real-life experiences emerging from MV Hospital's research provide more than institutional pride, they offer concrete evidence that psychological interventions, when applied thoughtfully and systematically, can profoundly influence the lives of people navigating complex, chronic illnesses. For patients with CKD or those at risk due to longstanding diabetes, such support is not just an adjunct but an essential component of comprehensive care.

BREAKING STIGMA WITHIN MEDICAL COMMUNITY ABOUT INTERVENTIONS

Despite clear benefits, psychological care is still underutilized due to *stigma,* both among patients and healthcare professionals.

In renal and endocrine care:
- Mental health symptoms are often seen as secondary.
- Referrals to psychologists are delayed or absent.
- Staff may feel unprepared to discuss psychological issues.

Addressing stigma requires:
- Training staff in trauma-informed care and active listening.
- Normalizing psychological screenings during ward rounds.
- Sharing success stories among medical teams.

Psychologists also facilitate staff reflective groups, helping team members recognize burnout and its impact on patient interactions, thereby creating more compassionate spaces for patients.[14]

Top Five Myths about Psychology in Medical Wards

1. *Myth:* Psychological issues are separate from physical health.
   Fact: Mental health significantly influences physical health outcomes.
2. *Myth:* Only patients with severe mental illness need psychological support.
   Fact: All patients can benefit from psychological support to manage stress, adherence, and coping strategies.
3. *Myth:* Discussing mental health will distress patients further.
   Fact: Open conversations about mental health can provide relief and improve patient engagement.
4. *Myth:* Psychological interventions are time-consuming.
   Fact: Brief interventions can be effective and time efficient.
5. *Myth:* Medical staff should handle all aspects of patient care.
   Fact: Collaborative care with psychologists enhances overall treatment effectiveness.

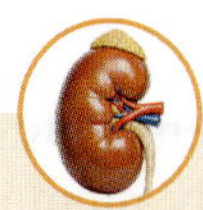

Stigma and misconceptions continue to hinder the integration of psychological care in medical wards, but targeted training, routine screenings, and collaborative approaches can normalize mental health support and improve patient and staff well-being.

OPPORTUNITIES FOR SCREENING, EARLY INTERVENTIONS, AND COLLABORATIVE CARE

Psychologists in DKD care offer unique opportunities for early detection of mental health issues and facilitate preventive interventions. Screening for depression, diabetes distress and cognitive impairments in newly admitted patients can significantly alter their treatment course.[15]

Recommended screening tools:
- Patient Health Questionnaire-9 (PHQ-9)
- Diabetes Distress Scale (DDS)
- Montreal Cognitive Assessment (Mo CA)

Models of collaborative care:
- Psychologists co-leading ward rounds
- Shared digital notes and feedback loops between psychology, dietetics and nephrology
- Joint family counseling sessions before initiating dialysis

These early interventions prevent psychological decomposition and improve discharge planning. For example, a patient flagged for depression early in their admission can be connected to outpatient services or peer support, increasing their long-term engagement with care.[16]

Furthermore, there is growing potential to incorporate expressive arts therapy and mindfulness-based interventions in renal wards. Pilot programs show promising results in reducing distress through journaling, drawing, or guided meditation.[17]

DAILY PSYCHOLOGICAL WELL-BEING CHECKLIST FOR INPATIENTS

This checklist is intended for use by psychologists or trained ward staff to facilitate daily mental health check-ins and ensure holistic care for patients with chronic conditions like DKD.
- Has the patient made eye contact and responded to greetings?
- Has the patient expressed their current mood or emotional state (positive/negative)?

- Have they expressed any signs of distress (withdrawal/agitation)?
- Have they engaged on any form of activity (reading, watching TV)?
- Have you documented their appetite and sleep patterns?
- Has the patient discussed about future goals/concerns?
- Would the patient be willing to participate in group sessions if made available?
- How has their interaction with family members been (if applicable)?
- Are they aware that psychological support is available?
- Any follow-up that is needed for mental health concerns flagged for today?

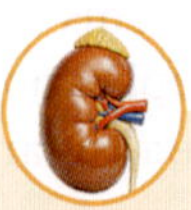

Early psychological screening and collaborative care models in DKD significantly enhance patient outcomes by identifying distress early, personalizing interventions, and promoting holistic, proactive treatment—supported by daily mental health check-ins and innovative therapies such as mindfulness and expressive arts.

SUMMARY

This chapter highlights the crucial integration of psychological care in managing DKD. It begins by exploring the mind-body loop and how mental health influences disease progression. Cognitive decline in CKD patients is emphasized, underlining the need for early screening. A central focus is the triadic relationship between HbA1c, depression/anxiety, and kidney function, showing how mental and metabolic health are intertwined. The brain–kidney axis and the role of stress hormones like cortisol are also discussed. The chapter examines how psychosomatic symptoms and emotional distress can disrupt treatment adherence. It details the evolving role of psychologists from postdischarge care to proactive inpatient support. Drawing from success stories at MV Hospital, it demonstrates how integrated psychological care improves adherence, reduces distress, and enhances quality of life. The chapter concludes with strategies to reduce stigma, tools for early screening, and models for collaborative, holistic care, including a practical inpatient well-being checklist.

CONCLUSION

The intricate relationship between psychological and physical health plays a crucial role in managing people with DKD. As we have explored, the mind-body loop demonstrates how mental health issues such as depression and anxiety can exacerbate kidney disease progression, while kidney dysfunction can worsen psychological well-being. Cognitive decline, psychosomatic symptoms, and the interplay of stress hormones all highlight the need for an integrated, holistic approach to care. By recognizing the significant impact of mental health on kidney disease outcomes, it becomes evident that multidisciplinary care, including psychological support, is essential for improving both physical and mental well-being. The evolving role of psychologists in renal care is a testament to the importance of addressing the psychological aspects of the disease along with medical treatment. Real-world success stories, such as those from MV Hospital, demonstrate that addressing mental health can lead to better patient outcomes, treatment adherence, and quality of life.

As we move forward, it is crucial to reduce the stigma surrounding psychological care among people with CKD and T2D and to implement effective screening and collaborative interventions. This approach can foster better compliance, reduce complications, and ultimately enhance patient outcomes.

TAKE HOME MESSAGES

- *Mental and physical health are interconnected:* Addressing both psychological and physical aspects of DKD is essential for optimal patient care and improved outcomes.
- *Early recognition and intervention are crucial:* Misattributions of symptoms can delay diagnosis and treatment. A comprehensive, multidisciplinary approach can help identify both physical and psychological issues early.
- *Collaboration is key:* Integrating nephrologists, psychologists, dietitians, and other specialists leads to better patient management and supports holistic care.
- *Reducing stigma is essential:* Creating an environment where psychological care is valued can improve treatment adherence, reduce distress, and enhance the overall quality of life for patients.

By embracing these principles, healthcare teams can significantly improve the well-being and treatment outcomes of individuals with DKD.

REFERENCES

1. Xie Z, Tong S, Chu X, Feng T, Geng M. Chronic kidney disease and cognitive impairment: Kidney Dis (Basel). 2022;8(4):275-85.
2. Zhang J, Wu L, Wang P, Pan Y, Dong X, Jia L, et al. Prevalence of cognitive impairment and its predictors among chronic kidney disease patients: A systematic review and meta-analysis. PLoS One. 2024;19(6):e0304762.
3. Tamura MK, Larive B, Unruh ML, Stokes JB, Nissenson A, Mehta RL, et al.; Frequent Hemodialysis Network Trial Group. Prevalence and correlates of cognitive impairment in hemodialysis patients: the Frequent Hemodialysis Network trials. Clin J Am Soc Nephrol. 2010;5(8):1429-38.
4. Afkarian M, Zelnick LR, Hall YN, Heagerty PJ, Tuttle K, Weiss NS, et al. Clinical manifestations of kidney disease among US adults with diabetes, 1988-2014. JAMA. 2016;316(6):602-10.
5. Gonzalez JS, Peyrot M, McCarl LA, Collins EM, Serpa L, Mimiaga MJ, et al. Depression and diabetes treatment nonadherence: a meta-analysis. Diabetes care. 2008;31(12):2398-403.
6. Sagmeister MS, Harper L, Hardy RS. Cortisol excess in chronic kidney disease - A review of changes and

impact on mortality. Front Endocrinol (Lausanne). 2023;13:1075809.

7. Muscat P, Weinman J, Farrugia E, Callus R, Chilcot J. Illness perceptions predict distress in patients with chronic kidney disease. BMC Psychol. 2021;9(1):75.

8. Simões E, Silva AC, Miranda AS, Rocha NP, Teixeira AL. Neuropsychiatric Disorders in Chronic Kidney Disease. Front Pharmacol. 2019;10:932.

9. Fisher L, Gonzalez JS, Polonsky WH. The confusing tale of depression and distress in patients with diabetes: A call for greater clarity and precision. Diabet Med. 2014;31(7):764-72.

10. Cukor D, Cohen SD, Peterson RA, Kimmel PL. Psychosocial aspects of chronic disease: ESRD as a paradigmatic illness. J Am Soc Nephrol. 2007;18(12):3042-55.

11. Hemavathi P, Satyavani K, Smina TP, Vijay V. Assessment of diabetes related distress among subjects with type 2 diabetes in South India. Int J Psychol Counsel. 2019;11(1):1-5.

12. Amalraj MJ, Viswanathan V. A study on positive impact of intensive psychological counseling on psychological well-being of type 2 diabetic patients undergoing amputation. Int J Psychol Counsel. 2017;9(2):10-6.

13. Arunraj M, Vijay V, Kumpatla S, Viswanathan V. The effect of progressive muscle relaxation therapy on diabetes distress & anxiety among people with type 2 diabetes. Indian J Med Res. 2025;161(1):72.

14. Gonzalez JS, Tanenbaum ML, Commissariat PV. Psychosocial factors in medication adherence and diabetes self-management: implications for research and practice. Am Psychol. 2016;71(7):539-51.

15. Anderson RJ, Freedland KE, Clouse RE, Lustman PJ. The prevalence of comorbid depression in adults with diabetes: a meta-analysis. Diabetes Care. 2001;24(6):1069-78.

16. Egede LE, Ellis C. Diabetes and depression: global perspectives. Diabetes Res Clin Pract. Diabetes Res Clin Pract. 2010;87(3):302-12.

17. Hilliard ME, Powell PW, Anderson BJ. Evidence-based behavioral interventions to promote diabetes management in children, adolescents, and families. Am Psychol. Am Psychol. 2016;71(7):590-601.

Key Research Takeaway

Vol. 11(1), pp. 1-5, January 2019
DOI: 10.5897/IJPC2018.0551
Article Number: D4E41C859902
ISSN 2141-2499
Copyright © 2019
Author(s) retain the copyright of this article
http://www.academicjournals.org/IJPC

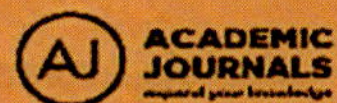

International Journal of Psychology and Counselling

Full Length Research Paper

Assessment of diabetes related distress among subjects with type 2 diabetes in South India

Hemavathi P., Satyavani K., Smina T. P. and Vijay V.*

M.V. Hospital for Diabetes and Prof. M. Viswanathan Diabetes Research Centre, WHO Collaborating Centre for Research, Education and Training in Diabetes and IDF Centre for Excellence in Diabetes Care, No 4, West Madha Church Street, Royapuram, Chennai – 600 013, India.

Received 26 October, 2018; Accepted 18 December, 2018

Diabetes is a complex chronic disease that affects not only an individual's physical health, but can also have a profound impact on mental wellbeing. The aim of this study was to assess the prevalence of DRD among subjects with type 2 diabetes (T2DM) using Diabetes Distress Scale-17 (DDS-17) and to see its correlation with glycemic control and treatment modalities. A cross-sectional study of 400 T2DM subjects (200 men and 200 women) aged between 25 to 65 years who visited the tertiary care centre for diabetes in South India between April 2017 and May 2018 were included in this study. Subjects with T1DM, gestational diabetes mellitus (GDM) and psychiatric illness were excluded. The total score of DDS-17 was calculated by taking a sum of the 17 items' results and then dividing the total by 17. Clinical validation of the DDS suggests that the following thresholds of severity should be applied when interpreting the scores: little or no distress < 2.0, moderate distress = 2.0 - 2.9, and high distress ≥ 3.0. The mean age of men and women was 52.0 ± 8.4 and 51.7 ± 8.1 years, respectively. The mean score in women was 2.79 ± 1.52 as compared to men (1.62 ± 0.83) (p<0.001). The study findings highlighted that women had high levels of distress in managing diabetes as compared to men. Diabetes distress should be considered as a significant health problem and steps should be taken for effective management by lifestyle modifications, coping with their stress and diabetes.

ORIGINAL ARTICLE

The effect of progressive muscle relaxation therapy on diabetes distress & anxiety among people with type 2 diabetes

Manjula Arunraj[1], Vaishnavi Vijay[1], Satyavani Kumpatla[1] & Vijay Viswanathan[2]

Departments of [1]Psychology, & [2]Diabetology, Prof. M. Viswanathan Diabetes Research Centre, Chennai, India

Received August 20, 2024; Accepted November 26, 2024; Ahead of print February 7, 2025; Published February 14, 2025

Background & objectives: Diabetes distress (DD) is a mental condition that can develop in people with diabetes and shares characteristics with stress, anxiety, and depression. The aim was to determine the effect of Jacobson's Progressive Muscle Relaxation (PMR) therapy on DD, anxiety, glycemic control, hemodynamic and lipid measures among people with type 2 diabetes (T2DM).

Methods: A total of 80 participants were recruited for this prospective randomised intervention study and divided into two groups equally; group 1 (Control) (n=40) received general counselling for stress reduction and group 2 (Intervention) (n=40) received PMR therapy and general counselling for stress reduction. A pre-, and post-test was done with diabetes distress Scale (DDS) and generalized anxiety disorder (GAD) Scales. Baseline data on anthropometric, hemodynamic, biochemical details were collected and repeated after three months. Thirty-six participants, with four dropouts in each group, reported for follow up. Diabetes medication regimens in both groups remained unchanged throughout the study period.

Results: There was a significant reduction in the total mean scores of DDS (Pre *vs.* Post) (3.8 *vs.* 1.6) and GAD Scale (17.9 *vs.* 6.3; $P<0.0001$) in the intervention group. The PMR therapy group showed a significant reduction in HbA1c, fasting and post prandial (PP) glucose levels with HbA1c (baseline *vs.* follow up; 9.2% *vs.* 7.6%), fasting (194.5 mg/dl *vs.* 142.4 mg/dl) and PP glucose levels (266.5 mg/dl *vs.* 175.5 mg/dl) ($P=0.001$) whereas control group showed an increase in HbA1c, fasting and PP glucose levels. The impact of PMR therapy was also reflected in the lipid profile. Seventy per cent of the intervention group participants followed PMR therapy regularly.

Interpretation & conclusions: Our study findings highlighted that PMR therapy had a positive effect on diabetes distress and anxiety among people with T2DM. It also improved glycemic control and can be used as an adjunctive to the medications for better management of T2DM.

Indiian J Med Res 161, January 2025, pp 72-80

DOI:10.25259/IJMR_1227_2024

academicJournals

Full Length Research Paper

Vol. 9(2), pp. 10-16, April, 2017
DOI: 10.5897/IJPC2016.0461
Article Number: 6A0E48164241
ISSN 2141-2499
Copyright © 2017
Author(s) retain the copyright of this article
http://www.academicjournals.org/IJPC

International Journal of Psychology and Counselling

"A study on positive impact of intensive psychological counseling on psychological well-being of type 2 diabetic patients undergoing amputation"

*Mary Jenifer Amalraj, Anitha Rani. A and Vijay Viswanathan**

M.V. Hospital for Diabetes, Diabetes Research Centre, WHO Collaborating Centre for Research, Education and Training in Diabetes, No. 4, Main Road, Royapuram Chennai – 600 013, India.

Amputation is one of the most dreadful complications in diabetes. Diabetic amputees are at elevated risk of psychological distress due to their disability. Thus, the current study aimed to evaluate the effect of intensive counseling on psychological outcomes among type 2 diabetic patients undergoing amputation. The study was conducted among 62 consecutive patients admitted in the diabetic centre and who underwent an amputation. These patients were randomly assigned to a routine counseling group (RCG-26) and intensive counseling group (ICG-36). World Health Quality of Life (WHQOL) was administered individually to all the patients based on inclusion criteria. In the RCG group, psychological therapy was given before amputation. For patients in the ICG group, psychological therapy was given before and every day after amputation, till the day of discharge. WHQOL questionnaire scores together with the demographic details were also recorded accordingly. The finding highlighted that the overall quality of the life improves in ICG group in both BKA and Toe amputation, as compared to the RCG group. ICG has better impact on QOL than RCG in amputation patients. Thus, intensive assessment and intervention has to be included as part of routine management among patients with diabetes when they undergo a surgical amputation.

6

Advent of New Drugs and Their Effect on Diabetic Kidney Disease

Prashanth Arun

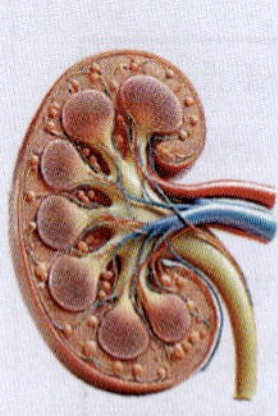

- ➤ Optimal use of RAAS inhibitors
- ➤ Pathophysiology of DKD and targets of newer therapies
- ➤ Finerenone
- ➤ SGLT2 inhibitors
- ➤ GLP-1 receptor agonists
- ➤ Comparative efficacy and synergistic use in DKD
- ➤ Practical considerations in clinical practice

Abstract

Diabetic kidney disease (DKD) is considered one of the major reasons for end-stage renal disease (ESRD) and is also a leading cause for significant cardiovascular morbidity as well as mortality. Despite standard therapies such as renin–angiotensin–aldosterone system (RAAS) blockade, many patients experience progressive kidney function decline. This chapter highlights the emergence of novel therapeutic agents—finerenone, sodium-glucose cotransporter-2 (SGLT2) inhibitors, and glucagon-like peptide-1 receptor agonists (GLP-1 RAs)—that target key pathogenic mechanisms beyond glycemic control, including inflammation, oxidative stress, and fibrosis. Clinical trials such as FIDELIO-DKD (FInerenone in reducing kiDnEy faiLure and disease prOgression in Diabetic Kidney Disease), CREDENCE (Canagliflozin and Renal Events in Diabetes with Established Nephropathy Clinical Evaluation), and LEADER (Liraglutide Effect and Action in Diabetes: Evaluation of cardiovascular outcome Results) have demonstrated their efficacy in slowing DKD progression and improving cardiovascular outcomes. The chapter also discusses practical considerations for their use and the role of emerging biomarkers and ongoing trials in shaping a personalized, multitargeted approach to DKD management.

Keywords: DKD, finerenone, RAAS blockade, SGLT2 inhibitor, glycemic control.

INTRODUCTION

Diabetic kidney disease (DKD), or diabetic nephropathy, is a major health issue that arises when diabetes coexists with chronic kidney impairment. It often goes undiagnosed for 4–7 years, with noticeable symptoms typically appearing only in later stages.[1] Globally, DKD affects approximately 40% of individuals with diabetes, making it a leading cause of kidney failure and a key driver of cardiovascular complications. This condition poses a growing challenge to public health systems and economies. During 1990 and 2021, the disability-adjusted life years (DALYs) for DKD increased significantly—by 74% in type 1 diabetes mellitus (T1DM) and

173.6% in type 2 diabetes mellitus (T2DM). By 2030, these are expected to exceed 4.4 million and 14.6 million, respectively, driven by aging and population growth.[2]

In India, the burden of DKD is particularly concerning. Multicenter studies have found that the prevalence of DKD among individuals with diabetes ranges from 34.4% to as high as 62.3%.[1] Alarmingly, according to global data on diabetes-related kidney deaths, India—alongside China—has recorded the highest numbers. Specifically, deaths attributed to type 1 DKD are estimated at 15.47 million, while those related to type 2 DKD amount to approximately 56.2 million.[3] DKD stands as the foremost cause of end-stage renal disease (ESRD), contributing significantly to increased morbidity and mortality, while severely impairing patients' quality of life.[4] Micro-albuminuria serves as a critical early indicator of kidney involvement in type 2 diabetes, with reported prevalence ranging from 12% to nearly 29%. Even patients with normal albumin levels at diagnosis remain at high risk of progression, emphasizing the need for routine screening to enable timely intervention and prevent DKD.[5] The primary strategies for managing DKD have traditionally involved stringent control of blood glucose levels and blood pressure, alongside the use of renin–angiotensin–aldosterone system (RAAS) blockers as monotherapy.

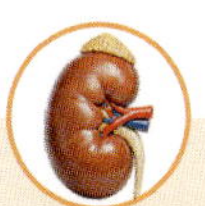

The primary strategies for managing DKD have traditionally involved stringent control of blood glucose levels and blood pressure, alongside the use of RAAS blockers as monotherapy.

OPTIMAL USE OF RENIN–ANGIOTENSIN–ALDOSTERONE SYSTEM INHIBITORS

Clinical trials have consistently demonstrated that angiotensin-converting enzyme (ACE) inhibitors and angiotensin receptor blockers (ARBs) are effective in slowing the progression of kidney dysfunction. The rationale behind combining RAAS inhibitors—such as ACE inhibitors with ARBs or adding mineralocorticoid receptor antagonists (MRAs) or direct renin inhibitors (DRIs)—was to provide more complete blockade of the RAAS pathway, aiming to improve cardiovascular and kidney outcomes.[6] However, major clinical studies and professional guidelines now advise against dual or triple RAAS blockade in patients with chronic kidney disease (CKD), regardless of diabetes status. This is due to the lack of long-term renal or cardiovascular benefit and the elevated risk of adverse events, particularly hyperkalemia and acute kidney injury (AKI), associated with such combinations.[7]

Despite adherence to recommended treatment protocols, a considerable risk of CKD progression remains, emphasizing the necessity for novel therapeutic approaches. Recent insights have highlighted the pathological role of MR overactivation in the development of cardiorenal syndromes—including DKD—primarily via mechanisms involving chronic inflammation and fibrosis, which further compromise kidney and heart function. While a meta-analysis indicated a 31% reduction in urinary protein or albumin excretion with steroidal MRAs in patients with CKD, the evidence for benefits on long-term clinical outcomes remains insufficient.[8]

In a review article by Viswanathan et al., it was suggested that hypertension remains the predominant risk factor that increases the progression of DKD. There are several drugs which can be used to treat hypertension, such as β-blockers, calcium-channel blockers (CCB), and α-blockers that can be second or third line of drugs. RAAS blockers such as ACE inhibitors and ARB remain the first line of therapy. Several studies, such as HOPE and Steno, have proved the effectiveness of ACE inhibitor in reducing the albumin excretion rate apart from its essential role in lowering the blood pressure.[5]

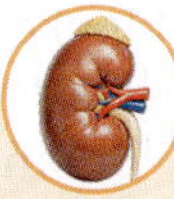

Despite adherence to recommended treatment protocols, a considerable risk of CKD progression remains, emphasizing the necessity for novel therapeutic approaches.

PATHOPHYSIOLOGY OF DIABETIC KIDNEY DISEASE AND TARGETS FOR NEWER THERAPIES

Diabetic kidney disease is a major microvascular complication of diabetes mellitus,[9] driven by a complex interplay of metabolic, hemodynamic, inflammatory, and fibrotic mechanisms. Chronic hyperglycemia initiates a cascade of cellular and molecular events that lead to progressive structural and functional damage in the kidney. In the early stages, increased sodium-glucose co-transport via sodium-glucose cotransporter-2 (SGLT2) in the proximal tubule reduces sodium delivery to the macula densa, disrupting tubuloglomerular feedback (TGF). This results in afferent arteriole vasodilation and efferent arteriole constriction, leading to glomerular hyperfiltration and elevated intraglomerular pressure, contributing to mechanical stress, podocyte injury, and proteinuria (**Flowchart 1**).[10]

Simultaneously, sustained hyperglycemia activates multiple pathways, including the polyol, hexosamine, and protein kinase C (PKC) pathways, along with excessive production of advanced glycation end-products (AGEs). These metabolic disturbances increase oxidative stress through reactive oxygen species (ROS), leading to deoxyribonucleic acid (DNA) damage,

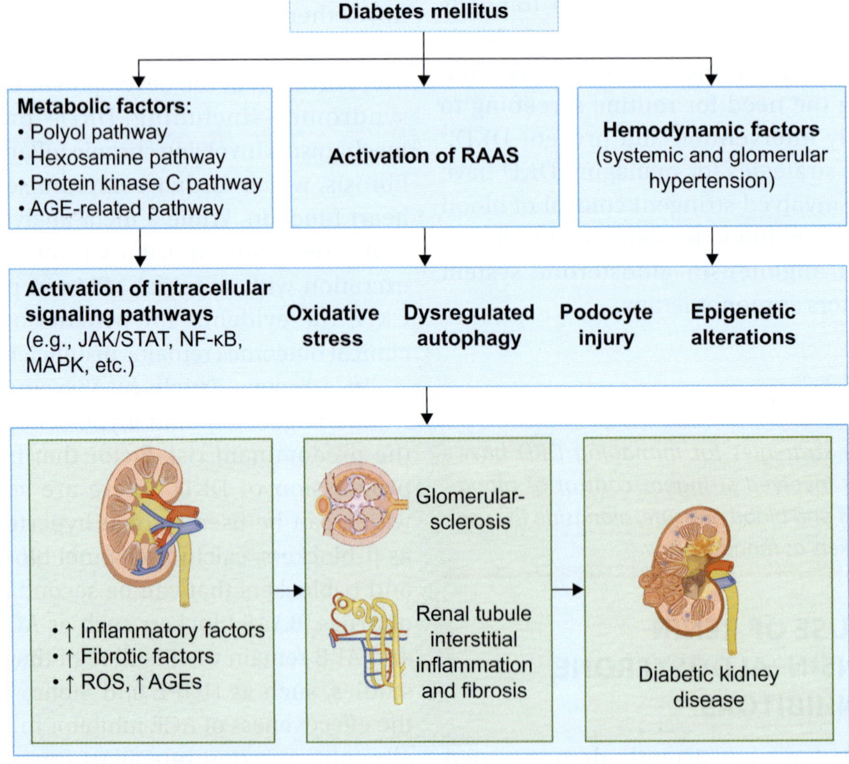

FLOWCHART 1: Mechanistic overview of diabetic kidney disease (DKD) pathogenesis.[14]

(AGEs: advanced glycation end-products; RAAS: renin–angiotensin–aldosterone system; ROS: reactive oxygen species)

mitochondrial dysfunction, and nitric oxide (NO) depletion. These effects stimulate transcription factors such as nuclear factor kappa B (NF-κB) and signaling cascades such as Janus kinase (JAK)–signal transducers and activators of transcription (STAT) and mitogen-activated protein kinases (MAPKs), triggering sustained production of proinflammatory cytokines [e.g., interleukin-6 (IL-6) and tumor necrosis factor-alpha (TNF-α)] and profibrotic mediators [e.g., transforming growth factor beta-1 (TGF-β1)], which promote glomerulosclerosis and tubulointerstitial fibrosis.[11,12]

Beyond classical mechanisms, recent evidence highlights the roles of impaired autophagy, endothelial dysfunction, and epigenetic modifications in sustaining renal injury. These changes contribute to "metabolic memory," where kidney damage progresses despite adequate glycemic control.[10,13]

Moreover, overactivation of the RAAS and MR signaling exacerbates sodium retention, inflammation, and fibrotic remodeling. Nonclassical MR activation in podocytes, mesangial, and endothelial cells can increase damage to the kidneys.[10]

Certain therapeutic approaches for diabetes management, such as thiazolidinediones, have demonstrated certain limitations; for instance, a previous study reported that approximately 70% of patients on thiazolidinediones developed plasma volume expansion. Consequently, the emergence of newer therapeutic options holds promise for enhancing the management of diabetic patients with diverse clinical profiles and comorbid conditions. In a study by Viswanathan et al., the effect of spironolactone and amiloride was studied on thiazolidinedione-induced fluid retention and it was found that there was a high prevalence of rosiglitazone-induced fluid retention. Amiloride, but not spironolactone reduced the protracted fluid retention among South Indian people living with T2DM.[15]

The development of new therapies for DKD is driven by a deeper understanding of the underlying pathophysiological mechanisms beyond glucose and blood pressure control. Contemporary treatment approaches now focus on targeting critical drivers of disease progression such as glomerular hyperfiltration, renal inflammation, oxidative stress, endothelial dysfunction, and fibrosis. These mechanisms are closely linked to structural and functional damage in the glomeruli and tubulointerstitium. Consequently, newer agents have been designed to intervene at these specific points. Finerenone, a novel ns-MRA, attenuates proinflammatory and profibrotic signaling within the kidneys, thereby reducing the risk of disease progression and cardiovascular events.[16] SGLT2 inhibitors act on the proximal tubules to enhance TGF, lower intraglomerular pressure, and mitigate oxidative and inflammatory stress.[17] Similarly, glucagon-like peptide-1 receptor (GLP-1R) agonists provide renal protection by promoting natriuresis, improving endothelial function, and suppressing renal inflammation and fibrosis.[16] These therapies represent a paradigm shift, offering targeted, organ-protective effects that go beyond glycemic regulation and establish new standards for comprehensive DKD management.

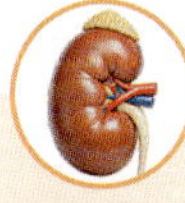

Diabetic kidney disease stems from chronic hyperglycemia causing metabolic, hemodynamic, and inflammatory changes, leading to glomerular stress and renal damage. Key drivers include oxidative stress, PKC/AGE activation, and fibrosis.

FINERENONE

Finerenone acts by selectively and passively blocking the MR, impairing MR signaling at multiple levels—including inhibition of MR-mediated sodium reabsorption and overactivation—without exhibiting the partial agonistic effects seen with steroidal MRAs such as spironolactone and eplerenone. Apart from the beneficial effects of Finerenone in reducing the blood pressure, it reduces endothelial cell apoptosis, inhibits smooth muscle cell proliferation, and decreases leukocyte recruitment and inflammation. These effects support endothelial repair, prevent vascular remodeling, and reduce proteinuria. Finerenone's unique MR binding enables it to downregulate hypertrophic, proinflammatory, and profibrotic gene expression regardless of aldosterone levels. It also downregulates gene expression related to renal hypertrophy and inflammation, decreases fibroblast accumulation and collagen deposition, and reduces tubulointerstitial fibrosis—ultimately preserving renal structure and function **(Fig. 1)**. Unlike steroidal MRAs, which accumulate more in the kidney, finerenone distributes equally between the heart and kidney, is cleared primarily via nonrenal pathways, and does not produce biologically active metabolites. These properties contribute to its potent, dose-dependent renal, and cardiovascular protective effects, without affecting blood pressure. Finerenone also demonstrates higher MR selectivity than spironolactone and greater receptor binding affinity than eplerenone, with at least comparable potency to spironolactone.[18,19]

Finerenone Phase III Study Program: Outcomes from the FIDELIO-DKD and FIGARO-DKD Trials and FIDELITY Meta-analysis

The FIGARO-DKD (Finerenone in reducing cardiovascular mortality and morbidity in diabetic kidney disease) and FIDELIO-DKD (FInerenone in reducing kiDnEy faiLure and disease prOgression in Diabetic Kidney Disease trials) are two pivotal phase-III studies assessing the efficacy of finerenone in patients with T2DM and CKD, with primary endpoints focused on cardiorenal outcomes. In FIGARO-DKD, finerenone significantly reduced the risk of renal composite outcomes—including kidney failure, sustained ≥57% decline in estimated glomerular filtration rate (eGFR), or renal death—by 23%. Similarly, in FIDELIO-DKD, finerenone demonstrated an 18% risk reduction in renal composite events compared to placebo when added to standard therapy [hazard ratio (HR) 0.82; 95% confidence interval (CI) 0.73–0.93; $p = 0.0001$]. While finerenone has been shown to decrease albuminuria in short-term interventions among T2DM patients with CKD, long-term data continue to build on its impact on hard renal and cardiovascular endpoints.

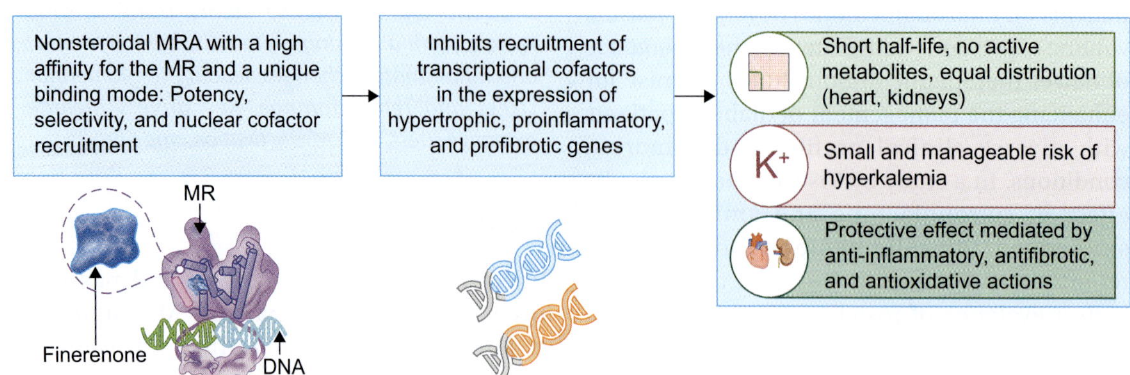

FIG. 1: Mechanism of action of finerenone.[19]
(DNA: deoxyribonucleic acid; MR: mineralocorticoid receptor; MRA: mineralocorticoid receptor antagonists)

Importantly, finerenone's adverse event profile was comparable to placebo. The FIDELITY pooled analysis of both trials confirmed a 23% reduction in renal composite risk (HR 0.77; 95% CI 0.67–0.88; p = 0.0002) and a 32% reduction in urinary albumin-to-creatinine ratio (UACR). Finerenone also decreased the incidence of nonfatal renal outcomes, including ESRD, and conferred cardiovascular protection across all UACR and eGFR strata in T2DM with CKD. Subgroup analyses showed a 29% reduction in renal composite risk in patients with a history of atherosclerotic cardiovascular disease (ASCVD) and a 19% reduction in those without ASCVD, with renal and mortality benefits observed irrespective of ASCVD status.[8,20,21]

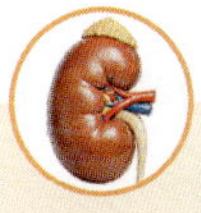

Finerenone is an ns-MRA that blocks MR signaling without partial agonist activity, unlike traditional steroidal MRAs. It offers cardiorenal protection by reducing inflammation, fibrosis, and vascular remodeling, while preserving kidney structure and function. With high MR selectivity and balanced tissue distribution, it provides potent effects independent of blood pressure changes.

SODIUM-GLUCOSE COTRANSPORTER-2 INHIBITORS

Sodium-glucose cotransporter-2 inhibitors are a novel class of antidiabetic drugs that have demonstrated strong kidney-protective effects, particularly in patients with DKD. These agents act by selectively blocking SGLT2 proteins located in the S1 segment of the proximal renal tubules, which normally reabsorb around 90% of filtered glucose. Their inhibition results in increased glucose and sodium excretion through urine,[22] reducing blood glucose levels independently of insulin and lowering intraglomerular pressure by improving TGF. This helps counteract glomerular hyperfiltration, a key factor in DKD progression.[23] Furthermore, SGLT2 inhibitors transiently activate the systemic RAAS due to fluid loss, yet suppress intrarenal RAAS, offering renal protection by reducing fibrosis and glomerular injury.[24] They also improve energy metabolism by enhancing fatty acid oxidation and ketone utilization and exert antioxidant and anti-inflammatory effects via the AGE-RAGE-TGF-β pathway **(Fig. 2)**.[25] These combined actions significantly slow DKD progression, even in advanced cases.

Clinical Studies Related to Sodium-glucose Cotransporter-2 Inhibitors

Several key clinical trials—DAPA-CKD (dapagliflozin and prevention of adverse outcomes in chronic kidney disease), EMPA-KIDNEY (study of heart and kidney protection with empagliflozin), and CREDENCE (Canagliflozin and Renal Events in Diabetes with Established Nephropathy Clinical Evaluation)—have shown that these drugs can slow the progression of CKD and reduce the risk of serious heart-related complications.[27-29]

The DAPA-CKD trial studied over 4,300 patients with moderate-to-severe kidney damage and high levels of protein in the urine. Patients receiving dapagliflozin experienced a 39% relative risk reduction in the progression of kidney dysfunction, onset of kidney failure, or mortality attributable to renal or cardiovascular causes. Importantly, these benefits were seen in people with and without T2DM, suggesting that the drug helps beyond blood sugar control.[27] The EMPA-KIDNEY trial included a broader group of CKD patients, many of whom had earlier stages of kidney disease. Empagliflozin lowered the risk of kidney disease progression or cardiovascular death by 28%. The findings support the idea that SGLT2 inhibitors can be useful even in those without high blood sugar levels but who are still at risk of worsening kidney function—such as people with early metabolic kidney changes.[28] The CREDENCE trial focused on people with both reduced kidney function and underlying metabolic conditions. Treatment with canagliflozin led to a 30% reduction in major kidney-related outcomes, such as the need for dialysis or a

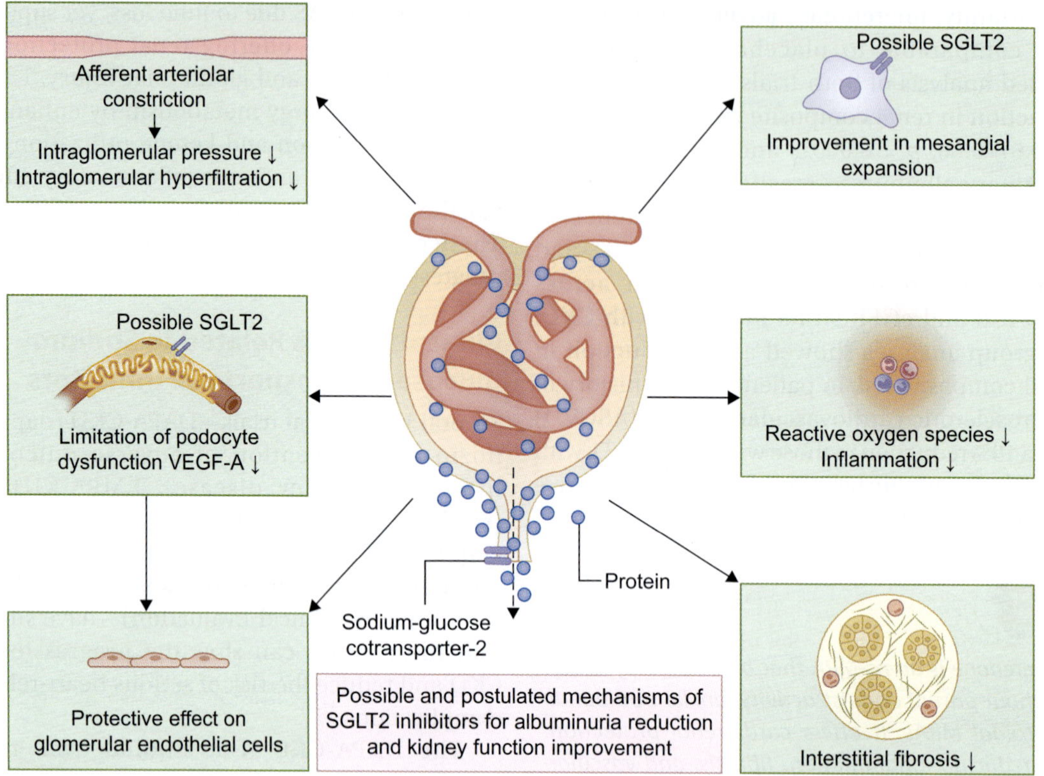

FIG. 2: Postulated mechanisms for the beneficial effect of SGLT2 inhibitors in patients with nephrotic-range proteinuria.[26]

(SGLT2: sodium-glucose cotransporter-2; VEGF-A: vascular endothelial growth factor A)

significant drop in kidney function. While some safety concerns were noted, the overall benefits for kidney and heart health were clear.[29]

Together, these studies highlight that SGLT2 inhibitors are a valuable option for slowing kidney damage in patients with CKD, especially when metabolic risk factors are present. SGLT2 inhibitors, while beneficial for kidney and heart health, are associated with some adverse effects. Common side effects include genital infections due to increased urinary glucose[30] and rare cases of euglycemic diabetic ketoacidosis.[31] Mild volume depletion and hypoglycemia may occur, especially when combined with diuretics or insulin.[31] The CREDENCE trial identified a potential association between canagliflozin use and an increased risk of lower-limb amputations; however, this finding has not been consistently replicated across other studies.[29] With proper education and monitoring, these risks are generally manageable.

The SGLT2 inhibitors are now recognized as a cornerstone in the treatment of DKD, as emphasized in the 2025 American Diabetes Association (ADA) guidelines.[32] These agents are recommended for all patients with T2DM and CKD with an eGFR of 20 mL/min/1.73 m^2 or higher, regardless of glycemic control.[32] Clinical trials have shown that SGLT2 inhibitors significantly reduce the risk of kidney disease progression, lower albuminuria, and offer robust cardiovascular protection. The incorporation of SGLT2 inhibitors marks a paradigm shift, offering a disease-modifying approach in DKD therapy.

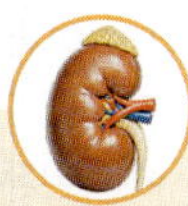

Sodium-glucose cotransporter-2 inhibitors, while primarily used for glycemic control, also exhibit significant renoprotective properties in the context of DKD. They reduce glucose and sodium reabsorption, improve TGF, lower intraglomerular pressure, and suppress intrarenal RAAS.

GLUCAGON-LIKE PEPTIDE-1 RECEPTOR AGONISTS

Glucagon-like peptide-1 receptor agonists mimic the action of endogenous GLP-1, an incretin hormone, exerting multiple effects through activation of GLP-1 receptors in the pancreas, gastrointestinal tract, brain, heart, and kidneys. They increase the insulin secretion based on the glucose levels, suppress glucagon release, and delay gastric emptying. All these actions eventually result in normalized postprandial glucose levels. In addition to glycemic regulation, GLP-1 RAs promote weight loss by acting on central appetite-regulating pathways, leading to reduced caloric intake. Emerging evidence also supports anti-inflammatory and anti-oxidative effects, which may contribute to their cardiovascular and renal protective properties.[33]

Multiple randomized controlled trials have assessed the safety and efficacy of GLP-1 analogs, one of the cardiovascular outcome trials being the LEADER (Liraglutide Effect and Action in Diabetes: Evaluation of cardiovascular outcome Results). Liraglutide was studied in more than 9,340 patients with T2DM and significant cardiovascular risk in the LEADER study. Liraglutide significantly reduced (13% compared to placebo) the risk of major adverse cardiovascular events (MACE). It also showed a trend toward reduced progression of nephropathy, primarily by decreasing new-onset persistent macroalbuminuria by 22%.[34]

The REWIND (Researching cardiovascular Events with a Weekly INcretin in Diabetes) trial assessed dulaglutide in a broader population, including patients with and without established cardiovascular disease. Dulaglutide demonstrated a statistically significant reduction in MACE (12% risk reduction compared to placebo), emphasizing its role in primary and secondary cardiovascular prevention. Moreover, the trial observed a reduction in the composite renal outcome, including decline in eGFR, progression to end-stage kidney disease, and worsening albuminuria, reinforcing the renal benefits of GLP-1 RAs.[35]

The AWARD-7 (Assessment of Weekly AdministRation of Dulaglutide in Diabetes-7) trial specifically addressed renal outcomes in patients with T2DM and moderate-to-severe CKD. Dulaglutide was compared to insulin glargine over a 1-year period. The trial found that dulaglutide preserved eGFR better than insulin and was associated with a lower risk of decline in renal function. Furthermore, dulaglutide demonstrated comparable glycemic control to insulin but with additional benefits in reducing body weight and hypoglycemia risk.[36]

Glucagon-like peptide-1 receptor agonists consistently show favorable effects on albuminuria and preservation of kidney function. Reductions in UACR have been documented across several trials, suggesting a role in slowing DKD progression.[37] These benefits are believed to result from improved metabolic control, reduction in systemic and intrarenal inflammation, and direct renal effects such as natriuresis and modulation of renal hemodynamics.[38]

Some of the most common adverse effects of using GLP-1 RA are gastrointestinal, including nausea, vomiting, and diarrhea, which are usually dose-dependent and can also diminish over time. These symptoms can be alleviated by gradual dose escalation. Concerns about acute pancreatitis have been raised; however, large-scale trials and meta-analyses have not established a definitive causal relationship. However, in those with a history of pancreatitis, caution needs to be exercised. Rare adverse events include gallbladder disease and, with certain agents, concerns about medullary thyroid carcinoma, though this is based primarily on rodent data.[39]

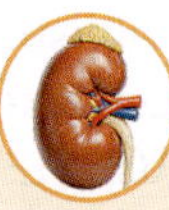

Glucagon-like peptide-1 receptor agonists improve blood glucose and support weight loss while offering cardiovascular and renal protection, as shown in major trials like LEADER, REWIND, and AWARD-7. They are generally well tolerated, with common gastrointestinal side effects.

COMPARATIVE EFFICACY AND SYNERGISTIC USE IN DIABETIC KIDNEY DISEASE

Combination therapies targeting multiple pathogenic pathways in DKD offer promising strategies for enhanced cardiorenal protection. While SGLT2 inhibitors are well established in slowing CKD progression, GLP-1 RAs also confer cardiorenal benefits in individuals with diabetic kidney disease. GLP-1 RAs are particularly suitable for patients with established ASCVD. GLP-1 RAs are recognized as disease-modifying therapies for T2DM, demonstrating efficacy in improving glycemic control, promoting weight loss, lowering blood pressure, and reducing cardiovascular events. Their potential renal protective effects are hypothesized to involve mechanisms such as natriuresis via inhibition of proximal tubular sodium reabsorption mediated by Na^+/H^+ exchanger 3 (NHE3), along with reductions in albuminuria through anti-inflammatory and antioxidant actions.[12,40]

Although SGLT2 inhibitors are preferred for slowing CKD progression regardless of cardiovascular disease status and are effective in heart failure, some patients, especially those with residual albuminuria, may derive additional benefit from adjunctive GLP-1 RA therapy. Furthermore, GLP-1 RAs may serve as viable alternatives in patients with low eGFR where SGLT2 inhibitors or RAAS inhibitors cannot be titrated. In real-world settings, many T2DM patients may meet criteria for both classes, supporting a sequential or combined therapeutic approach.[41]

Glucagon-like peptide-1 receptor agonists may be especially advantageous in individuals with obesity or obesity-related comorbidities and in those with prior stroke, as SGLT2 inhibitors have not demonstrated efficacy in reducing stroke risk.[42] For patients with CKD and persistent albuminuria or suboptimal control of metabolic risk factors such as hyperglycemia, hypertension, or excess weight, GLP-1 RAs should be considered as the preferred adjunctive treatment. In summary, for patients with CKD and an eGFR ≥20 mL/min/1.73 m², SGLT2 inhibitors remain the first-line agents to delay renal disease progression, with GLP-1 RAs providing complementary benefits when indicated.[43] Finerenone, a nonsteroidal selective MRA, also significantly benefits DKD, as shown in the FIDELITY pooled analysis. While each agent is effective alone, evidence on their combined use is still emerging. Animal studies suggest that SGLT2 inhibitor plus finerenone may provide synergistic renal benefits, with greater proteinuria reduction than monotherapy. However, trials such as FIDELIO-DKD show that finerenone reduces UACR independently of GLP-1 RA or SGLT-2 inhibitor use, and meta-analyses suggest that it does not significantly boost cardiovascular benefit when added to them. Combining finerenone with RAAS inhibitors also lowers albuminuria further, though with a modest increase in serum creatinine. Importantly, the risk of hyperkalemia is lower with finerenone than with older MRAs like spironolactone.[8,18,20,21]

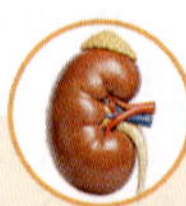

Combination therapy in DKD offers enhanced cardiorenal protection. SGLT2 inhibitors are first-line for CKD, while GLP-1 RAs add value in ASCVD, obesity, or residual albuminuria. Finerenone further reduces albuminuria, with emerging data on combined use.

PRACTICAL CONSIDERATIONS IN CLINICAL PRACTICE

In clinical practice, SGLT2 inhibitors are initiated in T2DM patients with CKD when eGFR is ≥20 mL/min/1.73 m^2, and therapy can be continued below this threshold unless kidney replacement therapy begins. Regular monitoring of renal function and volume status is essential, especially early in treatment, with close attention to adverse effects such as genital infections, dehydration, and rare cases of euglycemic diabetic ketoacidosis. In elderly and advanced CKD patients, cautious use and hydration monitoring are advised. GLP-1 RAs are mostly started at low doses and titrated gradually to reduce side effects of gastrointestinal system such as nausea and vomiting. Kidney function and status of the fluid levels should be continuously monitored, especially in people with pre-existing impairment. These agents are well-suited for T2DM patients with kidney disease, including the elderly, but are less effective in T1DM or severe beta-cell dysfunction. Finerenone, an ns-MRA, should be initiated only if serum potassium is <5.0 mmol/L and eGFR is ≥25 mL/min/1.73 m^2, with potassium and renal function monitored closely during treatment. Its primary risk is hyperkalemia, requiring dietary counseling and possible dose adjustment. It is effective and generally well-tolerated in elderly patients but contraindicated in those with significantly reduced eGFR or elevated potassium.[17]

FUTURE DIRECTIONS

Ongoing research in DKD is expanding beyond traditional approaches, reflecting a growing focus on therapies that address the complex, multifactorial nature of the disease. Taurine along with N-acetylcysteine played a key role in reducing microalbuminuria and soluble transforming growth factor-beta 1 (sTGF-β1) levels in people with T2DM. The glomerular damage that occurs in diabetes can be prevented or reduced if supplemented with taurine and N-acetyl cysteine.[44] While renin–angiotensin system (RAS) inhibitors have long been the foundation of DKD management, newer classes such as SGLT2 inhibitors and ns-MRAs have emerged as effective disease-modifying agents.[45] Trials like FIDELIO-DKD and FIGARO-DKD have shown that finerenone significantly reduces both renal and cardiovascular risks in this population. The ongoing CONFIDENCE (COmbinatioN effect of FInerenone anD EmpaglifloziN in participants with chronic kidney disease and type 2 diabetes using a UACR Endpoint) trial is an innovative direction in the field of combination therapy for DKD, which has been designed to assess the safety and efficacy of combined effect of administration of finerenone and SGLT2 inhibitor. Additionally, GLP-1 RAs are being explored for their potential renoprotective benefits, with the FLOW (Evaluate Renal Function with Semaglutide Once Weekly) trial aiming to clarify their role as a possible third therapeutic pillar in DKD.[46] Beyond these, a promising drug pipeline includes anti-inflammatory agents such as pentoxifylline and its analogs, chemokine receptor antagonists such as CCX140 (CCR2 inhibitor), and endothelin receptor blockers such as atrasentan, which target renal fibrosis and inflammation.[47] While some compounds, such as bardoxolone methyl, encountered setbacks due to safety concerns, ongoing development highlights a broader therapeutic strategy—targeting oxidative stress, fibrotic remodeling, and metabolic dysfunction—to delay DKD progression and improve long-term outcomes.[47] Traditional markers such as albuminuria and eGFR have limitations, particularly in patients who do not present with proteinuria. Recent advances have led to the discovery of novel biomarkers that reflect injury to different parts of the nephron, such as the glomeruli, tubules, and interstitial tissues. Biomarkers such as urinary type-IV collagen, fibronectin, cystatin C, neutrophil gelatinase-associated lipocalin (NGAL), and kidney injury molecule-1 (KIM-1) have shown promise in detecting early renal changes before clinical signs appear. Additionally, markers of oxidative stress and inflammation, such as 8-hydroxy-2'-deoxyguanosine (8-oxodG), monocyte chemoattractant protein-1 (MCP-1), and TNF-α, may help predict disease progression and treatment response. These emerging tools offer a more accurate and earlier window into DKD diagnosis, allowing for timely interventions and personalized therapy.[48]

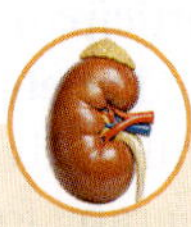

Ongoing DKD trials explore combination therapies such as finerenone with SGLT2 inhibitors (CONFIDENCE trial) and GLP-1 RAs (FLOW trial) for enhanced renoprotection. The innovative drugs target inflammation, fibrosis and oxidative stress.

SUMMARY

The key preventive strategy lies in identifying DKD at an early stage to delay its progression and thereby improve outcomes. SGLT2 inhibitors, GLP-1 RAs, and finerenone require careful dosing and monitoring, especially in elderly or CKD patients, to balance efficacy and side effects. Emerging biomarkers offer earlier DKD detection and personalized treatment beyond traditional markers such as albuminuria and eGFR. Finerenone, an ns-MRA, should be initiated only if serum potassium is <5.0 mmol/L and eGFR is ≥25 mL/min/1.73 m², with potassium and renal function monitored closely during treatment. SGLT2 inhibitors are initiated in T2DM patients with CKD when eGFR is ≥20 mL/min/1.73 m², and therapy can be continued below this threshold unless kidney replacement therapy begins. Regular monitoring of renal function and volume status is considered quintessential.

CONCLUSION

The emergence of finerenone, SGLT2 inhibitors, and GLP-1 RAs has reshaped DKD treatment, offering benefits beyond traditional RAAS blockade. These agents target hyperglycemia, inflammation, and fibrosis—key drivers of DKD. Finerenone protects kidneys and the heart; SGLT2 inhibitors slow eGFR decline and reduce albuminuria; and GLP-1 RAs aid in glycemic control and offer renocardiovascular benefits, especially in ASCVD or obesity. Trials like FIDELIO-DKD, CREDENCE, and LEADER confirm their efficacy. Combining these therapies may provide added protection, and they are now key elements of personalized DKD care.

TAKE HOME MESSAGES

- New therapies such as finerenone, SGLT2 inhibitors, and GLP-1 RAs have transformed DKD treatment beyond traditional RAAS blockade.
- These agents target key disease drivers—hyperglycemia, inflammation, and fibrosis.
- Finerenone offers renal and cardiovascular protection.
- SGLT2 inhibitors reduce albuminuria and slow eGFR decline.
- GLP-1 RAs improve glycemic control and provide additional cardiovascular and renal benefits, especially in patients with ASCVD or obesity.
- Major clinical trials (e.g., FIDELIO-DKD, CREDENCE, and LEADER) validate their efficacy.
- Combination therapy may enhance organ protection.
- The key preventive strategy lies in identifying DKD at an early stage to delay its progression and thereby improve outcomes.

REFERENCES

1. Upadhye KS, Patidar H. Decoding diabetic kidney disease: In-Depth analysis of prevalence, risk factors, biomarkers, and management strategies. J Med Sci Health. 2024;10(2):204-12.

2. Li J, Guo K, Qiu J, Xue S, Pi L, Li X, et al. Epidemiological status, development trends, and risk factors of disability-adjusted life years due to diabetic kidney disease: A systematic analysis of Global Burden of Disease Study 2021. Chin Med J (Engl). 2025;138(5):568-78.

3. Ma X, Liu R, Xi X, Zhuo H, Gu Y. Global burden of chronic kidney disease due to diabetes mellitus, 1990-2021, and projections to 2050. Front Endocrinol. 2025;16:1513008.

4. Wang J, Xiang H, Lu Y, Wu T, Ji G. New progress in drugs treatment of diabetic kidney disease. Biomed Pharmacother. 2021;141:111918.

5. Viswanathan V, Tilak P. Prevalence, aetiology and management of diabetic nephropathy: Indian overview. J Gen Med. 2010;22(1):25-9.

6. Whitlock R, Leon SJ, Manacsa H, Askin N, Rigatto C, Fatoba ST, et al. The association between dual RAAS inhibition and risk of acute kidney injury and hyperkalemia in patients with diabetic kidney disease: A systematic review and meta-analysis. Nephrol Dial Transplant. 2023;38(11):2503-16.

7. Mukoyama M, Kuwabara T. Role of renin-angiotensin system blockade in advanced CKD: To use or not to use? Hypertens Res. 2022;45(6):1072-5.

8. Bakris GL, Agarwal R, Anker SD, Pitt B, Ruilope LM, Rossing P, et al. Effect of finerenone on chronic kidney disease outcomes in type 2 diabetes. N Engl J Med. 2020;383(23):2219-29.

9. Kim MK, Kim DM. Current status of diabetic kidney disease and latest trends in management. J Diabetes Investig. 2022;13(12):1961-2.

10. Piko N, Bevc S, Hojs R, Ekart R. Finerenone: From the mechanism of action to clinical use in kidney disease. Pharmaceuticals. 2024;17(4):418.

11. Dai ZC, Chen JX, Zou R, Liang XB, Tang JX, Yao CW. Role and mechanisms of SGLT-2 inhibitors in the treatment of diabetic kidney disease. Front Immunol. 2023;14.

12. Kawanami D, Takashi Y. GLP-1 receptor agonists in diabetic kidney disease: From clinical outcomes to mechanisms. Front Pharmacol. 2020;11:967.

13. Sugahara M, Pak WLW, Tanaka T, Tang SCW, Nangaku M. Update on diagnosis, pathophysiology, and management of diabetic kidney disease. Nephrology (Carlton). 2021;26(6):491-500.

14. Sinha SK, Nicholas SB. Pathomechanisms of Diabetic Kidney Disease. J Clin Med. 2023;12(23):7349.

15. Viswanathan, Mohan V, Poongothai S, Parthasarathy N, Subramaniyam G, Manoharan D, et al. Effect of spironolactone and amiloride on thiazolidinedione-induced fluid retention in South Indian patients with type 2 diabetes. Clin J Am Soc Nephrol. 2012;8(2):225-32.

16. Huang W, Chen YY, Li ZQ, He FF, Zhang C. Recent advances in the emerging therapeutic strategies for diabetic kidney diseases. Int J Mol Sci. 2022;23(18):10882.

17. Zhao M, Cao Y, Ma L. New insights in the treatment of DKD: Recent advances and future prospects. BMC Nephrol. 2025;26(1):72.

18. Lv R, Xu L, Che L, Liu S, Wang Y, Dong B. Cardiovascular-renal protective effect and molecular mechanism of finerenone in type 2 diabetic mellitus. Front Endocrinol. 2023;14:1125693.

19. Arici M, Altun B, Araz M, Atmaca A, Demir T, Ecder T, et al. The significance of finerenone as a novel therapeutic option in diabetic kidney disease: a scoping review with emphasis on cardiorenal outcomes of the finerenone phase 3 trials. Front Med. 2024;11:1384454.

20. Agarwal R, Filippatos G, Pitt B, Anker SD, Rossing P, Joseph A, et al. Cardiovascular and kidney outcomes with finerenone in patients with type 2 diabetes and chronic kidney disease: The FIDELITY pooled analysis. Eur Heart J. 2022;43(6):474-84.

21. Pitt B, Filippatos G, Agarwal R, Anker SD, Bakris GL, Rossing P, et al. Cardiovascular events with finerenone in kidney disease and type 2 diabetes. N Engl J Med. 2021;385(24):2252-63.

22. Yamazaki T, Mimura I, Tanaka T, Nangaku M. Treatment of diabetic kidney disease: Current and future. Diabetes Metab J. 2021;45(1):11-26.

23. Vallon V, Verma S. Effects of SGLT2 inhibitors on kidney and cardiovascular function. Annu Rev Physiol. 2021;83:503-28.

24. Schork A, Saynisch J, Vosseler A, Jaghutriz BA, Heyne N, Peter A, et al. Effect of SGLT2 inhibitors on body composition, fluid status and renin-angiotensin-aldosterone system in type 2 diabetes: A prospective study using bioimpedance spectroscopy. Cardiovasc Diabetol. 2019;18(1):46.

25. Tsai KF, Chen YL, Chiou TTY, Chu TH, Li LC, Ng HY, et al. Emergence of SGLT2 inhibitors as powerful antioxidants in human diseases. Antioxidants. 2021;10(8):1166.

26. Kalay Z, Sahin OE, Copur S, Danacı S, Ortiz A, Yau K, et al. SGLT-2 inhibitors in nephrotic-range proteinuria: Emerging clinical evidence. Clin Kidney J. 2022;16(1):52-60.

27. Heerspink HJL, Stefánsson BV, Correa-Rotter R, Chertow GM, Greene T, Hou FF, et al. Dapagliflozin in patients with chronic kidney disease. N Engl J Med. 2020;383(15):1436-46.

28. The EMPA-KIDNEY Collaborative Group; Herrington WG, Staplin N, Wanner C, Green JB, Hauske SJ, et al. Empagliflozin in patients with chronic kidney disease. N Engl J Med. 2023;388(2):117-27.

29. Perkovic V, Jardine MJ, Neal B, Bompoint S, Heerspink HJL, Charytan DM, et al. Canagliflozin and renal outcomes in type 2 diabetes and nephropathy. N Engl J Med. 2019;380(24):2295-306.

30. Gorgojo-Martínez JJ, Górriz JL, Cebrián-Cuenca A, Castro Conde A, Velasco Arribas M. Clinical recommendations for managing genitourinary adverse effects in patients treated with SGLT-2 inhibitors: A multidisciplinary expert consensus. J Clin Med. 2024;13(21):6509.

31. Wang KM, Isom RT. SGLT2 inhibitor–induced euglycemic diabetic ketoacidosis: A case report. Kidney Med. 2020;2(2):218-21.

32. American Diabetes Association Professional Practice Committee. 11. Chronic kidney disease and risk management: Standards of care in diabetes—2025. Diabetes Care. 2024;48(1 Suppl 1):S239-51.

33. Zheng Z, Zong Y, Ma Y, Tian Y, Pang Y, Zhang C, et al. Glucagon-like peptide-1 receptor: Mechanisms and advances in therapy. Signal Transduct Target Ther. 2024;9(1):234.

34. Marso SP, Daniels GH, Brown-Frandsen K, Kristensen P, Mann JFE, Nauck MA, et al. Liraglutide and cardiovascular outcomes in type 2 diabetes. N Engl J Med 2016;375(4):311-22.

35. Gerstein HC, Colhoun HM, Dagenais GR, Diaz R, Lakshmanan M, Pais P, et al. Dulaglutide and cardiovascular outcomes in type 2 diabetes (REWIND): A double-blind, randomised placebo-controlled trial. The Lancet. 2019;394(10193):121-30.

36. Tuttle KR, Lakshmanan MC, Rayner B, Busch RS, Zimmermann AG, Woodward DB, et al. Dulaglutide versus insulin glargine in patients with type 2 diabetes and moderate-to-severe chronic kidney disease (AWARD-7): A multicentre, open-label, randomised trial. Lancet Diabetes Endocrinol. 2018;6(8):605-17.

37. Mann JFE, Ørsted DD, Brown-Frandsen K, Marso SP, Poulter NR, Rasmussen S, et al.; LEADER Steering Committee and Investigators. Liraglutide and renal outcomes in type 2 diabetes. N Engl J Med 2017;377(9):839-48.

38. Greco EV, Russo G, Giandalia A, Viazzi F, Pontremoli R, De Cosmo S. GLP-1 receptor agonists and kidney protection. Medicina. 2019;55(6):233.

39. Guo H, Guo Q, Li Z, Wang Z. Association between different GLP-1 receptor agonists and acute pancreatitis: Case series and real-world pharmacovigilance analysis. Front Pharmacol. 2024;15:1461398.

40. Gourdy P, Darmon P, Dievart F, Halimi JM, Guerci B. Combining glucagon-like peptide-1 receptor agonists (GLP-1RAs) and sodium-glucose cotransporter-2 inhibitors (SGLT2is) in patients with type 2 diabetes mellitus (T2DM). Cardiovasc Diabetol. 2023;22(1):79.

41. Yau K, Dharia A, Alrowiyti I, Cherney DZI. Prescribing SGLT2 inhibitors in patients with CKD: Expanding indications and practical considerations. Kidney Int Rep. 2022;7(7):1463-76.

42. Karlström P, Pivodic A, Fu M. Glucagon-like peptide 1 receptor agonist is associated with improved survival in overweight heart failure patients. JACC Heart Fail. 2025;13(5):754-66.

43. Goldenberg RM, Ahooja V, Clemens KK, Gilbert JD, Poddar M, Verma S. Practical considerations and rationale for glucagon-like peptide-1 receptor agonist plus sodium-dependent glucose cotransporter-2 inhibitor combination therapy in type 2 diabetes. Can J Diabetes. 2021;45(3):291-302.

44. Viswanathan V, Nair MB, Tilak P. Effect of taurine and acetyl cysteine in attenuating micoalbuminuria in type 2 diabetes. Indian J Nephrol. 2008;18(2):85.

45. Dekkers CCJ, Gansevoort RT, Heerspink HJL. New diabetes therapies and diabetic kidney disease progression: The role of SGLT-2 inhibitors. Curr Diab Rep. 2018;18(5):27.

46. Naaman SC, Bakris GL. Diabetic nephropathy: Update on pillars of therapy slowing progression. Diabetes Care 2023;46(9):1574-86.

47. Perez-Gomez MV, Sanchez-Niño MD, Sanz AB, Martín-Cleary C, Ruiz-Ortega M, Egido J, et al. Horizon 2020 in diabetic kidney disease: The clinical trial pipeline for add-on therapies on top of renin angiotensin system blockade. J Clin Med. 2015;4(6):1325-47.

48. Swaminathan SM, Rao IR, Shenoy SV, Prabhu AR, Mohan PB, Rangaswamy D, et al. Novel biomarkers for prognosticating diabetic kidney disease progression. Int Urol Nephrol. 2023;55(4):913-28.

Key Research Takeaway

Effect of taurine and acetylcysteine in attenuating microalbuminuria in type 2 diabetes

Sir,

It is shown that glomerular damage in diabetes can be prevented or at least attenuated by supplementation with taurine and *N*-acetylcysteine.[1] Diet supplemented with taurine was found to reduce the morphological damage in experimental models with diabetes. Hence, this study was conducted to determine the benefits of treatment with combination of taurine (500 mg) and acetylcysteine (150 mg) (Nefrosave™, Fourrts (India) Laboratories 2 diabetic subjects and to evaluate its potential in augmenting the renoprotective action of angiotensin-converting enzyme inhibitor (ACEI) or angiotensin receptor blocker (ARB).

The institutional ethics committee approved the study, and written informed consent was obtained from patients. Among the 41 well-controlled type 2 diabetic patients with microalbuminuria, 31 patients were given a combination of taurine and *N*-acetylcysteine along with an ACEI/ARB (treatment group) and 10 patients were treated with an ACEI/ARB alone (control group). Male:female ratio was 27:14. Both the treatment arms received similar doses of 5 mg of ACEI and 50 mg of ARB. Fasting plasma glucose, glycosylated hemoglobin triglycerides, cholesterol, urinary albumin/creatinine ratio (UACR), and serum transforming growth factor (sTGF-b1) were determined at baseline and at the end of 3 months of treatment period. The UACR was determined by immunoturbidimetry and sTGF-b1 was analyzed by sandwich enzyme linked immunosorbent assay.

group: 14 ± 7, control group: 17 ± 5 years), and weight (treatment group: 70 ± 14, control group: 69 ± 11 kg). At follow-up, significant reduction in diastolic blood pressure (DBP) (baseline: 82 ± 08 vs. follow-up: 78 ± 05 mmHg, $P = 0.021$), UACR (baseline: 85 ± 59 vs. follow-up: 45 ± 25 mg/mg creatinine, $P = 0.001$), and sTGF-b1 (baseline: 18.3 ± 12.4 vs. follow-up: 13.2 ± 9.9, $P = 0.002$) were seen in the treatment group. No such significant changes were noted in the control group [DBP - baseline: 79 ± 7 vs. follow-up: 79 ± 6 mmHg, $P = 0.2$; UACR - baseline: 61 ± 29 vs. follow-up: 92 ± 52 mg/mg creatinine, $P = 0.2$; and sTGF-β1 - baseline: 20 ± 4.2 vs. follow-up: 19.7 ± 8.1, $P = 0.6$)]. Along with the above parameters, glomerular filtration rate (GFR) was also estimated using Cockroft Gault Equation.[2] However, it was found that there was some increase in the GFR in the control group (baseline: 81.9 ± 23.9, follow-up: 95.5 ± 26.3; $P = 0.2$) compared with the treatment group (baseline: 84.0 ± 26.2, follow-up: 88.1 ± 30.3; $P = 0.6$) but the increase was not statistically significant.

This prospective study showed that taurine in combination with *N*-acetylcysteine was useful in attenuating UACR and sTGF-β1 levels in microalbuminuric type 2 diabetic patients. The benefits of taurine therapy on kidney function and blood pressure are noteworthy and may be useful in preventing the deterioration of microalbuminuria. The limitation of the study is its small sample size. A larger cohort with longer follow-up is needed to validate the findings of this study.

V. Viswanathan, M. B. Nair, P. Tilak
Diabetes Research Centre (WHO Collaborating Centre for Research, Education and Training in Diabetes), Chennai, Tamil Nadu, India

Address for correspondence:
Dr. Vijay Viswanathan, Diabetes Research Centre (WHO Collaborating Centre for Research, Education and Training in Diabetes), No. 4, Main Road, Royapuram, Chennai - 600 013, Tamil Nadu, India.
E-mail: dr_vijay@vsnl.com

**References

The Journal of General Medicine

Prevalence, Aetiology and Management of Diabetic Nephropathy: Indian overview

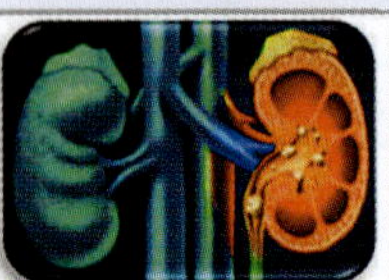

Viswanathan V, Tilak P

M.V Hospital for Diabetes and Diabetes Research Centre, [WHO collaborating centre for Research, Education and Training in Diabetes] No.5, West Mada Church Street, Royapuram, Chennai – 600013.

Type 2 diabetes is a diversified disease involving both impaired beta cell function and insulin resistance[1] and is associated with high morbidity and mortality mainly due to micro and macro vascular complications.[2] One such micro vascular complication of diabetes is diabetic nephropathy. Nearly 30% of chronic renal failures in India are due to diabetic nephropathy.[3] Nonetheless attention towards diabetic nephropathy is not directed until the patient has progressed towards the stage of renal failure. Nephropathy due to diabetes is the most common cause for end stage renal disease and for the patients undergoing dialysis. Diabetes is preventable and so are its complications.

This review article aims at describing diabetic nephropathy, origin and management in view of early prevention. Diabetic nephropathy is clinically defined by the presence of persistent proteinuria of >500 mg/day in a diabetic patient who has concomitant diabetic retinopathy and hypertension and in the absence of clinical or laboratory evidence of other kidney or renal tract disease.[4]

CURRENT SCENARIO OF DIABETIC NEPHROPATHY AMONG ASIANS

There are no population - based studies on the prevalence of diabetic nephropathy in India. However there are a few hospital-based data. The prevalence of microalbuminuria varies from 19.7% to 28.5% in type 2 diabetic subjects.[5-7] The prevalence of diabetic nephropathy in type 2 diabetic subjects is reported to be 5-9% from various Indian studies.[5,8,9]

In study of 205 newly diagnosed type 2 diabetic subjects, the prevalence of microalbuminuria was 12.2%.[10] However, another study by Vijay et al showed that 6.7% of newly diagnosed type 2 diabetic patients who were normoalbuminuric at diagnosis developed nephropathy within 6 years.[11] Even though a patient is normoalbuminuric at diagnosis, the risk of developing diabetic nephropathy is very high. Hence regular monitoring for microalbuminuria is very essential. Microalbuminuria is a condition where interplay of various complications occurs. The term "Microalbuminuria Syndrome" includes the following conditions,

- Elevated blood pressure
- Atherogenic lipid profile (increased very low density lipoprotein-triglycerides, decreased high-density lipoprotein-cholesterol, increased lipoprotein a)
- Elevated plasma fibrinogen and platelet activator inhibitor – I levels.
- Decreased insulin sensitivity
- Increased total-body exchangeable sodium
- Impaired basal endothelium-dependent vasorelaxation
- High sodium-lithium counter transport activity
- "Silent" ischaemic heart disease.

ORIGIN OF DIABETIC NEPHROPATHY

The pathophysiology of diabetic nephropathy is multi factorial and genetic susceptibility has been proposed to be an important factor in the development and progression of diabetic nephropathy. Diabetes produces qualitative and quantitative changes in the composition of the capillary basement membrane and this altered material undergoes accelerated glycosylation and further rearrangement to form advanced glycosylation end-products (AGE), which stimulate protein synthesis,[12] further decrease degradability of

ORIGINAL ARTICLE

Effect of Spironolactone and Amiloride on Thiazolidinedione-Induced Fluid Retention in South Indian Patients with Type 2 Diabetes

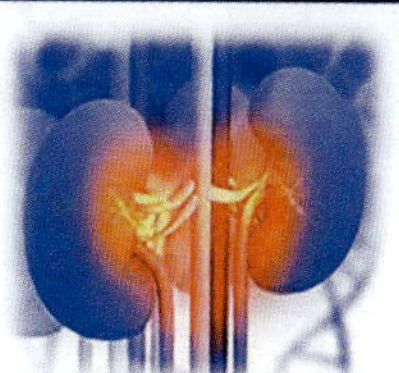

Vijay Viswanathan, * *Viswanathan Mohan,*[†] *Poongothai Subramani,*[†] *Nandakumar Parthasarathy,*[†] *Gayathri Subramaniyam,*[†] *Deepa Manoharan,*[†] *Chandru Sundaramoorthy,* * *Luigi Gnudi,*[‡] *Janaka Karalliedde,*[‡] *and Giancarlo Viberti*[‡]

Summary

Background and objectives Thiazolidinediones (pioglitazone and rosiglitazone) induce renal epithelial sodium channel (ENaC)–mediated sodium reabsorption, resulting in plasma volume (PV) expansion. Incidence and long-term management of fluid retention induced by thiazolidinediones remain unclear.

Design, setting, participants, & measurements In a 4-week run-in period, rosiglitazone, 4 mg twice daily, was added to a background anti-diabetic therapy in 260 South Indian patients with type 2 diabetes mellitus. Patients with PV expansion (absolute reduction in hematocrit in run-in, $1.5 percentage points) entered a randomized, placebo-controlled study to evaluate effects of amiloride and spironolactone on attenuating rosiglitazoneinduced fluid retention. Primary endpoint was change in hematocrit in each diuretic group versus placebo (control group).

Results Of the 260 patients, 70% (n=180) had PV expansion. These 180 patients (70% male; mean age, 47.8 years [range, 30–80 years])were randomly assigned to rosiglitazone, 4mg twice daily, plus spironolactone, 50mg once daily; rosiglitazone, 4 mg twice daily, plus amiloride, 10 mg once daily; or rosiglitazone, 4 mg twice daily, plus placebo for 24weeks. Hematocrit continued to decrease significantly in control and spironolactone groups (mean absolute change, 21.2 [P=0.01] and 20.7 [P=0.02] percentage points, respectively), suggesting continued PV expansion. No change occurred with amiloride (mean change, 0.0 percentage points). Amiloride, but not spironolactone, was superior to control (mean hematocrit difference [95% confidence interval] relative to control, 1.27 [0.21--2.55] and 0.49 [20.79--1.77] percentage points [P=0.04 and P=0.61], respectively).

Conclusions Prevalence of rosiglitazone-induced fluid retention in South Indian patients with type 2 diabetes is high. Amiloride, a direct ENaC blocker, but not spironolactone, prevented protracted fluid retention in these patients.

*Department of Diabetes, M.V. Hospital for Diabetes and Prof M.Viswanathan Diabetes Research Centre, Chennai, India; Department of Diabetes, Dr. Mohan's Diabetes Specialities Centre and Madras Diabetes Research Foundation, Chennai, India; and Cardiovascular Division, King's College of London, London, United Kingdom

Correspondence:
Dr. Janaka Karalliedde, Cardiovascular Division, King's College London, 3.33 Franklin Wilkins Building, 100 Stamford Street, London SE1 9RT, United Kingdom.
Email: j.karalliedde@kcl.ac.uk www.cjasn.

Clin J Am Soc Nephrol 8: 225–232, 2013. doi: 10.2215/CJN.06330612

<table>
<tr><td>

7

</td><td>

Complications and Comorbidities Associated with Diabetic Kidney Disease

</td></tr>
</table>

Sivashankari Selva Elavarasan, Vijay Viswanathan

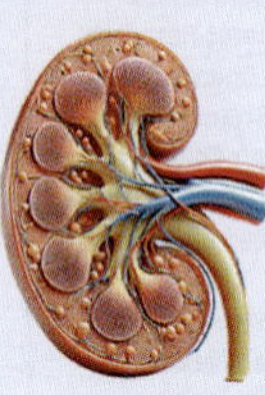

- ➤ Hypertension
- ➤ Dyslipidemia
- ➤ Cardiovascular complications
- ➤ Diabetic retinopathy
- ➤ Diabetic foot and amputations
- ➤ Sarcopenia
- ➤ Gout
- ➤ Osteoarthritis and renal osteodystrophy
- ➤ Anemia
- ➤ Metabolic acidosis

Abstract

Diabetic kidney disease (DKD) is a chronic, major, debilitating micro-vascular complication of type 2 diabetes mellitus (T2DM), which is associated with several comorbidities such as hypertension, dyslipidemia, obesity, ischemic heart diseases such as angina, myocardial infarction, and heart failure (HF), and peripheral vascular diseases, such as amputation and gangrene. The major complications that can arise from DKD are end-stage renal disease (ESRD) and cardiovascular morbidity, which can eventually lead to mortality. People with DKD are also prone to develop retinopathy, gout, osteoarthritis, and anemia. Renal function declines with worsening foot infection. An increase in urine albumin excretion is noted with the progression of DKD. Early diagnosis and staging based on Kidney Disease: Improving Global Outcomes (KDIGO) becomes impossible without urine albumin levels. Therefore, it becomes imperative to calculate the estimated glomerular filtration rate (eGFR) and urine albumin-creatinine ratio (UACR)/urine protein-creatinine ratio (UPCR) and diagnose DKD early to prevent the onset of comorbidities and complications of DKD. It is of paramount importance to understand these comorbidities so that we can prevent the potential serious life-threatening complications and reduce the substantial burden on the healthcare system of the nation. An integrated and comprehensive strategy is required to provide intensive glycemic and blood pressure control along with lifestyle modifications. This holistic approach can reduce the incidence of ESRD, HF, and even death, which is associated with the complications of DKD.

Keywords: Diabetic kidney disease, comorbidities, complications, end-stage renal disease, glycemic control.

INTRODUCTION

Diabetes mellitus is a vascular disease associated with several microvascular and macrovascular complications. Diabetic kidney disease (DKD) is a chronic, major, debilitating microvascular complication of type 2 diabetes mellitus (T2DM). Globally, it has been estimated that the prevalence of CKD in diabetes is 40% according to the IDF atlas 2025,[1] and the START-INDIA study also revealed that over 40% of people with diabetes are affected by CKD.[2] The most recent CITE study reported the prevalence of DKD to be 32% in India, and among those diagnosed with albuminuric CKD, 63% had microalbuminuria and 29% had macroalbuminuria. A significant association was noted between CKD and comorbidities such as HF, neuropathy, retinopathy, and atherosclerotic cardiovascular disease (CVD).[3] An increase in urine albumin excretion is observed with the progression of DKD. Early diagnosis and staging based on KDIGO becomes impossible without urine albumin levels. An early diagnosis of DKD requires calculation of eGFR using the chronic kidney disease epidemiology collaboration (CKD-EPI) equation and estimation of UACR/UPCR to prevent the onset of comorbidities and complications of DKD.

The major complications that can arise from DKD are ESRD and cardiovascular morbidity, which can eventually lead to mortality. The risk factors of DKD, which have been discussed in the previous chapters, are associated with several comorbidities, such as hypertension, dyslipidemia, obesity, and ischemic heart diseases, such as angina, myocardial infarction, and HF, peripheral vascular diseases, and cerebrovascular accidents. People with DKD are also prone to develop retinopathy, gout, osteoarthritis, and anemia. Renal function declines with worsening foot infection **(Fig. 1)**. It is of paramount importance to understand these comorbidities so that we can prevent the potential serious life-threatening complications and reduce the substantial burden on the healthcare system of the nation.

A significant association was noted between CKD and comorbidities, such as HF, neuropathy, retinopathy, and atherosclerotic CVD. An early diagnosis of DKD requires calculation of eGFR using the CKD-EPI equation and estimation of UACR/UPCR to prevent the onset of comorbidities and complications of DKD.

HYPERTENSION

Hypertension is often called a silent killer and a major public health problem, and the World Health Organization (WHO) states that every one in four adults in the South-East Asian region is affected by hypertension.[4] The prevalence of hypertension in the Southeast Asian region is 25%, which seems to be a little higher than the prevalence of hypertension worldwide, which is 22%. In a meta-analysis by Udaya et al., the prevalence of hypertension in India was 31.4%.[5] The European Society of Cardiology (ESC) 2024 defines hypertension as systolic blood pressure (BP) of ≥140 mm Hg and a diastolic BP of ≥90 mm Hg.[6] The Indian guidelines in 2024 recommend a systolic BP of ≥130 mm Hg and a diastolic BP of >80 mm Hg, like most other guidelines.[7]

The Indian Council of Medical Research–India Diabetes (ICMR-INDIAB) study reported the prevalence of hypertension as 35.5% among the general Indian population.[8] Several studies reported that the prevalence of hypertension in people with diabetes increased 1.5–2 times more when compared to people without diabetes.[9] It is alarming to understand that among people with diabetes, those diagnosed with hypertension are likely to spend 1.4 times more than people without hypertension.[10] The prevalence of hypertension among people with newly diagnosed diabetes was around 45%, as reported by Metri et al.[11]

Hypertension can itself be recognized as an independent risk factor that contributes significantly to the progression of DKD. Studies indicate that maintaining a lower blood

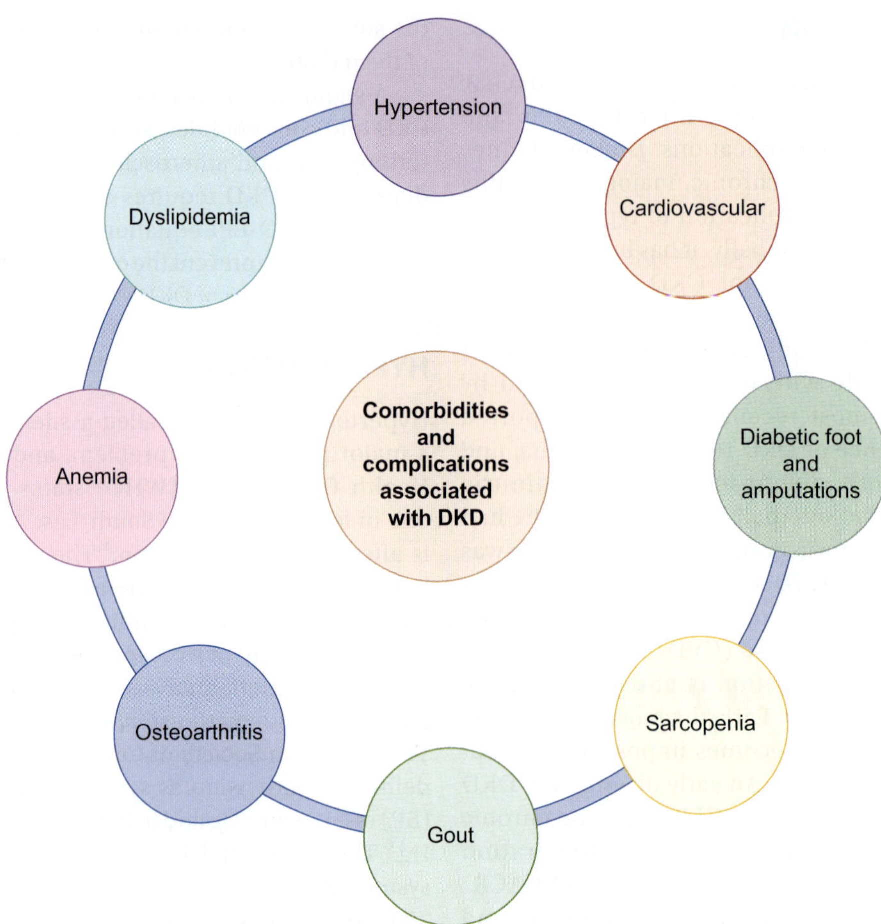

FIG. 1: Various comorbidities and complications associated with diabetic kidney disease.

pressure helps in reducing the progression of albuminuria and preventing ESKD.[12] Several reasons can be attributed to hypertension in diabetes, some of them are metabolic syndrome, or it can develop as a complication of diabetes or endocrine disorders. In some cases, it may be coincidental, for example, essential arterial hypertension, or it could be isolated systolic hypertension. The pathophysiology for the development of hypertension among people with DKD revolves around the concept of sodium retention and increased peripheral vascular resistance. In India, there is a high association of DKD and hypertension, which is collectively called DHKD syndrome, which is considered a complex of diabetes, hypertension, and kidney disease. In a study by Dash et al. in India, they reported that there was a high prevalence of 78.7% for all diabetes, hypertension, and kidney disease collectively, which justified the use of the term "DHKD syndrome."[13] The MAP (Micro Albuminuria Prevalence) study done in 10 Asian cohorts showed a high prevalence of microalbuminuria (58%) among people with diabetes.[14] The microalbuminuria is recognized as the earliest evidence of DKD and also a risk of cardiovascular morbidity and mortality in people with diabetes.[15]

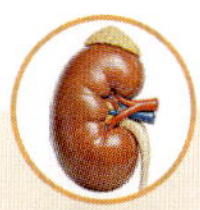

Hypertension can be recognized as an independent risk factor that contributes significantly to the progression of DKD. The pathophysiology for the development of hypertension among people with DKD revolves around the concept of sodium retention and increased peripheral vascular resistance. In India, there is a high association of DKD and hypertension, which is collectively called DHKD syndrome, which is considered a complex of diabetes, hypertension, and kidney disease. The microalbuminuria is recognized as the earliest evidence of DKD and also a risk of cardiovascular morbidity and mortality in people with diabetes.

DYSLIPIDEMIA

Dyslipidemia, which is characterized by abnormal lipid levels in the blood, is a major comorbidity associated with DKD. Dyslipidemia is associated with DKD, and even the presence of DKD can exacerbate dyslipidemia, which in turn can cause CVD. In diabetic dyslipidemia, the action of lipoprotein lipases in the endothelial cells is impaired, and this results in the accumulation of triglycerides (TGs) and reduced high-density lipoprotein cholesterol (HDL-C).[16] Apart from this, low-density lipoprotein cholesterol (LDL-C) can be normal or elevated in people with DKD. Innumerable studies state that dyslipidemia is associated with increased risk of declining kidney function, showing a decline in eGFR and an increase in albuminuria.[17] The insulin resistance in people with diabetes motivates the hormone-sensitive TG lipase, which in turn stimulates the release of free fatty acids (FFA) from the peripheral adipose tissue. Increased FFA causes the liver to synthesize TGs and decreases HDL-C. Impaired antioxidant levels of HDL-Cs stimulate advanced glycation end products (AGEs) and growth factors. This causes thickening of the basement membrane, glomerular hypertrophy, and mesangial hyperplasia. Oxidative stress in

the kidneys can cause an increase in oxidized LDL (oxLDL), which can cause damage to the glomeruli. An increase in the production of extracellular matrix (ECM) proteins increases the production of DKD. The mechanism of action of dyslipidemia causing DKD is depicted in **Figure 2**.[18]

Carotid intimal medial thickness (IMT) measured by ultrasonography can be used as a noninvasive marker of atherosclerosis. A study was conducted in South India to find out the effect of varying degrees of albuminuria on atherosclerosis, and it was found that an increase in carotid IMT was observed before the onset of albuminuria, and no deterioration in IMT was observed after the presence of albuminuria was detected.[19] Obesity can cause insulin resistance and is a risk factor for the onset and progression of CKD among people with diabetes. A strong association exists between high body mass index (BMI) and DKD in the Indian population. Viswanathan et al. reported that increased BMI is an independent risk factor among people with CKD and diabetes. It was observed that overweight and obese individuals diagnosed with T2DM were at four to five times the risk of progression of CKD.[20]

Figure 2 shows the mechanism of action of dyslipidemia leading to the progression of DKD.[18]

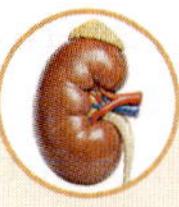

Dyslipidemia, which is characterized by abnormal lipid levels in the blood, is a major comorbidity associated with DKD. Dyslipidemia is associated with DKD, and even the presence of DKD can exacerbate dyslipidemia, which in turn can cause CVD. Dyslipidemia is associated with increased risk of declining kidney function, showing a decline in eGFR and an increase in albuminuria. The insulin resistance in people with diabetes motivates the hormone-sensitive TG lipase, which in turn stimulates the release of FFA from the peripheral adipose tissue.

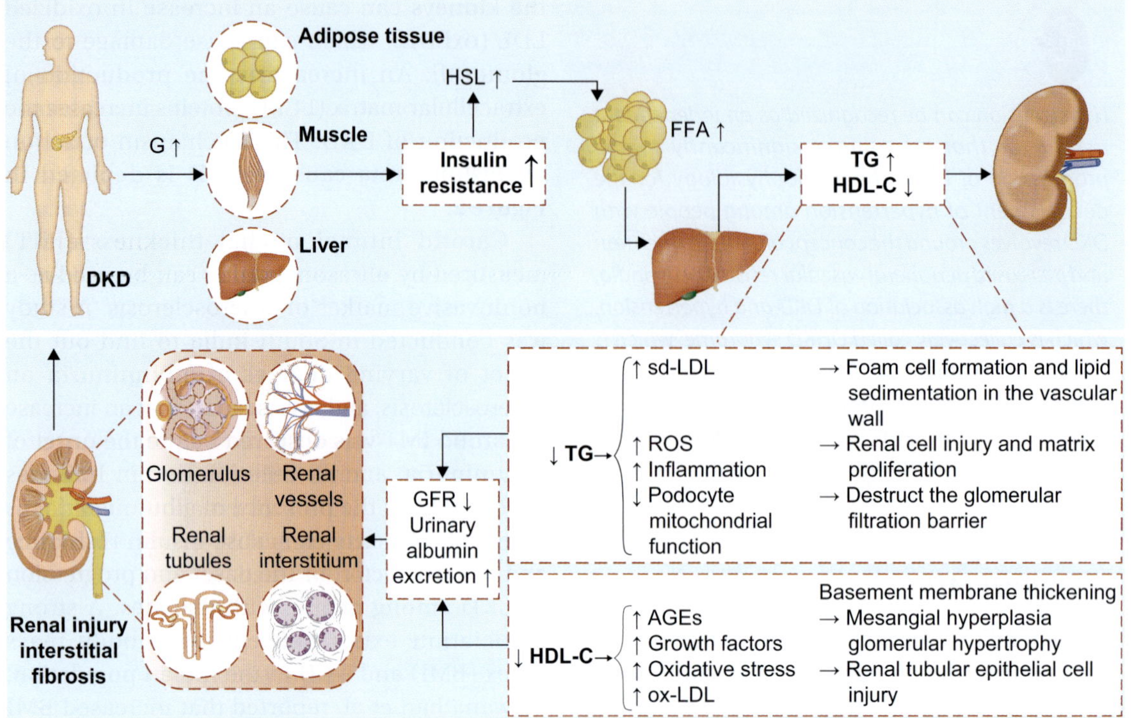

FIG. 2: Pathophysiological mechanisms of dyslipidemia in diabetic kidney disease (DKD).

CARDIOVASCULAR COMPLICATIONS IN DIABETIC KIDNEY DISEASE

There exists a bidirectional relationship between the kidney and heart, which implies that maintaining the fluid and acid–base balance, as well as keeping the blood pressure under control, highlights the interaction between CKD and coronary artery disease (CAD).

In a study by Viswanathan et al., a high prevalence and early onset of cardiac autonomic neuropathy were observed among South Indian people living with diabetes and nephropathy. Cardiac dysautonomia was diagnosed using autonomic function tests (AFTs). This study indicated that nephropathy was associated with an increased risk of developing cardiac autonomic neuropathy (CAN) among people with T2DM.[21] People diagnosed with DKD have high rates of cardiovascular morbidity and mortality, and death

occurs in these patients due to CVD rather than ESRD.[22] A decline in eGFR and albuminuria are both considered an independent risk factors for CVD and its associated mortality. The coexistence of traditional risk factors coupled with the other nontraditional risk factors is recognized as a potential reason for the underlying cardiovascular complications manifesting in DKD, as explained in **Figure 3**. Though the exact mechanism of action is unknown, these are some of the common risk factors that can contribute to CVD in DKD. In a study by Viswanathan et al, the cardiovascular morbidity was studied among the groups with proteinuria and normoalbuminuria. The study groups were evaluated for the presence of CVDs like myocardial infarction, ischemic heart disease, and a history of coronary bypass surgery. The risk of CVD was three times higher among people with proteinuria than in the nonproteinuric group. Hypertension was also more prevalent among

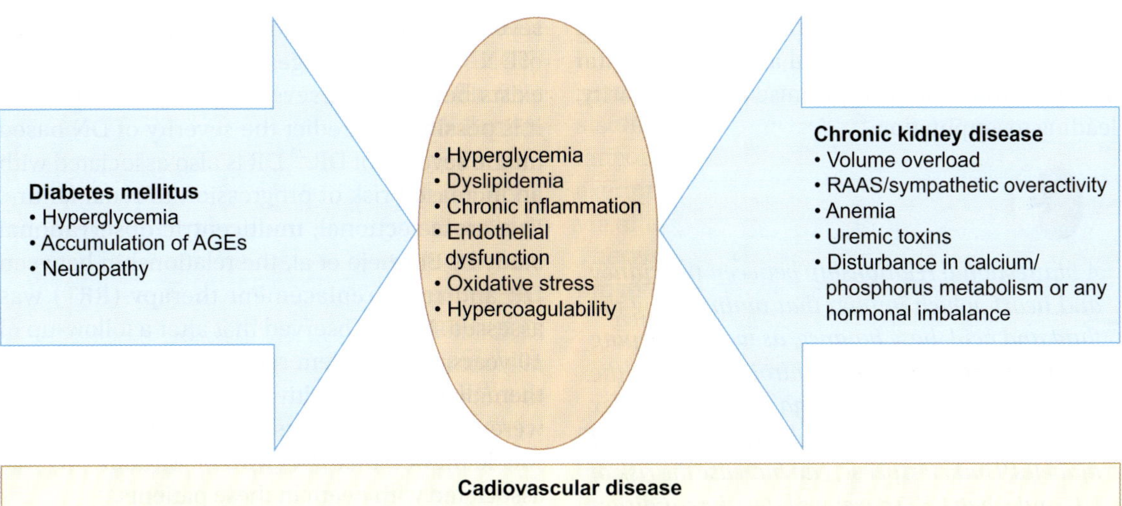

FIG. 3: Various risk factors and mechanisms of action for CVD in people with CKD and diabetes. (AGEs: advanced glycation end products; CKD: chronic kidney disease; CVD: cardiovascular disease; RAAS: renin–angiotensin–aldosterone system)

people with proteinuria. Multivariate logistic regression revealed age, proteinuria, and BMI to be independently associated with CKD among people with diabetes.[23]

Figure 3 depicts the various risk factors and mechanisms of action for CVD in people with CKD and diabetes.

When there is an imbalance between the oxygen that is being supplied and required due to a decrease in cardiac blood flow, it can lead to ischemic heart disease, and the most common reason is CAD. Studies reveal that there is a greater risk of atrial fibrillation, chronic coronary syndrome, and HF when the kidney function declines, and the eGFR begins to decline below 60. The management should target the modifiable risk factors such as hypertension, insulin resistance, smoking, and dyslipidemia, which are the principal risk factors for atherosclerosis, for both the underlying pathologies.[24]

A complex interplay is evident among HF, CKD, and diabetes. Diabetes, per se, can increase the risk of HF, and when CKD develops later, the condition worsens and the risk of mortality increases **(Fig. 4)**. In some cases, there can be

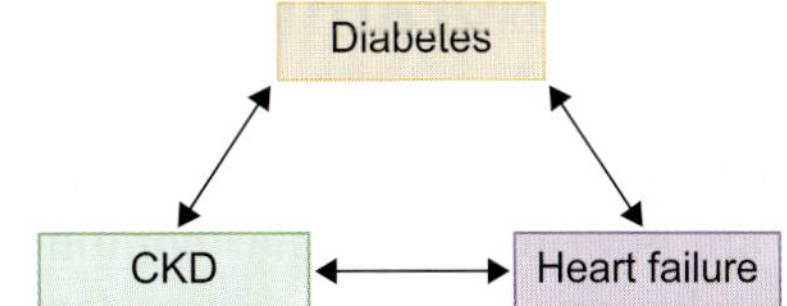

FIG. 4: Bidirectional links between diabetes, chronic kidney disease (CKD), and heart failure.

impaired kidney function, which can develop secondary to heart disease called *cardiorenal syndrome*. Left ventricular hypertrophy (LVH), which is an important risk factor for HF, occurs in around 70–80% of people with CKD. LVH is considered an independent risk factor for arrhythmias, IHD, HF, and even death.[25]

Figure 4 shows the complex interplay among heart failure, diabetes, and CKD.

Peripheral Arterial disease (PAD) is characterized by the narrowing of the peripheral arteries, leading to lower limb ischemia and amputation. It is six to eight times more common among people with CKD than in the general population.[26] The classic "Renal Foot" has been described in people with ESRD and chronic limb-threatening ischemia

(CLTI). This condition is characterized by arterial damage to the posterior tibial and lateral plantar arteries, which can compromise the vascularity, leading to amputation.[27]

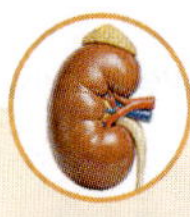

A bidirectional relationship between the kidney and heart, which implies that maintaining the fluid and acid–base balance, as well as keeping the blood pressure under control, highlights the interaction between CKD and CAD. A complex interplay is evident among HF, CKD, and diabetes. Diabetes, per se, can increase the risk of HF, and when CKD develops later, the condition worsens and the risk of mortality increases. The classic "Renal foot" has been described in people with ESRD and CLTI.

DIABETIC RETINOPATHY

There is a significant correlation between diabetic nephropathy (DN) and diabetic retinopathy (DR) as they are both microvascular complications, and hyperglycemia in both cases can damage the small blood vessels in the kidney and in the retina. DR can be classified as nonproliferative and proliferative retinopathy based on the changes in the retina and the process of neovascularization or formation of new blood vessels. Routine screening for retinopathy by an ophthalmologist at least annually is recommended. A comprehensive eye examination, which includes a dilation of the retina, fundus photography, optical coherence tomography (OCT), and, more recently, Fluorescein angiography, can be used to assess DR. A dilated eye examination can be used to detect abnormalities in the retina, such as microaneurysms, macular edema, neovascularization, and retinal hemorrhages. An OCT can produce three-dimensional, detailed photography of the retina and can also be used to determine leakage in the retina or its degree of swelling. DR is a good predictor of DN, and the severity of DR is linked to the pathological severity of DN.[28] Saini et al. suggest that a strong correlation exists between the severity of DR and DN, and it is possible to predict the severity of DN based on the severity of DR.[29] DR is also associated with an increased risk of progression to renal failure. In a cross-sectional, multicentric observational study by Bermejo et al, the relationship between DR and renal replacement therapy (RRT) was assessed. It was observed that after a follow-up of 10 years, 40% of them required RRT, and 21% of them died. In the multivariate analysis, DR or DN were independently associated with RRT, and it was identified that DN (with or without DR) was associated with death in these patients.[30]

Some studies proposed that there is some concordance and discordance between DKD and DR. In a study by Vijay et al., the severity of DR was associated with the severity of DN. The mortality rates were also high when both DR and DN occurred together.[31] In a Mexican study, discordance was found between the progression of DR and nephropathy. 65% of participants in ESRD have proliferative diabetic retinopathy (PDR), and 18% had no DR or nonproliferative retinopathy.[32] Tang et al. suggested that DR can accurately predict DN,[33] and some found no association between DR and ESRD. Longitudinal studies are warranted to understand the exact cause-and-effect relationship between DR and DN.

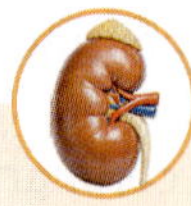

A strong correlation exists between the severity of DR and DN, and it is possible to predict the severity of DN based on the severity of DR. DR is also associated with an increased risk of progression to renal failure. Some studies proposed that there is some concordance and discordance between DKD and DR and found no association between DR and ESRD. Longitudinal studies are warranted to understand the exact cause-and-effect relationship between DR and DN.

DIABETIC FOOT AND AMPUTATIONS

Bonnet et al. suggested that declining kidney function is associated with podiatric risk among people with diabetes.[34] There exists a pathophysiological link between CKD and diabetic foot ulcers (DFUs). People with DKD are at an increased risk of developing infections due to chronic inflammation, impaired immunity, and metabolic changes. Uremia is considered an independent cause of neuropathy in ESRD. A link between a history of DFU and albuminuria was found by Aragon et al.[35] Those in ESRD are at a higher risk of developing DFUs, and this risk further increases once RRT begins. PAD is higher among people with ESRD, and tissue oxygenation becomes worsened by tissue edema and anemia. Dialysis also induces circulatory changes in the foot. The other factors that can contribute to DFUs are inappropriate footwear, patients' inability to access podiatry services during dialysis, the prescribed footwear becoming ill-fitting due to edema peri dialysis and immobilization, and pressure on the vulnerable areas like the heel during dialysis. The development of a foot ulcer can also accelerate the decline in kidney function.[36] The relationship between diabetic foot infection (DFI) and renal function was evaluated at the time of onset of DFI, and a significant reduction in eGFR was noted among people with CKD and DFI and people without CKD but with DFI.[37] It becomes important to prevent and treat DFUs appropriately to impede a decline in kidney function.

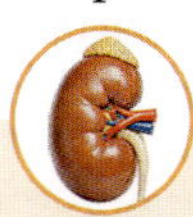

Dialysis induces circulatory changes in the foot and other factors, which can contribute to DFUs, such as inappropriate footwear, patients' inability to access podiatry services during dialysis, the prescribed footwear becoming ill-fitting due to edema peri dialysis and immobilization, and pressure on the vulnerable areas like the heel during dialysis. The development of a foot ulcer can also accelerate the decline in kidney function.

SARCOPENIA

Some studies suggested that sarcopenia and DKD are closely associated with each other. Sarcopenia is a condition characterized by a decrease in skeletal muscle mass (SMM), strength, and/or function. The insulin resistance in diabetes can reduce protein synthesis and degradation in the muscle, making it one of the most likely reasons for the development of sarcopenia among people with diabetes. Increase in inflammation and oxidative stress, combined with uremic toxins and reduced physical activity among people with CKD and diabetes, are some of the reasons that can contribute to sarcopenia. The Asian Working Group of Sarcopenia in 2019 developed an algorithm for the diagnosis of sarcopenia among Asians **(Flowchart 1)**.[38] Huang et al proposed that sarcopenia can be considered as an independent risk factor for severe DN.[39] A decrease in protein intake can also contribute to sarcopenia, but a low-protein diet can decrease the progression of DKD and also worsen a person's nutritional status.

Flowchart 1 shows the diagnostic algorithm for the diagnosis of sarcopenia, adapted from the Asian working group of sarcopenia 2019.

The protein degradation decreases with the increase in insulin resistance and chronic inflammation, uremic toxins, metabolic acidosis, protein energy wasting, and physical inactivity are some of the other factors that are responsible for the disruption of the balance between protein synthesis and degradation, thereby resulting in sarcopenia. The SMM or the skeletal muscle index (SMI) can be calculated either using bioelectric impedance analysis (BIA) or a dual X-ray absorptiometer, or more accurately using magnetic resonance imaging (MRI) or computed tomography (CT). The hand grip strength can be assessed using a hand dynamometer, and the gait speed can be evaluated using a pedometer. Gait speed can highlight the frailty and prognosis of people with CKD and diabetes. In a study by Selva Elavarasan et al., the prevalence and severity of sarcopenia were found to be higher among people with increasing grades of CKD based on KDIGO guidelines.[40] Another

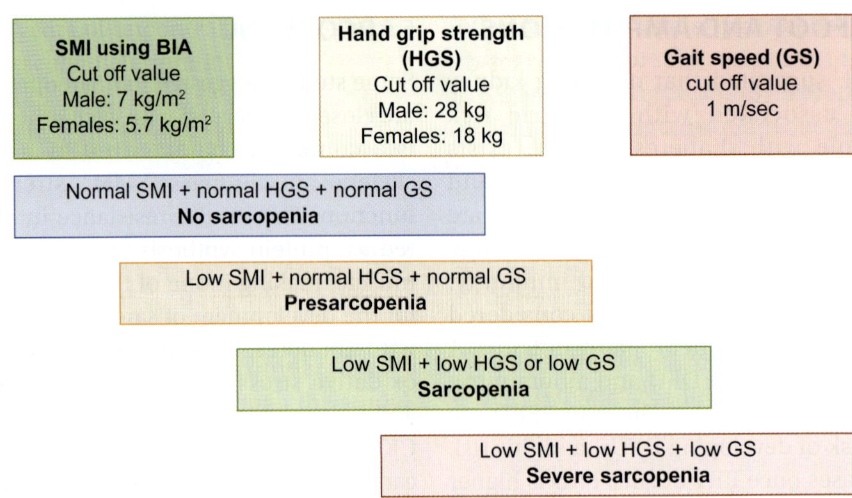

FLOWCHART 1: Diagnostic algorithm for sarcopenia.
Source: ASIAN Working Group; 2019.[39]

study by Lin et al. reported that a significant association existed between DKD, lower limb mass, and visceral fat area. The progression of DKD was strongly associated with increased visceral fat area and reduced lower limb mass.[41] It becomes imperative to diagnose this condition early and prevent its potential complications.

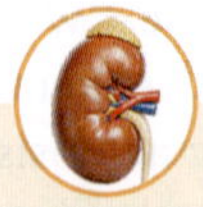

Sarcopenia is characterized by a decrease in SMM, strength, and/or function. The insulin resistance in diabetes can cause a decrease in protein synthesis and degradation in the muscle, making it one of the most likely reasons for the development of sarcopenia among people with diabetes. The protein degradation decreases with the increase in insulin resistance and chronic inflammation, uremic toxins, metabolic acidosis, protein energy wasting, and physical inactivity contribute to Sarcopenia.

GOUT

Insulin resistance, hypertension, and obesity are some risk factors that are common to both diabetes and gout, thereby creating a potential link between them. The coexistence of both diabetes and gout can increase the risk of progression to ESRD. Gout is a clinical condition characterized by the accumulation and deposition of monosodium urate crystals in the joints. It is also recognized as a common form of inflammatory arthritis. In people with DKD, there is an increased accumulation of uric acid due to the inability of the kidneys to filter out uric acid, which is a waste product. This, in turn, accumulates in the bloodstream, resulting in the formation of urate crystals in the joints, leading to pain, swelling, and redness. In a study by Li et al., diabetes and hyperuricemia were strongly related to increased all-cause mortality and ESRD in advancing grades of CKD.[42]

OSTEOARTHRITIS AND RENAL OSTEODYSTROPHY

People with CKD and diabetes have a higher prevalence of osteoarthritis (OA) due to similar risk factors like obesity, metabolic dysfunction, and chronic inflammation. The incidence of OA remained higher in females when compared to males. CKD-mineral bone disorder (MBD) affects the bone quality and resilience of the cartilage, and the accumulation of uremic toxins, coupled with the accumulation of AGEs, accelerates the progression of OA. Yang et al., in their review on OA and CKD, have quoted the findings of a survey which revealed that 54% of people with CKD who underwent long-term hemodialysis were diagnosed with OA.[43] People with DKD are also at an increased risk of developing fractures and bone problems due to CKD-MBD. There is a systemic imbalance of hormones and minerals, making the bones more brittle and prone to fractures. This type of abnormal bone remodeling is called renal osteodystrophy. Thus, early screening and diagnosis of OA and CKD-MBD, along with integrated management of CKD and diabetes, can decrease the progression of these conditions.

ANEMIA

Anemia is quite a prevalent clinical condition seen in people with CKD due to a decrease in erythropoietin production, iron deficiency, and chronic inflammation. Nephrotic syndrome and the use of ACE inhibitors and Angiotensin receptor antagonists cause a reversible reduction in hemoglobin among people with CKD and diabetes. Anemia can contribute to the progression of DKD and is also an independent risk factor for the development of HF, LVH, and cardiovascular mortality.[44] Management of anemia among people with CKD and diabetes can improve the treatment outcomes as well as their quality of life.

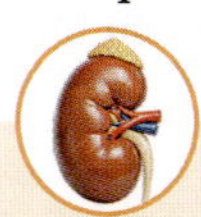

CKD-MBD affects the bone quality and resilience of the cartilage, and the accumulation of uremic toxins, coupled with the accumulation of AGEs, accelerates the progression of Osteoarthritis. Anemia can contribute to the progression of DKD and is also an independent risk factor for the development of HF, LVH, and cardiovascular mortality.

METABOLIC ACIDOSIS

This condition is quite common among people with CKD, and it occurs when the kidneys are not able to excrete the acid load. This can result in an increased accumulation of H^+ and a low CO_2 concentration, leading to poor outcomes such as loss of muscle mass, demineralization of bone, and decline in kidney function. Sodium bicarbonate is given to treat metabolic acidosis based on the recommendations of the current guidelines. However, consumption of fruits and vegetables and supplementation with oral alkali can be used to treat metabolic acidosis. More recently, Veverimer, a novel proton-binding polymer, can be used to treat metabolic acidosis.[45,46] If untreated, it can worsen the progression of CKD and can also lead to serious complications, such as cardiac arrhythmias and even death.

SUMMARY

Diabetes is a vascular disease associated with micro- and macrovascular complications. One such microvascular complication is DKD. Around 40% of people with diabetes are affected by CKD. Some of the important comorbidities and complications associated with DKD are hypertension, dyslipidemia, obesity, ischemic heart diseases such as angina, myocardial infarction, and HF, and peripheral vascular diseases. Hypertension is often called a silent killer and a major public health problem among people with diabetes. Hypertension can cause CKD, and CKD can worsen the hypertension, thereby creating a vicious cycle. The coexistence of these conditions can increase the risk of CVD and also increase the progression of CKD. Regular monitoring of blood pressure and kidney function is essential to prevent further complications. Abnormal lipid levels, such as high TG, LDL, and low HDL, can cause a decline in kidney function and are also a major contributor to cardiovascular risk. Hypertriglyceridemia is one of the earliest findings of CKD, and management of dyslipidemia can improve the cardiovascular outcomes and delay the progression of CKD. Obesity can cause insulin resistance and is a risk factor for the onset and progression of CKD among people with diabetes. Excess body fat in obesity can trigger glomerular hyperfiltration, causing a decline in kidney function and eventually leading to ESRD. There exists a bidirectional relationship between the kidney and heart, maintaining the fluid and acid–base balance as well as keeping the blood pressure under control, which highlights the interaction between CKD and CAD.

CKD can cause HF through fluid overload, the presence of uremic toxins, and anemia, and the blood flow is reduced in HF. The association is very complex and requires a specialized approach to address the challenges. Renal function is strongly associated with diabetic foot and podiatric risk. PAD is higher among people with ESRD, and tissue oxygenation worsens due to tissue edema and anemia. The "Renal Foot" is described in people with ESRD and CLTI. The insulin resistance in diabetes causes a decrease in protein synthesis and degradation in the muscle, which can lead to sarcopenia. Other conditions, such as

gout, anemia, osteoarthritis, metabolic acidosis, increased risk of fractures, and infections, are also associated with DKD. It becomes imperative to diagnose DKD early and also prevent the onset of associated comorbidities and complications related to DKD.

CONCLUSION

Diabetic Kidney Disease is associated with several comorbidities such as hypertension, dyslipidemia, obesity, and ischemic heart diseases such as angina, myocardial infarction, and HF, and peripheral vascular diseases, such as amputation and gangrene. Some of the major complications are ESRD, cardiovascular morbidity, and even death. People with DKD are also prone to develop retinopathy, gout, osteoarthritis, and anemia. A comprehensive, integrated, and systematic approach is required for the prevention and management of DKD for early diagnosis, to identify the risk factors associated with the onset and progression of DKD, decrease or prevent the onset of potential complications, and thereby improve the quality of life of people living with DKD.

TAKE HOME MESSAGES

- DKD is associated with several comorbidities and complications.
- Early diagnosis of DKD by calculating eGFR and measuring UACR/UPCR and staging based on KDIGO is essential to prevent the onset of these comorbidities and complications of DKD.
- An integrated and comprehensive strategy is required to provide intensive glycemic and blood pressure control along with lifestyle modifications.
- We can prevent the potential serious life-threatening complications and reduce the substantial burden on the healthcare system of the nation.

REFERENCES

1. International Diabetes Federation. IDF Diabetes Atlas, 11th edition. Brussels, Belgium: International Diabetes Federation; 2025.

2. Prasannakumar M, Rajput R, Seshadri K, Talwalkar P, Agarwal P, Gokulnath G, et al. An observational, cross-sectional study to assess the prevalence of chronic kidney disease in type 2 diabetes patients in India (START -India). Indian J Endocrinol Metab. 2015;19(4):520-3.

3. Kumar A, Mazumdar A, Bhattacharjee AK, Gupta A, Dasgupta A, Sinha B et al. Risk factors associated with Indian type 2 diabetes patients with chronic kidney disease: CITE study, a cross-sectional, real-world, observational study. BMC Nephrol. 2025;26(1):245.

4. World Health Organization. (2024). SEAHEARTS: World's largest expansion of hypertension coverage through PHC 2024. [Online] Available from https://www.who.int/southeastasia/news/events/detail/2024/05/20/defaultcalendar/seahearts--world-s-largest-expansion-of-hypertension-coverage-through-phc-2024 [Last accessed March, 2029].

5. Udaya R. RAG-SACA-2: EPIDEMIOLOGY OF HYPERTENSION IN SOUTH ASIA. J Hypertens. 2023;41(Suppl 1):e169.

6. McEvoy JW, McCarthy CP, Bruno RM, Brouwers S, Canavan MD, Ceconi C, et al. 2024 ESC Guidelines for the management of elevated blood pressure and hypertension. Eur Heart J. 2024;45(38):3912-4018.

7. Wander GS, Panda JK, Pal J, Mathur G, Sahay R, Tiwaskar M, et al. Management of Hypertension in Patients with Type 2 Diabetes Mellitus: Indian Guideline 2024 by Association of Physicians of India and Indian College of Physicians. J Assoc Physicians India. 2024;72(F8):e1-25.

8. Anjana RM, Unnikrishnan R, Deepa M, Pradeepa R, Tandon N, Das AK, et al. Metabolic non-communicable disease health report of India: the ICMR-INDIAB national cross-sectional study (ICMR-INDIAB-17). Lancet Diabetes Endocrinol. 2023;11(7):474-89.

9. International Diabetes Federation. IDF Diabetes Atlas, 9th edition. Belgium: International Diabetes Federation; 2019.

10. Tharkar S, Devarajan A, Kumpatla S, Viswanathan V. The socioeconomics of diabetes from a developing country: a population based cost of illness study. Diabetes Res Clin Pract. 2010;89(3):334-40.

11. G Metri K, Raghuram N, S Ram CV, Singh A, Patil SS, Mohanty SS, et al. The deadly duo of hypertension and diabetes in India: further affirmation from a new epidemiological study. J Assoc Physicians India. 2022;70(7):14-7.

12. Roy S, Schweiker-Kahn O, Jafry B, Masel-Miller R, Raju RS, O'Neill LMO, et al. Risk Factors and Comorbidities Associated with Diabetic Kidney Disease. J Prim Care Community Health. 2021;12:21501327211048556.

13. Dash SC, Agarwal SK, Panigrahi A, Mishra J, Dash D. Diabetes, Hypertension and Kidney Disease Combination "DHKD Syndrome" is common in India. J Assoc Physicians India. 2018;66(3):30-3.

14. Wu AY, Kong NC, de Leon FA, Pan CY, Tai TY, Yeung VT, et al. Diabetologia. 2005;48(1):17-26.

15. Viswanathan V, Smina TP. Blood pressure control in diabetes-the Indian perspective. J Hum Hypertens. 2019;33(8):588-93.

16. Djordjevic V. Hypertension and nephropathy in diabetes mellitus: what is inherited and what is acquired? Nephrol Dial Transplant. 2001;16:92-3.

17. Kawanami D, Matoba K, Utsunomiya K. Dyslipidemia in diabetic nephropathy. Ren Replace Ther. 2016;2:16.

18. Tu QM, Jin HM, Yang XH. Lipid abnormality in diabetic kidney disease and potential treatment advancements. Front Endocrinol. 2025;16:1503711.

19. Viswanathan V, SelvaElavarasan S, Kumpatla S. Increased Body Mass Index is Independently Associated with Chronic Kidney Disease among People with Type 2 Diabetes. Indian J Nephrol. 2025;35(Suppl 4):670-6.

20. Viswanathan V, Snehalatha C, Mohan RS, Mamtha Nair B, Ramachandran A. Increased carotid intimal media thickness precedes albuminuria in South Indian type 2 diabetic subjects. The British Journal of Diabetes & Vascular Disease. 2003;3(2):146-9.

21. Viswanathan V, SelvaElavarasan S, Kumpatla S. Increased Body Mass Index is Independently Associated with Chronic Kidney Disease among People with Type 2 Diabetes. Indian J Nephrol. 2025;35: 670-6.

22. Viswanathan V, Prasad D, Chamukuttan S, Ramachandran A. High prevalence and early onset of cardiac autonomic neuropathy among South Indian type 2 diabetic patients with nephropathy. Diabetes Res Clin Pract. 2000;48(3):211-6.

23. Keith DS, Nichols GA, Gullion CM, Brown JB, Smith DH. Longitudinal follow-up and outcomes among a population with chronic kidney disease in a large managed care organization. Arch. Intern. Med. 2004; 164(6):659-63.

24. Viswanathan V, Snehalatha C, Mathai T, Jayaraman M, Ramachandran A. Cardiovascular morbidity in proteinuric South Indian NIDDM patients. Diabetes Res Clin Pract. 1998;39(1):63-7.

25. Cepoi MR, Duca ST, Chetran A, Costache AD, Spiridon MR, Afrăsânie I, et al. Chronic Kidney Disease Associated with Ischemic Heart Disease: To What Extent Do Biomarkers Help? Life (Basel). 2023;14(1):34.

26. Taddei S, Nami R, Bruno RM, Quatrini I, Nuti R. Hypertension, left ventricular hypertrophy and chronic kidney disease. Heart Fail Rev. 2011;16(6):615-20.

27. Huish S, Nawaz S, Bellasi A, Diaz-Tocados JM, Haarhaus M, Sinha S. Clinical management of peripheral arterial disease in chronic kidney disease—a comprehensive review from the European Renal Association CKD-MBD Working Group. Clinical Kidney J. 2025;18(5):sfaf089.

28. Baghdasaryan PA, Bae JH, Yu W, Rowe V, Armstrong DG, Shavelle DM, et al. "The Renal Foot"- Angiographic Pattern of Patients with Chronic Limb Threatening Ischemia and End-Stage Renal Disease. Cardiovasc Revasc Med. 2020;21(1):118-21.

29. Wang Q, Cheng H, Jiang S, Zhang L, Liu X, Chen P, et al. The relationship between diabetic retinopathy

and diabetic nephropathy in type 2 diabetes. Front Endocrinol (Lausanne). 2024;15:1292412.

30. Saini DC, Kochar A, Poonia R. Clinical correlation of diabetic retinopathy with nephropathy and neuropathy. Indian J Ophthalmol. 2021;69(11):3364-8.

31. Bermejo S, González E, López-Revuelta K, Ibernon M, López D, Martín-Gómez A, et al. The coexistence of diabetic retinopathy and diabetic nephropathy is associated with worse kidney outcomes. Clin Kidney J. 2023;16(10):1656-63.

32. Viswanathan V, Kumpatla S, Tilak P, Kuppusamy A. Relationship Between Retinal-Renal Complications Among Type 2 Diabetic Subjects in India. Int J Diabetol Vasc Dis Res. 2013;1(2):8-14.

33. Fitzgerald A, Das R, Moezzi CJ, Salazar SR, Mankad R, Qualls CR, et al. Discordance of diabetic retinopathy severity in a cohort of diabetic nephropathy patients: a cross-sectional case-control study in a new Mexican population of type 2 diabetes. Front Endocrinol (Lausanne). 2025;16:1638415.

34. Tang S, An X, Sun W, Zhang Y, Yang C, Kang X, et al. Parallelism and non-parallelism in diabetic nephropathy and diabetic retinopathy. Front Endocrinol (Lausanne). 2024;15:1336123.

35. Bonnet JB, Szwarc I, Avignon A, Jugant S, Sultan A. Renal function is highly associated with podiatric risk in diabetic patients. Clin Kidney J. 2023;16(11):2156-63.

36. Aragón-Sánchez J, Lázaro-Martínez JL, García-Álvarez Y, Morales EG, Hernández-Herrero MJ. Albuminuria is a predictive factor of in-hospital mortality in patients with diabetes admitted for foot disease. Diabetes Res Clin Pract. 2014;104:e23-5.

37. Game F. The diabetic foot and renal disease. Br J Diabetes. 2025;25(1):38-40.

38. Anitha Rani A, Viswanathan V. Diabetic Foot Infection and Worsening Kidney Function: Implication for Health Care in the Developing World. Int J Diabetol Vasc Dis Res. 2017;5(5):208-13.

39. Chen LK, Woo J, Assantachai P, Auyeung TW, Chou MY, Iijima K, et al. Asian Working Group for Sarcopenia: 2019 Consensus Update on Sarcopenia Diagnosis and Treatment. J Am Med Dir Assoc. 2020;21(3):300-7.e2.

40. Huang YM, Chen WM, Chen M, Shia BC, Wu SY. Sarcopenia Is an Independent Risk Factor for Severe Diabetic Nephropathy in Type 2 Diabetes: A Long-Term Follow-Up Propensity Score-Matched Diabetes Cohort Study. J Clin Med. 2022;11(11):2992.

41. Elavarasan SS, Kumpatla S, Viswanathan V. Prevalence of different stages of Sarcopenia across various stages of kidney disease based on KDIGO among people with Type 2 Diabetes. Kidney Int Rep. 2025;10(2):S119.

42. Lin X, Chen Z, Huang H, Zhong J, Xu L. Diabetic kidney disease progression is associated with decreased lower-limb muscle mass and increased visceral fat area in T2DM patients. Front Endocrinol (Lausanne). 2022;13:1002118.

43. Li CH, Lee CL, Hsieh YC, Chen CH, Wu MJ, Tsai SF. Hyperuricemia and diabetes mellitus when occurred together have higher risks than alone on all-cause mortality and end-stage renal disease in patients with chronic kidney disease. BMC Nephrol. 2022;23(1):157.

44. Yang RS, Chan DC, Chung YP, Liu SH. Chronic Kidney Disease and Osteoarthritis: Current Understanding and Future Research Directions. Int J Mol Sci. 2025;26(4):1567.

45. Mehdi U, Toto RD. Anemia, diabetes, and chronic kidney disease. Diabetes Care. 2009;32(7):1320-6.

46. Kim HJ. Metabolic Acidosis in Chronic Kidney Disease: Pathogenesis, Clinical Consequences, and Treatment. Electrolyte Blood Press. 2021;19(2):29-37.

Key Research Takeaway

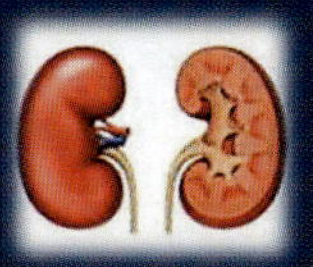

Increased carotid intimal media thickness precedes albuminuria in South Indian type 2 diabetic subjects

VIJAY VISWANATHAN, CHAMUKUTTAN SNEHALATHA, RANGAMOORTHY SURESH MOHAN, BALAKRISHNAN MAMTHA NAIR, AMBADY RAMACHANDRAN

Abstract

Introduction Intimal media thickness (IMT) of common carotid artery (CCA) is used as an index of atherosclerosis. IMT is increased in subjects with diabetes and also with diabetic nephropathy.

Aim
The study was undertaken in South Indian type 2 diabetic patients with different degrees of albuminuria to see whether albuminuria worsened IMT.

Material and methods
IMT was measured by ultrasonography in 273 diabetic subjects with normoalbuminuria (n=91), microalbuminuria (n=92), clinical proteinuria (Prot) (n=90) and in age-matched non-diabetic subjects (n=99). The diabetic subjects were older than the non-diabetic subjects hence IMT was age-adjusted using a linear regression formula.

Results
Age-adjusted IMT value in diabetic subjects was significantly higher (0.88+0.3 mm) than in non-diabetic subjects (0.57+0.34 mm) (p<0.001). Mean IMT in normoalbuminuria (0.87+0.26 mm), microalbuminuria (0.90+0.33 mm) and Prot (0.86+0.39 mm) patients were not significantly different from each other. Male gender, age, diabetes and total cholesterol were independently associated with IMT, while duration of diabetes, hypertension and HbA1C were not.

Conclusion
Increased carotid IMT occurred in type 2 diabetes prior to the presence of albuminuria. Further deterioration in IMT did not occur with the presence of albuminuria. *Br J Diabetes Vasc Dis* 2003;**3**:146–9

High prevalence and early onset of cardiac autonomic neuropathy among South Indian Type 2 diabetic patients with nephropathy

*Vijay Viswanathan *, Durga Prasad, Snehalatha Chamukuttan, Ambady Ramachandran*

Diabetes Research Centre, No. 4 Main Road, Royapuram, Madras 600 013, India

Received 26 July 1999; received in revised form 9 December 1999; accepted 14 January 2000

Abstract

Objective: This study was conducted to assess the adverse effects of diabetic nephropathy on cardiovascularautonomic neuropathy (CAN) in South Indian Type 2 diabetic patients. *Methods*: Comparison was made between Type 2 diabetic patients with nephropathy (group 1, $n25$), Type 2 diabetic patients without nephropathy (group 2, $n25$) and non-diabetic, non-hypertensive control subjects ($n20$). All had a detailed clinical and biochemical work-up and cardiac assessment by ECG. Cardiac dysautonomia was assessed by a battery of five non invasive autonomic function tests (ANF) as recommended by Ewing and Clarke [D.J. Ewing, B.F. Clarke, Diagnosis and Management of autonomic neuropathy. Br. Med. J. 285 (1982) 916–918]. *Results*: Group 1 patients showed a higher percentage of abnormal CAN function and a more severe form of CAN compared with patients in group 2. Group 1 patients showed early development of the abnormalities. They also had a higher prevalence of peripheral neuropathy compared with the patients without nephropathy. *Conclusions*: The present study showed that the presence of nephropathy was associated with the risk of cardiac autonomic neuropathy in Type 2 diabetic patients and it probably had an earlier onset also in them. © 2000 Elsevier Science Ireland Ltd. All rights reserved.

Diabetes Research and Clinical Practice 48 (2000) 211–216

Cardio vascular morbidity in proteinuric South Indian NIDDM patients

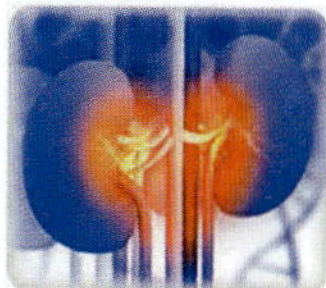

Vijay Viswanathan *, C. Snehalatha, Terin Mathai, Muthu Jayaraman, A. Ramachandran

Diabetes Research Centre, No. 5, Main Road, Royapuram, Chennai, 600 013, India

Received 21 March 1997; received in revised form 8 July 1997; accepted 13 July 1997

Abstract

Proteinuria is a well known risk factor for cardiovascular morbidity. There has been no report on cardiovascular morbidity in Indian NIDDM patients with proteinuria. Hence this study has been undertaken to estimate the prevalence of cardiovascular diseases (CVD) in South Indian NIDDM with proteinuria. We studied two groups of NIDDM patients with diabetes for ≥ 5 years: group PR with persistent proteinuria of > 500 mg/day ($n = 297$) and group NPR with normoalbuminuria (albuminuria ≤ 30 μg/mg creatinine) ($n = 296$), who reported for review during the study period. They were matched for age, duration of diabetes and BMI. The prevalence of cardiovascular diseases, namely myocardial infarction, the presence of ischaemic heart disease and the history of coronary bypass surgery were compared in the two groups. The prevalence of hypertension was higher among the PR than the NPR patients (56.5 vs 24.7%, $\chi^2 = 61.3$, $P < 0.001$). CVD were detected in 39.2% ($n = 116$) of the PR and 13.2% ($n = 39$) of the NPR groups. ($\chi^2 = 54.85$, $P < 0.001$). The risk was thus three-fold higher in the PR group. Univariate analysis showed that in the proteinuric group, the prevalence of complications was higher in association with hypertension (45.8 vs 30.2%, $\chi^2 = 6.82$, $P = 0.009$). Multiple logistic regression analysis showed that the factors associated with CVD were proteinuria (odds ratio 5.03), age (OR 1.08) and BMI (OR 1.07) while sex, age at onset of diabetes, duration of diabetes, hypertension, smoking, HbA$_1$, serum creatinine, cholesterol and triglycerides did not show independent contribution. The study, highlights the high risk conferred by macroproteinuria in Indian NIDDM patients. This risk is found to be independent of the presence of associated hypertension. © 1998 Elsevier Science Ireland Ltd. All rights reserved.

International Journal of Diabetology & Vascular Disease Research(IJDVR) ISSN 2328-353X

Vijay Viswanathan
2013, Volume I Issue No.2

Relationship Between Retinal-Renal Complications Among Type 2 Diabetic Subjects in India

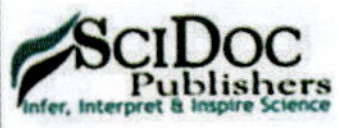

Vijay Viswanathan*, Satyavani Kumpatla*, Priyanka Tilak*, Archana Kuppusamy*
*CM. V Hospital for Diabetes and Prof M. Viswanathan Diabetes Research Centre, No. 5, Main Road, Royapuram,Chennai - 600 013. India.

Research Article

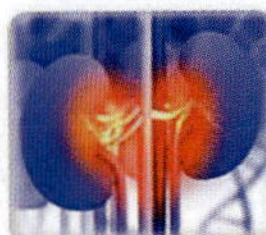

Abstract

Aim: The aim of this study was to determine the relationship between retinal-renal complications among type 2diabetic subjects in India.

Subjects and Methods: A total of 502 subjects with type 2 diabetes who underwent FundusPhotography and Fundus Fluorescein Angiography (FFA) for diabetic retinopathy (DR) and 24hr urinary creatinine clearance (Crcl) test for diabetic nephropathy (DN) on the same day were included in this analysis. They were divided into groups based on the severity of retinopathy and Crcl values. Out of 502 subjects, 272 subjects had subsequent follow-up details spanning 22 months. Anthropometric, haemodynamic and biochemical details at baseline and follow-up and mortality details were recorded.

Results: The mean Crcl values decreased significantly with increasing severity of DR (p<0.001). The percentage of subjects with non-proliferative diabetic retinopathy also decreased with decreasing Crcl. In the follow-up data, severity of DR increased compared to baseline as per stages of Crcl. There was a decline in survival when both the complications are present. Number of subjects who died was high at severe stages of these complications. Crcl was significantly associated with declining status of both the complications.

Conclusions: The degree of diabetic retinopathy and severity of diabetic nephropathy showed significant association among type2 diabetic subjects.

***Corresponding Author:**
Dr.Vijay Viswanathan, M.D., Ph.D.
FRCP (Lon)., FRCP (Glas)
Prof M. Viswanathan Diabetes Research Centre, WHO Collaborating Centre for Research, Education and Training in Diabetes, No. 5, Main Road, Royapuram, Chennai – 600 013, India.
E-mail: drvijay@mvdiabetes.com
Tel: +91-44-25954913-15 ; Fax: +91-44-25954919

Accepted: April 24, 2013
Published: April 26, 2013

Citation: Vijay Viswanathan (2013) Relationship Between Retinal-Renal Complications Among Type 2 Diabetic Subjects in India 1:202

WCN25-3869 

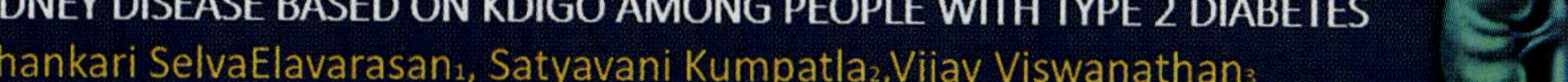
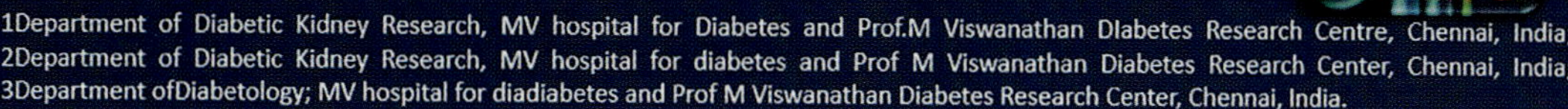

PREVALENCE OF DIFFERENT STAGES OF SARCOPENIA ACROSS VARIOUS STAGES OF KIDNEY DISEASE BASED ON KDIGO AMONG PEOPLE WITH TYPE 2 DIABETES

Sivashankari SelvaElavarasan[1], Satyavani Kumpatla[2],Vijay Viswanathan[3]

1Department of Diabetic Kidney Research, MV hospital for Diabetes and Prof.M Viswanathan DIabetes Research Centre, Chennai, India;
2Department of Diabetic Kidney Research, MV hospital for diabetes and Prof M Viswanathan Diabetes Research Center, Chennai, India;
3Department ofDiabetology; MV hospital for diadiabetes and Prof M Viswanathan Diabetes Research Center, Chennai, India.

Introduction: Sarcopenia is characterized by progressive decrease in the skeletal muscle mass, strength, and or function. Chronic Kidney Disease (CKD) progression can have an impact on the nutrition and lifestyle due to decrease in protein consumption and lack of physical activity, thereby affecting the skeletal muscle mass.Limited literature is available on the prevalence of the different stages of sarcopenia across the various stages of diabetic kidney disease. The aimof this study is to determine the prevalence of Sarcopenia among peoplewith type 2 diabetes and CKD based on KDIGO.

Methods: A total of 184 (M:F-111:73) participants were recruited for this cross sectional study from November 2023 to August 2024 at a tertiary care center, Chennai. The participants were screened according to KDIGO into: CKD stages 1- Low risk (n¼61), 2-Moderate risk (n¼64), 3-High risk (n¼59).Participants with artificial electrical implants such as a defibrillator or pacemaker and with diabetic foot ulcers were excluded.Skeletal muscle mass (SMM) was measured using Body Impedence Analysis (In Body 570) and Skeletal Muscle index (SMI) was calculated by dividing the SMM by square of the participants' height(in m2).Hand Grip strength (HGS) was estimated using Jamar hydraulic dynamometer in the dominant hand and a 6-minute walk test was used to assess the physical performance. The Asian Working Group criteria (2019) was used to diagnose Sarcopenia. Participants with only SMI <7 kg/m2 for males and <5.7 kg/ m2 for females but with normal hang grip strength and physical performance were diagnosed with Presarcopenia. Those with decreased SMI (with the above mentioned cut off) with either decreased muscle strength (M:<28 kg,F:<18 kg) or function (6 metre walk;<1 m/s) were diagnosed with Sarcopenia. Severe sarcopenia was associated with low SMI, low muscle strength as well as low physical performance.

Results: Participants in CKD stage 3 were older than the other stages (57vs 55,52;p¼0.034).SMM ,SMI and HGS were significantly lower in stage 3 than stage 1[(22.4 vs 24.9), (6.7 vs 7.2), (24 vs 31)];p<0.001 for all. The median duration of diabetes andHbA1cwere significantly higher in stage 3 than stage 1(18 vs 10) years, (8.7 vs 7.2) %whereas the eGFR and the amount of protein estimated were significantly lower in stage 3 when compared to stage 1[(39 vs 78), (7.9 vs 9)];p<0.001 for all. The prevalence of presarcopenia across the stages were 32.8%,18.8%,10.2% respectively (p¼0.008). The prevalence of sarcopenia and severe sarcopenia in stages 2 and 3 were 10.9%,4.7% and 18.6%,10.2% respectively. The BMI and eGFR of participants with sarcopenia and severe sarcopenia were significantly lower than participants without sarcopenia.(25.8,23.1vs28.8)and (46,32vs60);p<0.001.SMI was positively correlated with BMI and Egfr but negatively correlated with age, duration of diabetes and HbA1c.

Conclusions: Our study findings showed that the prevalence and severity of sarcopenia was higher among people with advancing stages of CKD and type 2 diabetes. Thus, it is essential to diagnose this condition early to prevent muscle loss and its associated potential complications.

<table>
<tr><td>**8**</td><td></td></tr>
</table>

Nutritional Recommendations for People with Diabetic Kidney Disease

Patricia Trueman

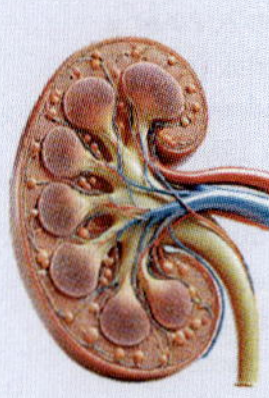

- Glycemic control in people with diabetes
- Kidney Disease: Improving Global Outcomes guidelines
- Modifications/restrictions to be made in the diet
- Protein intake
- Water intake
- Foods rich in potassium
- Sample diet

Abstract

Chronic kidney disease (CKD) is characterized by estimated glomerular filtration rate (eGFR) < 60 mL/min/1.73 m². Good glycemic control is significant in maintaining kidney function. The Kidney Disease: Improving Global Outcomes (KDIGO) guidelines 2024 recommend an ideal body weight energy intake of 25–35 kcal/kg. A total fat intake of 25–35% of the total calories is recommended. CKD patients' diet should include fiber, which helps prevent constipation. 25–30 g/day of fiber intake is recommended. High-fiber vegetables and recommended fruits can be included. Sodium, potassium, protein, water intake, and phosphorus should be restricted. In CKD, the kidneys are unable to remove excess sodium from the body, so sodium intake should be decreased. The sodium level should not exceed 2,000 mg/day. Potassium in the diet should be restricted when potassium levels increase in the blood above normal values. We can consume vegetables and fruits which are low in potassium. Recommended levels of protein intake according to guidelines are 0.6–0.8 g/day. Vegetable protein is a better choice than animal proteins as it contains less phosphorus. In South Indian setting, a drastic reduction in protein intake may not be advisable. Restrictions are to be made in the diet that should be based on the stage of CKD and the nephrologist's advice.

Keywords: Chronic kidney disease, diet, sodium, water restriction, Kidney Disease: Improving Global Outcomes.

INTRODUCTION

Chronic kidney disease (CKD) is a condition characterized by a gradual decrease in kidney function and the estimated glomerular filtration rate (eGFR) declines below 60 mL/min/1.73 m². It is also diagnosed when there is albuminuria, hematuria, or abnormalities detected through laboratory testing.[1] It is projected that nearly 10% of the adults globally are affected by CKD which can cause 1.2 million deaths and 28 million years of life lost every year.[2,3] The kidneys filter waste from the blood. This helps in maintaining the right balance of minerals and salts in the blood. In kidney disease, the kidney loses their capacity to maintain this balance. The most important factor that helps maintain a healthy balance in CKD is diet.

Undernutrition is very common in CKD due to decreased intake. Many factors, such as decreased appetite, reduced food intake, and dietary restrictions, account for malnutrition. Due to a persistent inflammatory state, patients with CKD have higher resting energy expenditure, leading to protein breakdown and decreased anabolism.[4] Malnutrition results in increased mortality and morbidity in patients with CKD, which causes immunodeficiency and increased infections and hospitalization.[4]

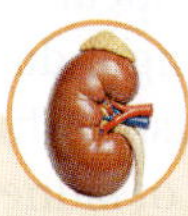

The CKD is characterized by eGFR < 60 mL/min/ 1.73 m². The kidneys maintain the right balance of nutrients in the body.

GLYCEMIC CONTROL IN PEOPLE WITH DIABETES

The quality, quantity as well as the timing of consumption of carbohydrates is considered crucial for people living with diabetes. The amount of carbohydrates consumed in each meal should be fixed to correspond with the dose of insulin or oral hypoglycemic agents, with regular meal timings. The carbohydrate fiber ratio should be balanced. Patients need to be educated about healthy food choices with knowledge of exchange lists, carbohydrate counting, and portion size. Patients should be helped to read food labels. Educating them regarding the glycemic index and glycemic load may be beneficial for sugar control.[5] The diet should be balanced with a good exercise pattern, or yoga, for 30 minutes each day for at least 5 days a week. Regular evaluation of biochemical parameters is very important. The patient should also be educated on self-monitoring of blood glucose and maintaining a record of values. Stress levels in the patient can also be evaluated and proper counseling should be done.

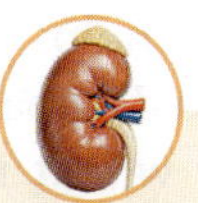

It is important to maintain good dietary habits, exercise and regular evaluation help to maintain glycemic control.

KDIGO GUIDELINES

Kidney Disease: Improving Global Outcomes (KDIGO) provides guidelines, recommendations, and practice points for clinical management of CKD. It highlights healthy lifestyles and their modifications with new medications, which gives improved treatment options. The guidelines highlight the implementation of healthy diet modifications in maintaining the diet. The guidelines emphasize the use of plant-based foods over animal-based foods and the prevention of processed foods. It provides important practice points for the clinical dietitian in restricting protein, sodium, potassium, etc., in the diet.[6]

Energy Intake

The CKD is usually characterized by low energy intake of <25 kcal/kg due to poor appetite. The KDIGO[6] guidelines 2024 recommend an energy intake of 25–35 kcal/kg ideal body weight in CKD patients based on age, gender, physical activity, weight, CKD stage, comorbidity, and inflammation to maintain nutritional status.[7]

Fat Intake

Patients with CKD develop lipid imbalance when eGFR begins to decline.[8] Recommended total fat intake of 25–35% of total calories, with a higher level of monounsaturated fatty acid (MUFA) up to 20%, and polyunsaturated fatty acids (PUFA) up to 10%, saturated fatty acid (SFA) < 7%, and transfats < 1% of total calorie intake.[9]

Carbohydrate Intake

Carbohydrate consumption must be sufficient to meet energy needs as per requirement, especially when the proteins are restricted. This helps to prevent ketosis and provides fibers. Mixed cereals such as rice and rice derivatives or wheat in combination with dals or milk to improve protein quality are recommended. Cereals should be used with pulses, peas, milk, and milk products to mutually complement proteins, which increases the quality of the protein. Small, frequent meals may be advised.[5]

Fiber Intake

Ideally, 25–30 g/day of fiber intake is recommended for people with CKD which can help prevent constipation.[5] High fiber vegetables and recommended fruits can be included.

Vitamin and Mineral Intake

Adequate vitamins and minerals, micronutrients, should be adequate in the diet as per the requirement.

Electrolytes Balance

A restricted diet in sodium, potassium, and protein is recommended when eGFR falls below normal values.[9]

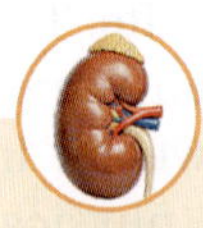

A renal diet is important in managing kidney disease and its related complications. It also helps in decreasing disease progression and the complete loss of kidney function. Energy intake of 25–35 kcal/ kg ideal body weight is recommended according to KDIGO guidelines of 2024. Total fat intake of 25–35% of total calories. Complex carbohydrates should be used with pulses or milk products. A daily fiber intake of 25–30 g/day is recommended.

MODIFICATIONS/RESTRICTIONS TO BE MADE IN THE DIET

Restrictions to be made in the diet should be based on the stage of CKD and the nephrologist's advice.

- Sodium
- Potassium
- Protein
- Water intake
- Phosphorus

Sodium

In CKD, the kidneys are unable to remove excess sodium from the body, so sodium intake should be decreased. Increased levels of sodium cause fluid build-up in the tissues and bloodstream, and symptoms such as increased thirst, swelling, high blood pressure and shortness of breath appear.[10,11] The sodium intake should be <2,000 mg a day. This equals about 5 g of salt (about 1 tsp). This value decreases depending on the stage of kidney disease.[6] The salt in the diet comes from added salt while cooking and from hidden sources in the form of preservatives, canned products, condiments, meats, baked products containing cooking soda or baking powder, cheese, and other processed food items, so it is best to avoid such foods and based on the level of sodium in the blood to limit sodium intake based on doctors' advice.[11]

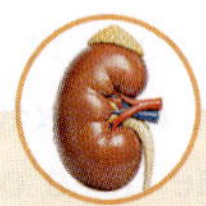

According to KDIGO guidelines, sodium intake should be < 2 g/day or 5 g of table salt.

Potassium

Potassium plays a crucial role in maintaining fluid and electrolyte balance. Normal potassium levels in the blood range from 3.5–5.3 mEq/L. In kidney disease, this level goes up. Kidneys provide the major route for the excretion of potassium. Therefore, in case of any kidney problem, it is necessary to monitor potassium levels in the body and take appropriate action as per the physician's advice.[6,12,13] **Table 1** gives the list of foods containing low, medium, and high potassium levels in food, which can be included or avoided based on potassium levels in the blood.

TABLE 1: The guidelines for low potassium diet.

Low potassium foods	Medium potassium foods	High potassium foods
Vegetables		
Snake gourd, beetroot, radish, bottle gourd, green peas, broad beans, cucumber, knol khol, ridge gourd, and fenugreek leaves	Onion, carrot, bitter gourd, brinjal, cauliflower, French beans, ladies finger, tomato, and cabbage	All dark green leafy vegetables, potato, sweet potato, drumstick mushrooms, coriander, yams, and pumpkin
Fruits		
Pineapple -1 slice papaya- 1 slice, half an apple, half an orange, guava, and half a pear	Pomegranate, watermelon, lime, and grapes	Mango, amla, plums, sapota, sweet lime, musk melon, banana, dried fruits, and dates
Cereals		
• Rice (cooked by straining method) • Semolina	• Rice flakes • Vermicelli	• Rice flakes • Ragi, jowar, and bajra
Nonveg		
Chicken (a small piece) boiled in excess water and drained, and egg white		Liver, fish, mutton, and prawns
		Drink: Cocoa, coffee, tender coconut water, most fruit juices
		Nuts and oilseeds: Almonds, walnuts peanuts, coconut, and cashew nuts

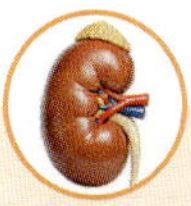

Normal values of potassium in the blood ranges from 3.5–5.3 mEq/L. Potassium intake should be restricted when levels go above the normal.

When potassium levels go very high foods listed in high potassium foods category should be limited or the foods can be leached to remove potassium

Leaching

Method 1

- Wash, peel, and cut vegetables into small pieces
- Soak in warm water for 2–3 hours
- Discard water

Method 2 (Double Boiling Method)

- Peel vegetables and cut them into small pieces
- Boil in large quantity of water
- Discard water

Protein

Amino acids are essential for building structures such as muscles and maintaining key body functions. However, kidneys which are affected will find it cumbersome to remove protein waste from the blood. This causes more stress on organs that do not function well, to begin with. Therefore, protein intake should be restricted. A plant-based diet with animal foods such as egg whites, low-fat milk and milk derivatives, and lean meat will often meet nutrient needs.[9] A plant-based diet is rich in anti-inflammatory nutrients, fiber, and phytochemicals, and has been shown to reduce proteinuria and decrease metabolic acidosis. Dietary patterns that include more plant-based, unprocessed protein are beneficial.[6]

The average Indian diet is usually low in (0.6–0.8 g/kg) protein intake.[13] Restricting common protein-containing items such as pulses without proper dietary advice to meet the daily requirements leads to protein energy malnutrition[14] and muscle wasting. Therefore, an appropriate balance should be maintained. The type of protein that is included in the diet is considered very important. Protein comes from plants and animals, and most people eat both types. Good quality protein intake is vital. Protein levels of 0.6–0.8 g/kg body weight are advised during kidney disease.[15]

Table 2 gives the average protein content of foods in grams. The average Indian diet is usually low in (0.6–0.8 g/kg) protein intake.[14] Restricting common protein-containing items such as pulses without proper dietary advice to meet the daily requirements leads to protein energy malnutrition[15] and muscle wasting. Therefore, a proper balance should be maintained. Exceeding the recommended dietary allowance (RDA) may increase the risk of health complications even for healthy adults allowance (RDA) may increase the risk of health complications even for healthy adults. The required level of protein for CKD patients depends on the stage of the disease based on the level of eGFR function.[7]

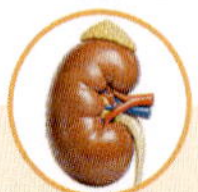

Protein levels of 0.6–0.8 g/kg body weight are advised during kidney disease. A plant-based protein diet is usually recommended.

Metabolic acidosis in CKD improves when low-protein diet (LPD) is followed. Acid is generated during the metabolism of proteins, including sulfur-containing acids. LPD also offers better control of CKD-mineral and bone disorder (MBD). Hyperphosphatemia in CKD can be controlled if an LPD is followed. Incorporating plant proteins in the diet is beneficial in lowering serum phosphorus, as they contain less phosphorus than animal protein.[16] Consequences of dietary protein restriction in advanced CKD include reduced proteinuria. Improves lipid control, reduces uremic toxins and acids, reduces oxidative stress, and improves insulin resistance[17] summarized in **Figure 1**.

But during dialysis, extraprotein may be needed to keep the body functioning properly and prevent muscle loss. The type of protein that is included in the diet is vital. Protein comes from plants and animals, and most people eat both types. Good quality protein intake is vital. Protein levels of 0.6–0.8 g/kg body weight are advised during kidney disease.[16]

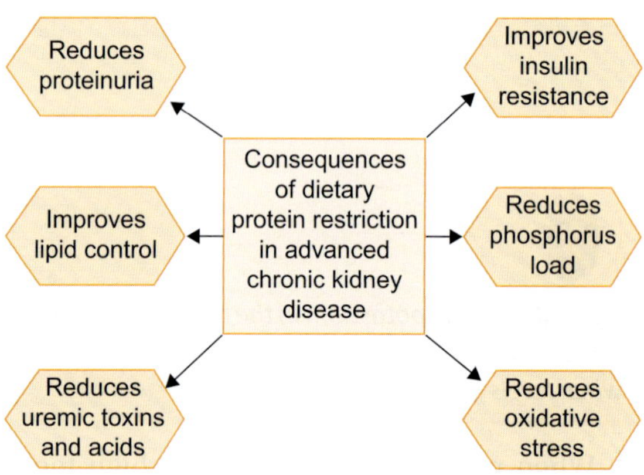

FIG. 1: The consequences of restricting dietary protein in chronic kidney disease.

TABLE 2: Good sources of protein for chronic kidney disease.		
Sources of protein	**Amount of protein to be consumed**	**Protein content present**
Animal protein		
Meat, fish poultry, and seafood	28 g	6–8 g
1 whole egg	50 g	6–8 g
Dairy, milk, and yogurt	250 mL	8–10 g
Plant proteins		
Legumes, dried beans, and nuts seeds	100 g cooked ½ cup	7–10 g
Whole grains and cereals	100 g cooked ½ cup	3–6 g
Starchy vegetables	100 g	2–4 g

In a study by Viswanathan et al., the prevalence of diabetic nephropathy was assessed among vegetarians and nonvegetarians; protein consumption was higher among nonvegetarians than vegetarians. However, there was a difference in microalbuminuria and macroproteinuria between the groups. It was concluded that protein restriction was required only among nonvegetarians with nephropathy, which can be done by limiting the intake of animal protein.

Another prominent study was conducted by Viswanathan et al. to assess the levels of serum albumin among South Indian patients with type 2 diabetes and CKD and to determine the extent of protein restriction that was required for people living with CKD. It was concluded that the serum albumin levels were significantly lower among people with heavy proteinuria. A drastic reduction in protein intake is not advisable among South Indians with diabetic kidney disease unless the patient has severe uremia.

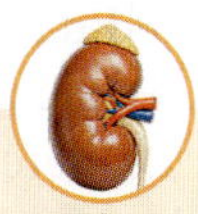

Protein restriction was required only among nonvegetarians with nephropathy which can be done by limiting the intake of animal protein. A drastic reduction in protein intake is not advisable among South Indians with diabetic kidney disease unless the patient has severe uremia.

Phosphorus

Phosphorus is a mineral that helps form bones and teeth and plays other important roles in the body. But in CKD, the kidneys are unable to remove excess phosphorus from the blood. Many foods have added phosphorus, or phosphate additives, that the body absorbs well. This can cause problems and is to be avoided.[17]

Foods that often contain phosphate additives include:

- Colas and other bottled beverages
- Baked goods
- Canned foods
- Fast food

Foods that contain phosphorus are:

- Cheese
- Cocoa
- Dried beans
- Ice cream

PROTEIN INTAKE AND PHOSPHORUS

Proteins are rich in phosphorus. Proteins contain about 1.3–1.5% phosphorus. 30–70% is absorbed. Thus, an intake of 100 g of protein a day results in a very high absorption of phosphorus daily.[17] Thus, there are two good reasons to restrict protein intake in chronic renal disease. A reduction in the intake of protein helps to slow kidney disease progression. Secondly, phosphorus intake is also reduced.

Nutritional Assessment in Low-protein Diet

The requirement of protein and energy differs under various clinical conditions and stages of disease, and actual intake is affected by the individual's condition. Therefore, the intake should be evaluated once every 2 or 3 months. Dietary intake can be assessed with dietary recalls, interviews, or a food frequency questionnaire. Physical measurements such as body weight and anthropometrics, or biochemical parameters, can be used and muscle wasting can be evaluated. Guidelines for healthy food choices that can be adopted in routine practice is given in **Box 1**.

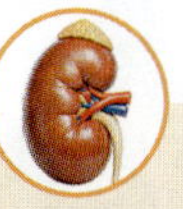

Anthropometric measurements and dietary recall with food frequency can be used to evaluate the nutritional status.

WATER INTAKE

The kidneys are the primary organ of water balance. Water intake should be restricted in the later stages of kidney disease. Drinking too much water may cause fluid to accumulate in the body because of decreased urine output. Increased fluid in the body puts excess pressure on the heart and lungs.[18,19]

Besides water and other drinks, the fluids used in cooking should also be taken into account, i.e., curries, rasam, buttermilk, etc.

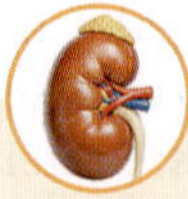

Intake of water quantity depends on the stage of CKD and has to be prescribed by the nephrologist.

The portion size that can be taken along with the type of foods to be included in CKD is given **Figures 2A and B**.

Table 3 shows the exact amount of food to be taken in the diet depends on the age and the stage of CKD.

Table 3 gives a sample menu for CKD. It includes the portion size of the food listed including water. The menu planned contains 48 g of protein. Protein and water intake is as per the advice of the nephrologist. A summary has been provided for better comprehension of nutritional recommendations in people with CKD in **Figure 3**.

The guidelines for dietary management of CKD are brought out clearly in the KDIGO guidelines as well as in various published data. However, research carried out in the MV Hospital for Diabetes and Prof M Viswanathan Diabetes Research Centre shows the actual intake of salt and other macronutrient consumption in patients with CKD. The urinary sodium excretion and dietary salt intake of type 2 diabetes mellitus group

---

BOX 1: The guidelines for healthy foods that can be followed for people with CKD.

Many healthy foods can be used:
- Vegetables such as cabbage, red bell peppers, cauliflower, and onions can be used
- Fruits—apples
- Lean meat, skinless poultry, eggs, and fish are healthy choices
- Fresh or dried herbs, spices, garlic, and olive oil can be used to add flavor in the diet
- Whole grains—barley, wheat, rice, etc., can be used
- Choose fresh foods and cook from scratch to avoid added ingredients
- Fast food and packaged foods are usually high in sodium and hence preferable to avoid such foods
- Keep protein serving sizes small A serving size of protein is 2–3 ounces of chicken, fish, or meat
- Read food labels
- Watch serving sizes
- Choose fresh over packaged foods
- Check manufacture and expiry dates

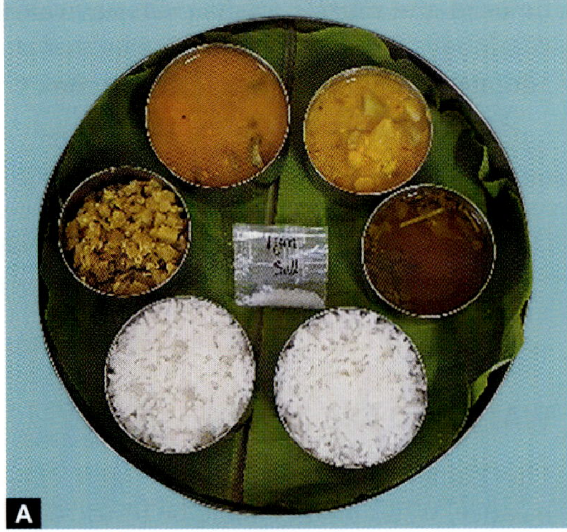

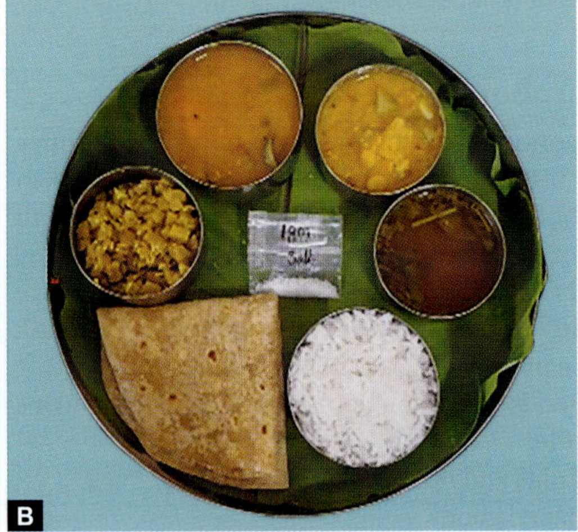

FIGS. 2A AND B: A picture of sample diet that can be given for people with chronic kidney disease.

TABLE 3: Sample menu for chronic kidney disease—1,400 Kcal.	
Meals	*Food items*
Early morning (6:00–6:30 AM)	Skim milk—100 mL
Breakfast (8:00–8:30 AM) Choose any one combination	• Idly/chapathi/wheat rava upma—3 nos/11/2 Cup • Dhal/onion chutney—1 cup/1/2 cup
Midmorning (10:00–11:00 AM) Choose any one	Fruits as per low potassium chart/skim milk
Lunch (1:00–2:00 PM) Choose any one combination	• Rice/chapathi—2 cup/3 nos • Dhal/nonveg (fish/chicken/egg white 50 g)—1/2 cup • Vegetable gravy/vegetable poriyal (low potassium)—1 cup • Skim milk curd—1/2 cup
Evening time (4:30 PM)	• Skim milk/buttermilk—100 mL • Red rice flakes khichdi/sabudana khichdi—1/2 cup
6:30 PM	Dhal soup—100 mL/buttermilk—100 mL
Dinner (8:00–8:30 PM)	• Idli/chapathi/wheat rava upma—3 nos/11/2 cup • Tomato chutney/onion chutney—1/2 cup
Bed-time (9:30–10:30 PM) Choose any one	Resource renal—100 mL

Calories: 1,485
Carbohydrates: 257 g (69%)
Protein: 48 g (13%)
Fat: 30 g (18%)
Note: Suggested resource renal supplement
Dilution: Mix two scoops in 100 mL of warm water to be taken at bedtime
Salt: As per doctors advice
Fluids: As per doctors advice

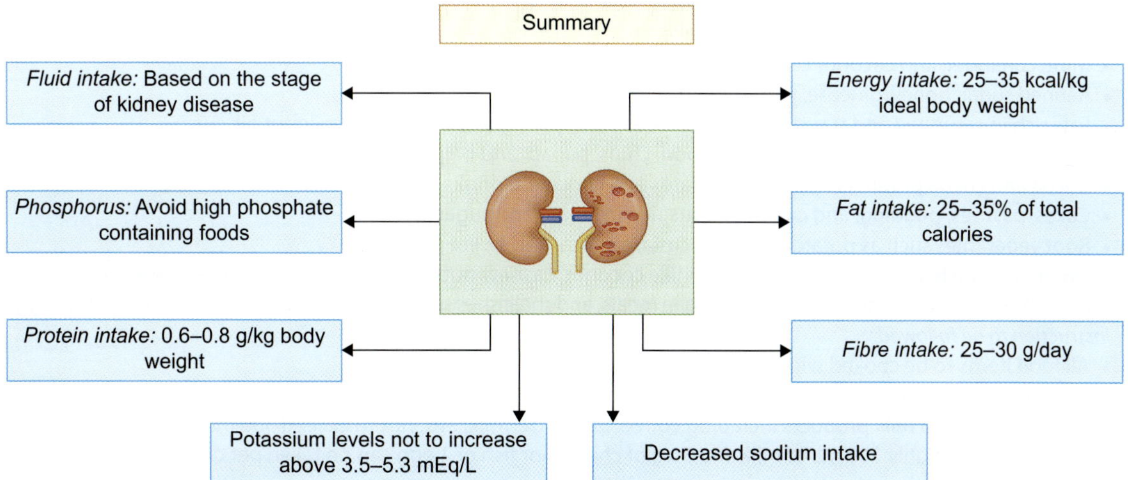

FIG. 3: Diet precautions and restrictions during chronic kidney disease.

subjects were found to be 250.8 ± 114 mmol/24 h and 14.5 ± 6 g/day, respectively. These values are way above the recommended values for CKD. The study showed that in the CKD group, only 22% were consuming <6 g of salt/day. The rest 30%, 36%, and 12% were consuming 6–12 g, 12–18 g and >18 g of the salt/day, respectively. It was also noted that the calorie consumption was less than the recommended values.[20]

CONCLUSION

The kidney helps in maintaining the normal balance of nutrients in the body. Disease prevents this normal balance. Therefore, diet is important for people with CKD because it helps maintain a healthy balance of minerals and salts in the body, which complements the kidneys' role in maintaining balance. Undernutrition is very common in CKD due to decreased intake. It is usually characterized by low energy intake of <25 kcal/kg, due to poor appetite. The KDIGO guidelines 2024 recommend an energy intake of 25–35 kcal/kg ideal body weight in CKD. Carbohydrate consumption must be sufficient to meet energy needs, especially when proteins are restricted. Complex carbohydrates should be used with pulses or milk. A daily fiber intake of 25–30 g/day is recommended. Adequate vitamins and minerals, micronutrients, should be adequate in the diet as per the requirement. Protein, sodium, potassium, and phosphorus water should be restricted based on the stage of CKD.

Box 2 gives us a summary of the foods to be avoided and healthy practices to be followed in people with CKD.

BOX 2: Summary of the foods to be avoided and healthy practices.

In a nutshell

Foods avoided:
- Salt, preserved chutneys, papads, and pickles
- Dry fish, salted preserved meat, bacon, ham, and sausages
- Baking powder, soda bicarbonate, and ajinomoto (monosodium glutamate)
- Canned food items (vegetables, meats, fish, etc.)
- Cheese and salted butter
- Salted snacks such as salted biscuits, nuts, popcorn, chips, and other savory items
- Commercial salad dressing, sauces and ketchups, and instant soups
- Raw vegetables, vegetable salads, and vegetable soup
- Fruit juice, squash, and tender coconut water
- Aerated drinks such as Fanta, Pepsi and Coke, etc.
- Mint, coriander, and coconut chutney
- Refined sugar, honey, glucose, jaggery, jam, and jellies
- Fats rich in saturated and transfatty acids such as vanaspati, ghee, butter, and coconut oil
- Deep fried foods such as samosa, vada, poori, chips, papad, and bajji
- Cocoa and cocoa products such as chocolates and chocolate drinks
- Cakes, pastries, pudding, and cream biscuits rich in cream and sugar
- Root vegetables such as potato, yam, colocasia, tapioca, and sweet potato
- Dried fruits such as dates, raisins, and nuts like coconut, cashew nuts, groundnuts, almonds, and walnuts
- Fatty meats such as mutton, ham, bacon, organ meats, and shellfishes such as crab, prawn, and shrimp and yolk of egg

Instruction to be followed:
- All food items to be cooked without salt and no extra salt to be added
- All vegetables to be cooked well before consumption
- Intake of milk and milk products including coffee, tea, buttermilk, etc., not to exceed 300 mL/day
- If nonvegetarian only 200 mL of milk and 50 g of chicken or fish or 1 egg can be taken per day

A word of caution about salt substitutes:
- Salt substitutes contain potassium and should be used with caution. Consult your physician before using salt substitutes

TAKE HOME MESSAGES

- The most important aspect is the maintenance of glycated hemoglobin (HbA1c) values below 7.0% in people with diabetes.
- It is imperative to maintain diet control and portion size.
- A healthy exercise pattern to maintain blood sugar levels should be followed.
- The patient should also follow the doctor's advice on protein intake, sodium, and potassium fluid intake.

REFERENCES

1. Webster AC, Nagler EV, Morton RL, Masson P. Chronic kidney disease. Lancet. 2017;389:1238-52.
2. GBD Chronic Kidney Disease Collaboration. Global, regional, and national burden of chronic kidney disease, 1990–2017: a systematic analysis for the Global Burden of Disease Study 2017. Lancet. 2020;395:709-33.
3. Xie Y, Bowe B, Mokdad AH, Xian H, Yan Y, Li T, et al. Analysis of the Global Burden of Disease study highlights the global, regional, and national trends of chronic kidney disease epidemiology from 1990 to 2016. Kidney Int. 2018;94:567-81.
4. Govindan S, Iyengar A, Mohanasundaram S, Priyamvada PS. Nutrition Compass: Guiding Patients with Chronic Kidney Disease Across Ages 2025. Indian J Nephrol. 2025;35(2):187-97.
5. Sinha A, Prasad N. How to Give Dietary Advice to Patients with Kidney Disease? Indian J Nephrol. 2025;35(2):178-86.
6. Kidney Disease: Improving Global Outcomes (KDIGO) CKD Work Group. KDIGO 2024 Clinical Practice Guideline for the Evaluation and Management of Chronic Kidney Disease. Kidney Int. 2024;105(4S):S117-314.
7. Naber T, Purohit S. Chronic kidney disease: Role of diet for a reduction in the severity of the disease. Nutrients. 2021;13:3277.
8. MacLaughlin HL, Friedman AN, Ikizler TA. Nutrition in kidney disease: Core curriculum 2022. Am J Kidney Dis. 2022;79:437-49.
9. Hayes K. Dietary fat and heart health: In search of the ideal fat. Asia Pac J Clin Nutr 2002;11Suppl 7:S394-400.
10. Sinnakirouchenan R, Kotchen TA. Role of sodium restriction and diuretic therapy for "resistant" hypertension in chronic kidney disease. Semin Nephrol. 2014;34:514-9.
11. Cobb M, Pacitti D. The Importance of Sodium Restrictions in Chronic Kidney Disease patient education. J Ren Nutr. 2018;28(5):e37-40.
12. Clegg DJ, Headley SA, Germain MJ. Impact of Dietary Potassium Restrictions in CKD on Clinical Outcomes: Benefits of a Plant-Based Diet Kidney Med. 2020;2(4):476-87.
13. De Nicola L, Garofalo C, Borrelli S, Minutolo R. Recommendations on nutritional intake of potassium in CKD: it's now time to be more flexible! Kidney Int. 2022;102(4):700-3.
14. Shah BV, Patel ZM. Role of low protein diet in management of different stages of chronic kidney disease - practical aspects. BMC Nephrol. 2016;17:156.
15. Obi Y, Qader H, Kovesdy CP, Kalantar-Zadeh K. Latest consensus and update on protein-energy wasting in chronic kidney disease. Curr Opin Clin Nutr Metab Care. 2015;18:254-6.
16. Ko GJ, Obi Y, Tortorici AR, Kalantar-Zadeh K. Dietary Protein Intake and Chronic Kidney Disease. Curr Opin Clin Nutr Metab Care. 2017;20(1):77-85.
17. González-Parra E, Gracia-Iguacel C, Egido J, Ortiz A. Phosphorus and Nutrition in Chronic Kidney Disease Int J Nephrol. 2012;2012:597605.
18. Wagner S, Merkling T, Metzger M, Bankir L, Laville M, Frimat L, et al; CKD-REIN study group, Water intake and progression of chronic kidney disease: the CKD-REIN cohort study. Nephrol Dial Transplant. 2022;37(4):730-9.
19. Choi HY, Park HC, Ha SK. High Water Intake and Progression of Chronic Kidney Diseases. Electrolyte Blood Press. 2015;13(2):46-51.
20. Smina TP, Kumpatla S, Viswanathan V. Higher dietary salt and inappropriate proportion of macronutrients consumption among people with diabetes and other co morbid conditions in South India: Estimation of salt intake with a formula. Diabetes Metab Syndr. 2019;13(5):2863-8.

Key Research Takeaway

Diabetes & Metabolic Syndrome: Clinical Research & Reviews 13 (2019) 2863–2868

Contents lists available at ScienceDirect

Diabetes & Metabolic Syndrome: Clinical Research & Reviews

journal homepage: www.elsevier.com/locate/dsx

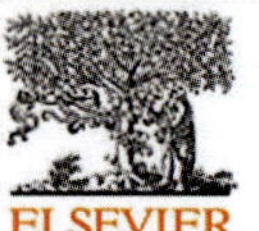

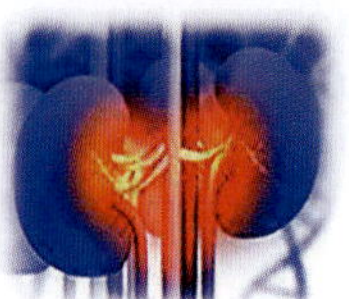

Original Article

Higher dietary salt and inappropriate proportion of macronutrients consumption among people with diabetes and other co morbid conditions in South India: Estimation of salt intake with a formula

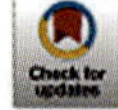

T.P. Smina, Satyavani Kumpatla, Vijay Viswanathan[*]

M.V. Hospital for Diabetes and Prof. M. Viswanathan Diabetes Research Centre, WHO Collaborating Centre for Research, Education, Training in Diabetes, IDF Centre for Excellence in Diabetes Care, No 4, West Madha Church Street, Royapuram, Chennai, 600 013, India

ARTICLE INFO

Article history:
Received 10 July 2019
Accepted 29 July 2019

Keywords:
Urinary sodium excretion
Dietary sodium
Dietary protein
Type 2 diabetes
Renal dysfunction

ABSTRACT

Aim: The present study analysed the regular salt and macronutrients consumption of South Indian population with diabetes, hypertension and renal dysfunction.

Methods: The cross sectional study was performed among 200 subjects, divided into four different groups consisted of control, subjects with type 2 diabetes (T2DM) without any other complications, T2DM subjects with chronic kidney disease (CKD) and T2DM subjects with hypertension (HTN). The dietary salt intake was estimated from 24-h urinary sodium excretion and the amount of macronutrients was calculated using 24-h dietary recall method.

Results: Out of 200 study subjects, only 28 (14%) were consuming salt as per the recommended levels by WHO (i.e., 5–6 g/day). Thirty-eight (19%) subjects were consuming more than 18 g of salt per day, 67 (33.5%) were consuming 12–18 g of salt per day and another 67 (33.5%) were found to be consuming salt in a range of 6–12 g/day. Calorie contribution from the carbohydrates was significantly high compared to the calories from the proteins. Fat consumption and its corresponding energy contribution were also high among HTN group subjects.

Conclusion: Observations of the study point out to the requirement of nationwide intensive and persistent efforts to enhance the public awareness on salt reduction.

© 2019 Published by Elsevier Ltd on behalf of Diabetes India.

* Corresponding author. M.V. Hospital for Diabetes and Prof. M. Viswanathan Diabetes Research Centre, Royapuram, Chennai, 600 013, India. E-mail address: drvijay@mvdiabetes.com (V. Viswanathan).

ARTICLE

Serum albumin levels in different stages of type 2 diabetic nephropathy patients

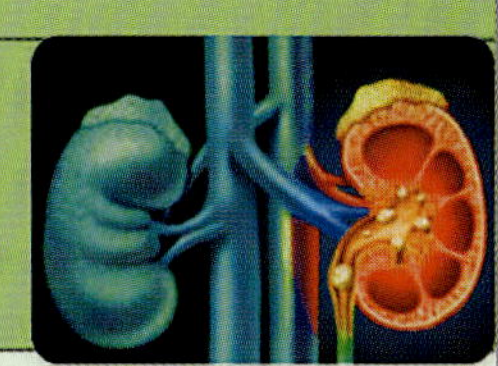

V Viswanathan, C Snehalatha, R Kumutha, M Jayaraman, A Ramachandran
Diabetes Research Centre, Chennai - India.

Abstract

Aim: To study the serum albumin concentration in South Indian type 2 diabetic patients with nephropathy to decide regarding the extent of protein restriction required in these patients.

Research design and methods: Type 2 diabetic patients (n=139) admitted for review in M.V. Hospital for Diabetes, Chennai consisting of 49 patients with normoalbuminuria (< 20 mg of albumin / min), 52 patients with macroalbuminuria (> 200 mg of albumin / min and proteinuria < 3.5 gm /day) and 38 patients with nephrotic syndrome (proteinuria > 3.5 gm /day) were studied. Blood pressure, anthropometry, fasting and post-prandial plasma glucose, HbA1c, total serum albumin, lipid profile, urea and creatinine were measured.

Results: Serum albumin level was significantly lower in the nephrotic syndrome group of patients ($p < 0.05$) when compared with the macroalbuminuric and normoalbuminuric group of patients. Patients with end-stage renal disease, severe renal failure and moderate renal failure showed lower serum albumin concentrations compared with patients having early renal insufficiency and early renal damage. Serum albumin level decreased significantly in patients with reduced creatinine clearance. Serum albumin showed a significant positive association with creatinine clearance ($p < 0.03$), negative association with macroalbuminuria ($p < 0.0001$) and nephrotic proteinuria ($p < 0.0001$) among the independent variables included in the multiple linear regression analysis.

Conclusion: Serum albumin was significantly lower in patients with heavy proteinuria. Unless there is severe ureamia, drastic reduction in protein intake in south Indian diabetic patients with nephropathy may not be advisable.

Indian J Nephrol 2004;14: 89-92

ARTICLE   Indian J Nephrol 2002;12: 73-76 7 3

Prevalence of albuminuria among vegetarian and non-vegetarian south Indian diabetic patients

V Viswanathan, C Snehalatha, MP Varadharani, BM Nair, M Jayaraman, A Ramachandran
Diabetes Research Centre, Chennai - India.

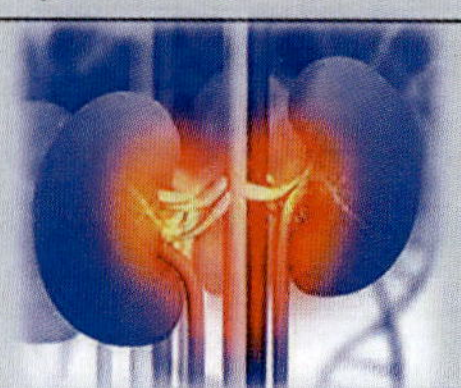

Abstract

Aim: To determine the prevalence of diabetic nephropathy among vegetarians and non- vegetarians.

Patients and methods: Type 2 diabetic subjects (n=405) from the Diabetes Research Centre & M.V. Hospital for Diabetes, Chennai consisting of vegetarians (group 1, n=155) and non-vegetarians (group 2, n=250) were studied. Blood pressure, anthropometry, fasting and post-prandial plasma glucose, HbA1C, urea, creatinine were measured. Protein intake was calculated by estimating 24 hour urinary nitrogen. Dietary recall method was used to assess the diet pattern. Subjects were classified as having normoalbuminuria (<20 µg / min), microalbuminuria (MAU) (20-200 µg /min) and clinical (macro) proteinuria (total proteinuria > 500 mg/day) based on 24 hour albumin excretion.

Results: Group 1 and Group 2 were matched for duration of diabetes. The prevalence of nephropathy (total protein >500 mg/day with diabetic retinopathy) was 11.6% (n=18) in group 1 and 13.6% (n=34) in group 2. Mean albuminuria (mg albumin/mg creatinine) in group 1 was 67.5+38.6 and in group 2, 72.5+45.9. Mean protein intake was significantly higher in non-vegetarians but was within the recommended limits. Multiple logistic regression analysis showed that only hypertension and duration of diabetes were associated with MAU and macro proteinuria; amount of protein intake or type of protein
did not show correlation.

Conclusions: Protein content of non-vegetarian diet was higher compared to the vegetarian diet. However, prevalence of MAU and macro proteinuria did not vary in these groups. Protein restriction may be required only in the non-vegetarians with nephropathy, and can be done by reducing the intake of animal protein.

9

Comprehensive Care for People Living with Diabetic Kidney Disease

Vijay Viswanathan, Reshma Mirshad

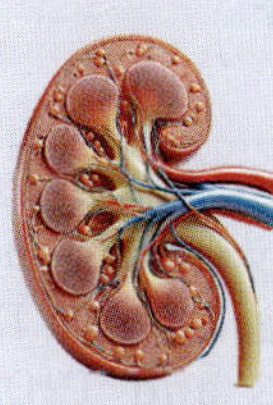

> ➢ Diagnosis and staging of diabetic kidney disease
> ➢ Comprehensive care for diabetic kidney disease
> ➢ Structured education program
> ➢ Shared decision-making
> ➢ Multidisciplinary care team
> ➢ Lifestyle modification
> ➢ Glycemic control
> ➢ Blood pressure management
> ➢ Lipid management
> ➢ Antiplatelet therapy
> ➢ CKD-mineral and bone disorder

Abstract

Diabetic kidney disease (DKD) is a serious microvascular complication of diabetes, accounting for a significant proportion of chronic kidney disease (CKD) and end-stage renal disease (ESRD) cases worldwide. Affecting nearly half of individuals with diabetes, DKD is linked to increased cardiovascular morbidity, premature mortality, and substantial healthcare costs. Early identification through routine screening for albuminuria and estimated glomerular filtration rate (eGFR) is essential for timely risk stratification and therapeutic intervention. Individualized glycemic targets offer renal and cardiovascular benefits, especially with novel antidiabetic agents such as sodium-glucose cotransporter-2 (SGLT2) inhibitors and glucagon-like peptide-1 (GLP-1) receptor agonists. Blood pressure control using renin–angiotensin–aldosterone system (RAAS) inhibitors is crucial for reducing proteinuria and slowing renal decline, while statins help mitigate cardiovascular risk. Structured diabetes self-management education and support (DSMES) programs, along with psychological support, help address the high prevalence of depression and anxiety in this population. A team-based approach comprising primary care physicians, endocrinologists, nephrologists, diabetes educators, dietitians, pharmacists, and social workers is fundamental to delivering personalized and coordinated care. This chapter deals with the goals of comprehensive care, which not only slows disease progression and reduces complications but also improves the quality of life and survival in people living with DKD.

Keywords: Diabetic kidney disease, comprehensive care, multidisciplinary approach, chronic kidney disease.

INTRODUCTION

Diabetic kidney disease (DKD) is a significant microvascular complication, affecting approximately half of the individuals with type 2 diabetes (T2D) and one-third of those with type 1 diabetes.[1] It is the leading cause of end-stage renal disease (ESRD), with about 700 million people affected.[2] Global epidemiological studies have reported varying prevalence rates of DKD. Diabetes-related ESRD incidence increased from 22.1 to 31.3% between 2000 and 2015, whereas its prevalence climbed continuously from 19.0 to 29.7%.[3] A cross-sectional study involving 15,856 patients with diabetes in China demonstrated a 38.8% prevalence of chronic kidney disease (CKD). In contrast, studies from India reported DKD prevalence rates of 34.4% and 62.3% in different multicenter cohorts.[4] DKD imposes a higher economic burden than people without complications (Median ₹12,664 vs. ₹3214).[5] The expense gradually increases as the disease progresses to advanced stages of DKD.[6]

Early diagnosis of DKD is essential by monitoring the albumin-to-creatinine ratio (ACR) values $\geq$ 30 mg/g and/or when the estimated glomerular filtration rate (eGFR) is <60 mL/min/1.73 m^2 in individuals with diabetes. The pathophysiology of DKD involves three major pathways—(1) hemodynamic, (2) metabolic, and (3) inflammatory. Diabetes can lead to hyperfiltration, which causes alterations in metabolism, hormones, hemodynamics, inflammation, and epigenetics, causing oxidative stress and hypoxia, leading to podocyte damage, mitochondrial distress, glomerulosclerosis, fibrosis, and tissue death. The risk factors of DKD are increased albuminuria, hyperglycemia, hypertension, dyslipidemia, and obesity, older age, family history of kidney disease, cardiovascular disease (CVD), smoking and other high-risk comorbidities, environmental exposure, or genetic factors.[4]

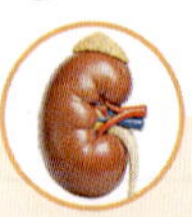

Comprehensive care for DKD is essential to managing multimorbidity, slowing the progression to end-stage kidney disease (ESKD), reducing premature mortality, and improving quality of life.

DIAGNOSIS AND STAGING OF DIABETIC KIDNEY DISEASE

Kidney Disease: Improving Global Outcomes (KDIGO) stated that persons with hypertension, diabetes, or CVD should be screened for CKD every 5 years in type 1 diabetes and T2D, irrespective of the duration. Screening is done based on assessing urinary albumin-creatinine ratio (UACR) to detect albuminuria, serum creatinine, and cystatin C to estimated GFR.[7]

There are few novel biomarkers for the early diagnosis of DKD, as timely diagnosis and appropriate interventions are the best way to approach these conditions. Evidence suggests elevated levels of galectin-3, growth differentiation factor 15, neutrophil gelatinase-associated lipocalin (NGAL), fibroblast growth factor-23 (FGF23), platelet-derived growth factor (PDGF), and kidney injury molecule-1 (KIM-1) show early signs of kidney damage.[8] The stages of DKD is explained in **Table 1**.[9]

TABLE 1: The stages of DKD.		
Stages	**Kidney function**	**eGFR/UAER**
1	Hyperfunction and hypertrophy	Microalbuminuria, eGFR $\geq$ 90 mL/min/1.73 m^2
2	Glomerular lesions without clinical disease	Microalbuminuria, eGFR 60–89 mL/min/1.73 m^2
3	Incipient DKD	UAER—30–299 mg/24 h, eGFR 30–59 mL/min/1.73 m^2
4	Overt DKD	UAER $\geq$ 300 mg/24 h, eGFR 15–29 mL/min/1.73 m^2
5	ESRD	eGFR < 15 mL/min/1.73 m^2

(DKD: diabetic kidney disease; ESRD: end-stage renal disease; eGFR: estimated glomerular filtration; UAER: urine albumin excretion rate)

Imaging techniques such as ultrasound, magnetic resonance imaging (MRI), computed tomography (CT), and renal scintigraphy provide valuable information on kidney size, volume, structure, function, metabolism, perfusion, oxygenation, and blood flow.[10]

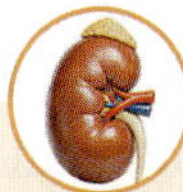

Screening is done based on assessing UACR to detect albuminuria, serum creatinine, and cystatin C to estimate eGFR.

COMPREHENSIVE CARE FOR DIABETIC KIDNEY DISEASE

The primary goal of comprehensive care, as per both the guidelines [American Diabetes Association (ADA) and KDIGO], is to treat the patients as a whole by incorporating multidisciplinary management, such as diet, lifestyle management, and structured education, to obtain primary and secondary prevention of diabetes-related complications [including CKD, atherosclerotic cardiovascular disease (ASCVD), and heart failure (HF)] and pharmacological therapy to improve risk factors **(Fig. 1)**.[11]

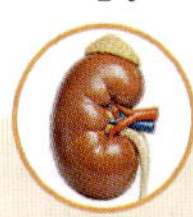

Treat patients as a whole by incorporating multidisci-plinary management.

STRUCTURED EDUCATION PROGRAM

To minimize the progression of kidney disease and promote glycemic control, the patient's self-care management or the ability to follow appropriate lifestyle modifications, medicine, and self-monitoring is highly dependent on them. Structured education and behavioral counseling are necessary to make the patient adhere to the complex regimens. Understanding DKD aids patients in comprehending their condition

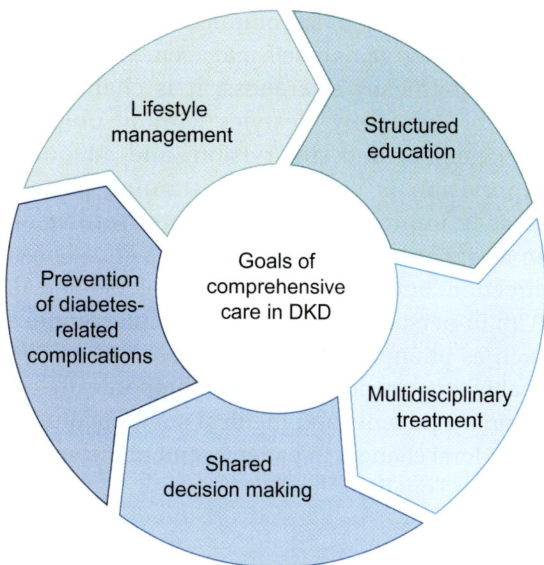

FIG. 1: Goals of comprehensive care in diabetic kidney disease (DKD).[12]

and the significance of preventative measures for hyperglycemia, hypertension, and DKD progression. For many years, much research has been conducted on the effectiveness of educational programs for people with diabetes. Research indicates that educational programs designed to enhance blood pressure (BP) regulation or improve dietary habits are beneficial for DKD.[12]

Diabetes self-management education and support (DSMES) services and behavioral intervention are thought to be essential for managing and preventing DKD as well as other diabetes-related complications. A study with African Americans' showed a significant improvement in eGFR at 36 months due to telephone educational sessions. Frequent phone calls and case management by researchers led to a lower rate of ESRD in the intervention group (13%) compared to the nonintervention group (28%) among patients who needed close monitoring in the Fogelfeld et al. trial.[13]

Patients were assessed by phone or email if there was a more than one-month gap between outpatient appointments. The findings demonstrated gains in self-management practices and self-efficacy awareness. It is challenging to alter unhealthy lifestyles without ongoing management and supervision, and adequate supervision is crucial to sustaining patient lifestyle improvements. Therefore, setting up an all-inclusive program that offers knowledge, direction, and ongoing assistance is beneficial. With in-person interviews, remote interventions such as phone calls, videophones, and mobile health apps provide continuous support with less strain on patients and medical staff, encourage behavioral changes in patients, and may improve eGFR and quality of life.[14]

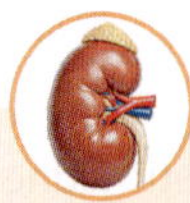

A well-structured education and behavioral counseling are necessary to make the patient adhere to the complex regimens.

SHARED DECISION-MAKING

Patients or surrogates and their practitioners are expected to use shared decision-making (SDM), considering medical evidence and the patient's values and preferences to make a medical decision. Patients on dialysis frequently express feelings that they were only passive participants in the choice to begin dialysis, which points to more chances to improve the use of SDM in kidney disease decision-making. Sensitive, culturally and equity-informed communication, and successful collaboration between the patient or surrogate and the doctor are the hallmarks of SDM. The patient's expertise in their values and priorities is elicited, and the clinician's medical expertise is shared.

Van der Horst found that several decisions about planning, medication adjustments, lifestyle modifications, treatment objectives, and diagnostic tests are commonly made during routine CKD checkups. Approximately, one-third of the patients favored a SDM role for all

of these decision subjects, another third favored leaving the decision primarily to the clinician, and the other third left the decision entirely up to the clinician. Except for some lifestyle modification options, patients rarely made the decision (mostly) alone. There is evidence that SDM improves patients' comprehension of their condition and their level of satisfaction, reduces anxiety, improves treatment compliance, and increases the quality of life with the choices they make between dialysis, conservative kidney management, and transplant.[15,16]

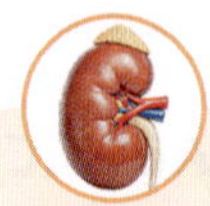

To reach a medical decision, SDM between patients and their practitioners is essential, as it considers medical evidence and patients' values and preferences.

MULTIDISCIPLINARY CARE TEAM

Diabetes is a chronic, long-term condition that can progress into various complications over time, depending on different contexts, demographics, and populations. Primary care physicians serve as coordinators and conduits for additional services and support, requiring a broad range of experience to facilitate person-centered care. To provide continuous, accessible, consistent, comprehensive, and effective care centered on each patient's priorities, needs, and goals, an interdisciplinary team comprises primary care and specialty clinicians, diabetologists, dietitians, podiatrists, and community-based providers.

To guarantee the best possible kidney health, referrals to specialists such as podiatry, sleep medicine, nephrology, cardiology, and mental health should be considered when more direction or assistance is required. Importantly, robust primary care, as outlined in the Chronic Care Model, is essential to reducing care fragmentation and ensuring that treatments are person-centered, non-conflicting, do not increase treatment burden, and do not surpass individuals' capacity for self-management because people with diabetes frequently have multiple comorbidities and thus require the care of various specialists.[11]

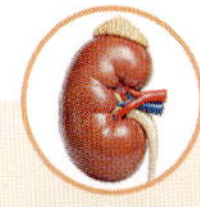

An interdisciplinary team comprising primary care and specialty clinicians, including diabetologists, dietitians, nephrologists, podiatrists, and community-based providers are required to treat multiple comorbidities.

LIFESTYLE MODIFICATION

A registered dietitian nutritionist should be integrated for optimal and individual-tailored nutrition management in DKD patients. Patients with DKD should include a balanced diet rich in vegetables, fruits, whole grains, fiber, legumes, plant-based proteins, unsaturated fats, nuts, low in refined carbohydrates, processed foods, and sweetened beverages. The recommended sodium intake, ADA (1,500 to < 2,000 mg/day), and KDIGO (<2,000 mg/day), helps in controlling BP and reducing cardiovascular risk in patients with DKD. The protein intake for DKD patients was recommended to be 0.8 g/kg/day to improve kidney and other health conditions. In patients undergoing dialysis, particularly peritoneal dialysis, it causes a catabolic response and is malnourished. Hence, a higher protein intake of 1.0–1.2 g/kg/day is advised. When providing dietary options to patients and their families, healthcare clinicians should consider comorbidities, expenses, cultural differences, food intolerances, disparities in food supplies, and cooking skills.

Body mass index (BMI) > 30 kg/m^2 indicates obesity, which is a risk factor for both CVD and the progression of renal disease. A BMI of >27.5 kg/m^2 raises the likelihood of negative consequences among Asian populations. According to pooled data from 40 nations, including almost 5.5 million adults, a higher BMI, waist circumference, and waist-to-height ratio appear to be independent

risk factors for renal function decline and death in those with normal or lowered levels of eGFR.

The physical activity recommendation for patients with DKD is moderate to intense activity with a cumulative duration of at least 150 min/week, depending on the cardiovascular status or physical tolerance. For the older age group, baseline and routine physical activity should be considered before making recommendations on the physical activity monitor for comorbid conditions (such as peripheral neuropathy and osteoarthritis). Smoking cessation is advised as it can reduce the risk of premature mortality from CVD, respiratory problems, or cancer.[11,17]

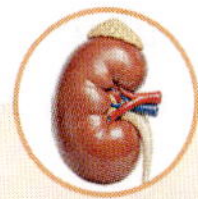

Patients with DKD should undergo lifestyle modifications, including a balanced diet, sodium intake (<2,000 mg/day), protein intake (0.8 g/kg/day), and physical activity at least 150 min/week.

GLYCEMIC CONTROL

Strict glycemic control can help people with diabetes to delay the onset and progression of DKD. A 6.5-year follow-up study, the Diabetes Control and Complications Trial (DCCT), showed that patients under intensive glycemic control had a marked decrease in the progression of DKD into moderate and severe albuminuria compared to standard care.[18,19] Viswanathan et al. showed that insulin resistance increases significantly with decline in renal function.[20] In individuals with diabetes with varying degrees of renal diseases, glycated albumin can be utilized as a marker to assess short-term glycemic state.[21]

According to two standard guidelines, the ADA (2018) recommended that the A1c target range be <7–8%, KDIGO recommends a target of <6.5% to <8.0% for patients with diabetes and CKD. A1c targets in this range have been linked to decreased risk of CKD progression and will benefit microvascular endpoints, cardiovascular outcomes, and survival. However, it is associated with several adverse effects, including an increased risk of hypoglycemia, polypharmacy, and a higher mortality rate. Hence, personalized glycemic control tailored to individual patient characteristics is essential.[22]

Among long-term type 1 and T2D, glycated hemoglobin (HbA1c) is the ideal measurement to monitor blood glucose levels. Glycemic assessment using HbA1c is performed twice a year for stable T2D patients fulfilling treatment goals and once a quarter for patients under close supervision whose therapy has changed or whose treatment goals are not met. For daily glucose monitoring, continuous glucose monitoring (CGM) and self-monitoring of blood glucose (SMBG) are used to prevent hypoglycemia and improve glycemic control.[17]

There is a list of glucose-lowering drugs with renoprotective action—metformin, dipeptidyl peptidase 4 (DPP-4) inhibitors, glucagon-like peptide-1 receptor agonists (GLP-1 RA), thiazolidinediones, and sodium-glucose cotransporter-2 (SGLT2) inhibitors. The GLP-1 RA and SGLT2 inhibitors are considered the first choice to combine with metformin in people with diabetes, cardiovascular risk, and DKD.[23]

For most patients with T2D and CKD, the ADA 2022 Standards of Care and the KDIGO 2022 guideline advise early introduction of metformin plus an SGLT2 inhibitor, which can reduce the risk of developing diabetes complications. Then, depending on patient-specific factors, additional glucose-lowering medications (GLP-1 RA is preferred) can be administered as necessary to achieve the glycemic target. Metformin is recommended for patients with DKD and eGFR $\geq$ 30 mL/min/1.73 m^2. Adjust the metformin dose depending on the eGFR drops below 60 mL/min/1.73 m^2. SGLT2 inhibitor can be added when eGFR $\geq$ 20 mL/min/1.7 m^2 to prioritize organ protection independent of baseline HbA1c and glycemic targets. A long-acting GLP-1 receptor agonist is added when DKD patients are not achieving the optimal glycemic targets despite using metformin and SGLT2 inhibitor

or who cannot withstand those medications. Insulin with proper titration and sulfonylurea can be recommended to reduce hypoglycemia in selected patients.[11,17]

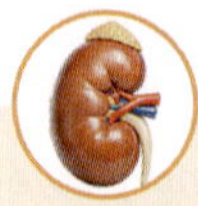

To achieve an A1c target range <8.0%, the first drug choice is metformin plus SGLT2 inhibitor; then, depending on patient-specific factors, additional glucose-lowering medications (GLP-1 RA is preferred) for patients with diabetes and CKD.

BLOOD PRESSURE MANAGEMENT

Blood pressure control plays a key role in the comprehensive care of patients with DKD as it prevents the progression of DKD, ASCVD, and HF. The recommended target by ADA for patients with diabetes, hypertension, and high cardiovascular risk is < 130/80, and for patients with low cardiovascular risk is < 140/90. Even at low BMI, BP is a significant risk factor for developing renal disease.[24]

The drug of choice to decrease the risk of DKD progression is a renin–angiotensin system (RAS) inhibitor, such as the angiotensin-converting enzyme (ACE) inhibitors and angiotensin receptor blockers (ARBs). RAS inhibitors are initiated in patients with diabetes, hypertension, and albuminuria. The ONTARGET (Ongoing Telmisartan Alone and in Combination with Ramipril Global Endpoint Trial) showed that the combination therapy of ACEI and ARB can cause hypotension, syncope, and renal failure; hence, they are not recommended.

Other agents, such as calcium channel blockers (CCBs) (amlodipine), are effective and safe in patients with DKD. Cilnidipine, a novel CCB agent, helps to improve both glucose metabolism and renal protection. β-blockers are not considered as the first-line therapy but have shown significant benefit in patients with postmyocardial infarction, atrial fibrillation, heart attack, and women of childbearing age.

Thiazide-like diuretics such as chlorthalidone and indapamide are effective during the early stages of CKD. Loop diuretics are preferred in the advanced cases of CKD as they show a significant effect in volume control. Combination therapy for people with DKD, ACEI, or ARB plus CCB is highly preferred. Studies show cilnidipine with ARB is considered safe and promising for Indian patients with DKD. If the BP targets are not achieved, adding a thiazide diuretic can be regarded as. In patients with hypertension and no albuminuria, dihydropyridine CCBs and thiazide-like diuretics can be considered. To attain BP targets, multiple drugs are often required in combination, such as RAS inhibitors, dihydropyridine CCBs, and diuretics.[25,26]

Another choice for reducing renal and cardiovascular risk in those with T2D and DKD is the finerenone, nonsteroidal mineralocorticoid receptor antagonist (NS-MRA). The US Food and Drug Administration has approved finerenone for use in individuals with T2D and CKD based on results from two large clinical trials. This medication lowers the risk of a sustained decline in eGFR, progression to ESKD, cardiovascular death, nonfatal myocardial infarction, and HF hospitalization. Although maximal tolerated RAS medication, finerenone is advised for individuals with T2D, an eGFR of ≥ 25 mL/min/1.73 m^2, normal serum potassium levels, and albuminuria (UACR ≥ 30 mg/g).[27]

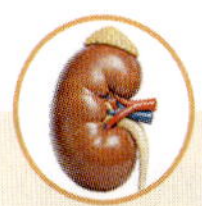

According to the ADA, the recommended blood pressure target for patients with diabetes, hypertension, and high cardiovascular risk is <130/80. The drug of choice to decrease the risk of DKD progression is an RAS inhibitor (ACEi and ARBs).

LIPID MANAGEMENT

Dyslipidemia increases the risk of ASCVD and significantly impacts the occurrence and progression of DKD. Among patients with DKD,

dyslipidemia is very common. It is diagnosed as elevated triglycerides (TG), reduced high-density lipoprotein cholesterol (HDL-C) and normal or mildly elevated low-density lipoprotein cholesterol (LDL-C). The Joint Association of British Clinical Diabetologists and Kidney Association suggested performing annual testing of complete lipid profile in patients with DKD, post kidney transplant, and in dialysis.

Statins, inhibitors of 3-hydroxy-3-methyl-glutaryl-coenzyme A (HMG-CoA) reductase, are considered the first drug of choice for patients with DKD and who are not undergoing dialysis to prevent the risk of ASCVD. This drug is recommended for patients aged ≥ 50 years with CKD and eGFR ≥ 60 mL/min/1.73 m^2 and for patients aged 18–49 years with DKD and with a history of coronary heart disease ischemic stroke.

Fibrates, peroxidase proliferator-activated receptor alpha (PPAR-α) agonists, help to reduce serum TG levels and increase HDL-C levels. Use lower doses of fibrates (fenofibrate and gemfibrozil) when eGFR falls below 60 mL/min/1.73 m^2. Fibrates should be discontinued if eGFR drops below 30 mL/min/1.73 m^2. Proprotein convertase subtilisin/kexin type 9 (PCSK9) inhibitors help in LDL-C catabolism and reduce plasma LDL-C levels. Long-term safety needs to be assessed before administering PCSK9 in patients with DKD. Depending on their ASCVD risk and LDL cholesterol levels, some patients may benefit from adding ezetimibe or a PCSK-9 inhibitor or intensifying their statin medication (for primary prevention).[28]

Among people with diabetes, lipid-lowering drugs are initiated in patients aged above 30 years with persistent albuminuria or patients aged 18–30 years (albuminuria with additional cardiovascular risk). Atorvastatin is the first drug of choice in patients with eGFR < 30 mL/min/1.73 m^2, and rosuvastatin is administered in patients with CKD stage 3 or lower. Lower doses of fibrates can be used when eGFR falls below 60 mL/min/1.73 m^2 but should be discontinued if eGFR falls below 30 mL/min/1.73 m^2.[29]

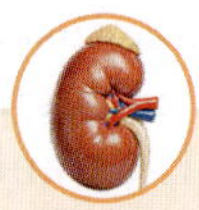

Statins, HMG-CoA reductase inhibitors, are considered the first drug of choice for patients with DKD and who are not undergoing dialysis to prevent the risk of ASCVD.

ANTIPLATELET THERAPY

Cardiovascular disease is a significant problem in the mild-to-severe stages of CKD and is the leading cause of morbidity and death. People with early-stage CKD have a twofold increased risk of CVD compared to the general population, and those who require dialysis have a 30- to 50-fold increased risk, which is responsible for half of all deaths. For individuals with CKD and established ischemic CVD, KDIGO guidelines recommend the use of oral low-dose aspirin to avoid repeated ischemic CVD episodes (also known as secondary prevention). As a secondary preventive measure, administer aspirin therapy (75–162 mg/day) to people with diabetes who have a history of ASCVD. People with ASCVD who have a history of aspirin allergies should take 75 mg of clopidogrel daily.

A multidisciplinary team approach involving a cardiovascular or neurological specialist should be used to decide how long diabetic patients should receive dual antiplatelet therapy using low-dose aspirin and a P2Y12 inhibitor following an acute coronary syndrome or acute ischemic stroke/transient ischemic attack. To avoid severe adverse limb and cardiovascular events, those with stable coronary and/or peripheral artery disease (PAD) and low bleeding risk should be evaluated for combination therapy with aspirin and low-dose rivaroxaban after a thorough conversation with the patient about the advantages versus the same increased risk of bleeding, aspirin therapy (75–162 mg/day) may be considered as the primary preventive strategy for people with diabetes who are at greater cardiovascular risk.

Low-dose aspirin has been shown to offer cardiovascular advantages in patients with established ASCVD, according to meta-analyses of trials. Any adverse effect of bleeding is far outweighed by the benefit.[30]

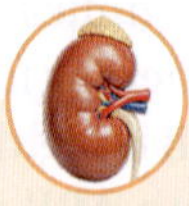

Aspirin therapy (75–162 mg/day) is recommended for people with diabetes who have a history of ASCVD as a secondary preventive measure.

CKD-MINERAL AND BONE DISORDER

One of the complications of CKD is CKD–mineral bone disease (CKD-MBD) is typified by abnormalities in the levels of calcium, phosphate, parathyroid hormone (PTH), vitamin D, and FGF23. Changes in bone morphology and systemic effects result from these disturbances, and cardiovascular problems are the leading cause of the increased mortality rates. Serum abnormalities of calcium, phosphorous, PTH, and vitamin D impact bone health and extraskeletal calcifications in CKD-MBD.

The degree of the underlying kidney impairment, the distinctive bone disease, and the prevailing metabolic abnormalities all influence the therapy of patients with CKD-MBD. Phosphate, calcium, vitamin D, and PTH levels must be strictly controlled to treat CKD-MBD.[31]

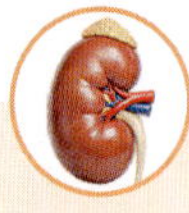

The CKD-MBD, a complication of CKD, is typified by abnormalities in the levels of calcium, phosphate, PTH, vitamin D, and FGF23.

SUMMARY

- Early screening for albuminuria and eGFR enables timely diagnosis, risk stratification, and initiation of targeted interventions to delay DKD progression.
- SGLT2 inhibitors and GLP-1 receptor agonists offer renal and cardiovascular protection.

- A multidisciplinary team approach that includes physicians, nephrologists, educators, and mental health professionals ensures holistic and comprehensive care for DKD patients.
- Empowering patients through structured diabetes self-management education and psychological support improves adherence, mental health, and overall quality of life in individuals with DKD.

CONCLUSION

Comprehensive care for individuals with DKD requires a multifaceted, patient-centered approach that integrates early detection, optimized glycemic and BP control, lipid management, and structured patient education. The use of novel therapeutic agents, along with a multidisciplinary team strategy, ensures tailored interventions that address both renal and cardiovascular outcomes. Empowering patients through education and psychosocial support is pivotal in enhancing adherence and quality of life. Early, coordinated, and holistic management can significantly slow disease progression, reduce morbidity and mortality, and improve overall outcomes in those affected by DKD.

TAKE HOME MESSAGES

- ❑ Regular monitoring of UACR and eGFR enables early identification and proactive management of DKD. Collaborative care involving specialists, educators, and dietitians supports comprehensive treatment and improves patient outcomes.
- ❑ To protect kidney and heart health, ensure tight glycemic and BP control through evidence-based therapies such as SGLT2 inhibitors, GLP-1 receptor agonists, and RAAS blockers.
- ❑ Structured diabetes education and SDM empower patients to participate in their self-care and improve adherence actively.
- ❑ Implement a holistic management strategy for lifestyle changes, mental health, cardiovascular risk, and bone health to prevent complications and enhance quality of life effectively.

REFERENCES

1. Hoogeveen EK. The epidemiology of diabetic kidney disease. J Clin Med. 2021;10(11):2462.
2. Roelofs JJ, Vogt L. Diabetic Nephropathy: Pathophysiology and Clinical Aspects; Springer: Cham, Switzerland, 2019.
3. Cheng HT, Xu X, Lim PS, Hung KY. Worldwide epidemiology of diabetes-related end-stage renal disease, 2000-2015. Diabetes Care. 2021;44:89-97.
4. Qazi M, Sawaf H, Ismail J, Qazi H, Vachharajani T. Pathophysiology of Diabetic Kidney Disease. EMJ Nephrol. 2022;10(1):102-13.
5. Satyavani K, Kothandan H, Jayaraman M, Viswanathan V. Direct costs associated with chronic kidney disease among type 2 diabetic patients in India. Indian J Nephrol. 2014;24(3):141-7.
6. Viswanathan V, Mirshad R. The burden of diabetic nephropathy in India: Need for prevention. Diabetic Nephropathy. 2023;3(2):25-8.
7. Shlipak MG, Tummalapalli SL, Boulware LE, Grams ME, Ix JH, Jha V, et al; Conference Participants. The case for early identification and intervention of chronic kidney disease: conclusions from a Kidney Disease: Improving Global Outcomes (KDIGO) Controversies Conference. Kidney Int. 2021;99(1):34-47.
8. Hussain S, Jamali MC, Habib A, Hussain MS, Akhtar M, Najmi AK. Diabetic kidney disease: An overview of prevalence, risk factors, and biomarkers. Clin Epidemiol Glob Health. 2021;9:2-6.
9. Gong L, Wang R, Wang X, Liu J, Han Z, Li Q, et al. Research progress of natural active compounds on improving podocyte function to reduce proteinuria in diabetic kidney disease. Ren Fail. 2023;45(2):2290930.
10. Friedli I, Baid-Agrawal S, Unwin R, Morell A, Johansson L, Hockings PD. Magnetic Resonance Imaging in Clinical Trials of Diabetic Kidney Disease. J Clin Med. 2023;12(14):4625.

11. de Boer IH, Caramori ML, Chan JCN, Heerspink HJL, Hurst C, Khunti K, et al. Diabetes management in chronic kidney disease: A consensus report by the American Diabetes Association (ADA) and Kidney Disease: Improving Global Outcomes (KDIGO). Diabetes Care. 2022;45(12):3075-90.

12. Li T, Wu HM, Wang F, Huang CQ, Yang M, Dong BR, et al. Education programmes for people with diabetic kidney disease. Cochrane Database Syst Rev. 2011;(6):CD007374.

13. Fogelfeld L, Hart P, Miernik J, Ko J, Calvin D, Tahsin B, et al. Combined diabetes-renal multifactorial intervention in patients with advanced diabeticnephropathy: proof-of-concept. J Diabetes Complicat. 2017;31(3):624-30.

14. Kemmochi T, Oka M, Inokuma A, Shirato N, Totsuka R. Effectiveness of educational programs for patients with diabetic kidney disease: a systematic review and meta-analysis. Ren Replace Ther. 2024;10(1):38.

15. Van der Horst DEM, Hofstra N, van Uden-Kraan CF, Stiggelbout AM, van den Dorpel MA, Pieterse AH, et al. Shared Decision Making in Health Care Visits for CKD: Patients' Decisional Role Preferences and Experiences. Am J Kidney Dis. 2023;82(6):677-86.

16. Miller LM, Schell JO, Weiner DE. Shared decision-making and patient communication in nephrology practice. Adv Kidney Dis Health. 2023;30(6):100125.

17. Kidney Disease: Improving Global Outcomes (KDIGO) Diabetes Work Group. KDIGO 2022 Clinical Practice Guideline for Diabetes Management in Chronic Kidney Disease. Kidney Int. 2022;102(5S):S1-S127.

18. Diabetes Control Complications Trial Research Group; Nathan DM, Genuth S, Lachin J, Cleary P, Crofford O, Davis M, et al. The effect of intensive treatment of diabetes on the development and progression of long-term complications in insulin dependent diabetes mellitus. N Engl J Med. 1993;329(14):977-86.

19. Diabetes Control Complications Trial/Epidemiology of Diabetes Interventions Complications Research Group. Sustained effect of intensive treatment of type 1 diabetes mellitus on development and progression of diabetic nephropathy: the epidemiology of diabetes interventions and complications (EDIC) study. JAMA. 2003;290(16):2159-67.

20. Viswanathan V, Tilak P, Meerza R, Kumpatla S. Insulin Resistance at different stages of Diabetic Kidney Disease in India. J Assoc Physicians India. 2010;58:612-5.

21. Viswanathan V, Kumpatla S, Tilak P, Muthukumaran P. Levels of Glycated albumin at different stages of diabetic nephropathy in India. Int J Diabetes Metabol. 2009;17:77-80.

22. Scilletta S, Di Marco M, Miano N, Filippello A, Di Mauro S, Scamporrino A, et al. Update on Diabetic Kidney Disease (DKD): Focus on Non-Albuminuric DKD and Cardiovascular Risk. Biomolecules. 2023;13(5):752.

23. De Bhailís ÁM, Azmi S, Kalra PA. Diabetic Kidney Disease: Update on Clinical Management and Non-Glycaemic Effects of Newer Medications for Type 2 Diabetes. Ther Adv Endocrinol Metab. 2021;12:20420188211020664.

24. Viswanathan VV, Snehalatha C, Ramachandran A, Viswanathan M. Proteinuria in NIDDM in south India: analysis of predictive factors. Diabetes Res Clin Pract. 1995;28:41-6.

25. Banerjee D, Winocour P, Chowdhury TA, De P, Wahba M, Montero R, et al. Management of hypertension in patients with diabetic kidney disease: summary of the joint Association of British Clinical Diabetologists and UK Kidney Association (ABCD-UKKA) guideline 2021. Kidney Int Rep. 2022;7(4):681-7.

26. Wander GS, Panda JK, Pal J, Mathur G, Sahay R, Tiwaskar M, et al. Management of Hypertension in Patients with Type 2 Diabetes Mellitus: Indian Guideline 2024 by Association of Physicians of India and Indian College of Physicians. J Assoc Physicians India. 2024;72(8):e1-e25.

27. ElSayed NA, Bannuru RR, Bakris G, Bardsley J, de Boer IH, Gabbay RA, et al. Diabetic Kidney Disease Prevention Care Model Development. Clin Diabetes. 2024;42(2):274-84.

28. Tu QM, Jin HM, Yang XH. Lipid abnormality in diabetic kidney disease and potential treatment advancements. Front Endocrinol (Lausanne). 2025;16:1503711.

29. Zac-Varghese S, Mark P, Bain S, Banerjee D, Chowdhury TA, Dasgupta I, et al. Clinical practice guideline for the management of lipids in adults with diabetic kidney disease: abbreviated summary of the Joint Association of British Clinical Diabetologists and UK Kidney Association (ABCD-UKKA) Guideline 2024. BMC Nephrol. 2024;25(1):216.

30. American Diabetes Association Professional Practice Committee. 10. Cardiovascular Disease and Risk Management: Standards of Care in Diabetes-2024. Diabetes Care. 2024;47(Suppl 1):S179-S218.

31. Shah A, Hashmi MF, Aeddula NR. Chronic Kidney Disease-Mineral Bone Disorder (CKD-MBD) [Internet]. In: StatPearls [Internet]. Treasure Island (FL): StatPearls Publishing; 2024.

Key Research Takeaway

Insulin resistance at different stages of diabetic kidney disease in India

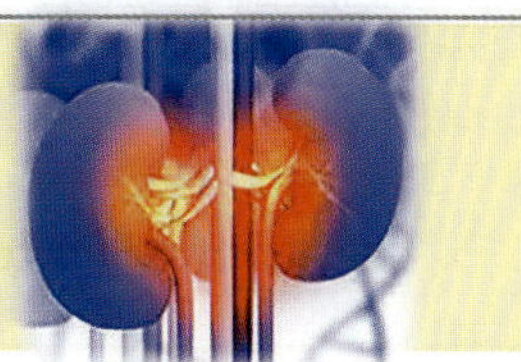

Vijay Viswanathan, Priyanka Tilak, Rafi Meerza, Satyavani Kumpatla

Abstract

Objective: Many studies showed that Insulin resistance (IR) is present in chronic renal failure and evidences suggest that IR can also occur in early stages of renal disease. There is paucity of data from India, hence this study was planned to assess the degree of Insulin resistance at different stages of diabetic nephropathy.

Study subjects and methods: This is a cross sectional study with a total of 128 subjects (M: F; 81:47) divided into 3 groups based on their renal function, Group 1 (control) n=32, group 2 (Normoalbuminuria) n=26, group 3 (Microalbuminuria) n=59 and group 4 (Macroalbuminuria) n=43. Subjects on insulin treatment were excluded. Insulin was estimated by chemiluminescence method. Biochemical investigations were done by enzymatic procedures. Insulin resistance was calculated using HOMA method. The normal cut off value for HOMA IR (2.4) was derived using mean+2SD of control group.

Results: There was no significant difference between the study groups with respect to age, BMI, duration of diabetes and glycemic control. Mean HOMA IR increased significantly with decreasing renal function (control: 1.30 +/- 0.53; Normo: 4.0 +/- 2.7; Micro: 5.8 +/- 4.1; Macro: 7.9 +/- 5.1, p < 0.0001). Larger percentage of subjects had HOMA IR (> or = 2.4) at different stages of diabetic kidney disease (Normoalb: 57.6%; Microalb: 76.2%, Macroalb: 90.6%) compared to normal (3.1%). The results of multiple logistic regression analysis showed an association between HOMA IR and diabetic nephropathy.

Conclusion: This cross-sectional study demonstrated an association between IR and diabetic kidney disease in Indian population with type 2 diabetes. Further prospective studies are needed to look for causative relationship between IR and renal function.

JAPI OCT 2010 Vol.58 Page612-615.

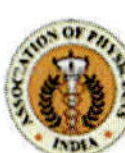

Int J Diabetes & Metabolism (2009) 17:77- 80

Levels of glycated albumin at different stages of diabetic nephropathy in India

Vijay Viswanathan, Satyavani Kumpatla, Priyanka Tilak, Parthiban Muthukumaran.
M V Hospital for Diabetes and Diabetes Research Centre, WHO Collaborating Centre for Research, Education and Training in Diabetes, Chennai, India

Abstract

Aims: Glycated haemoglobin (HbA1c) which is an index of long term glycaemic control in diabetic patients is measured in majority of patients worldwide. Glycated albumin (GA) is useful for the evaluation of short term glycaemic control (2 weeks) in patients with diabetes. The aim of this study was to assess the GA levels at different stages of diabetic nephropathy in Indian population. **Materials and Methods:** A total of 147 subjects (M:F; 95:52) were selected for this study and were divided into three groups based on their renal function and compared with a non diabetic control group (n = 50, M:F; 14:36). The groups were as follows; group1 (control) n = 50, group2 (normoalbuminuria) n = 42, group 3 (microalbuminuria) n = 55, group 4 (proteinuria) n = 50. GA was measured by enzymatic procedure using the Lucica GA – L kit (Asahi Kasei Pharma Corp, Japan). **Results:** The normal cutoff value for GA was derived using control group and it was found to be 15% (range 7-17%). GA was significantly higher in diabetic patients at different stages of diabetic nephropathy compared to non diabetic control group [cont: 12.9 ± 1.8, normo: 20.8 ± 5.8, micro: 26.1 ± 8.6, macro: 23.5 ± 8.3). Microalbuminuric patients had significantly higher GA levels than normoalbuminuric patients (p< 0.05). Proteinuric subjects had slightly lower GA levels compared to microalbuminuric group but it was not statistically significant. **Conclusion:** GA was found to be a better marker for evaluating short term glycaemic status among diabetic patients with different degree of renal impairment prior to ESRD.

10

Primary Prevention of Diabetic Kidney Disease

*Arutselvi Devarajan, Rizwana Parveen,
Sivashankari Selva Elavarasan, Vijay Viswanathan*

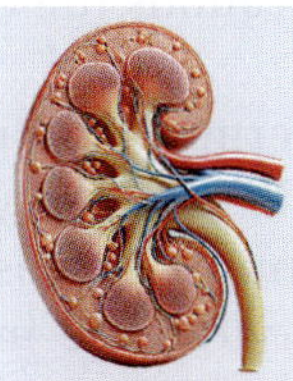

- ➤ Existing evidence on prevention or nonprogression of DKD
- ➤ Screening and early diagnosis of DKD
- ➤ Importance of patient education and support
- ➤ Primary care model for the prevention of DKD
- ➤ Strategies for implementation of community-based prevention program

Abstract

Diabetes is increasing worldwide, which is considered a major public health problem mainly in low- and middle-income countries. Given the substantial rise in the prevalence of type 2 diabetes (T2D), it is anticipated that diabetic kidney disease (DKD) will also increase unless immediate preventive measures are implemented. Primary prevention of DKD aims to prevent the initial onset of kidney damage in people with diabetes, which is possible by treating and managing diabetes to avoid the devastating effects on an individual's physical health. Critical strategies include maintaining optimal glycemic control, strict blood pressure management, lifestyle modifications (diet, exercise, weight control, and smoking cessation), and early detection of risk factors such as hyperfiltration and albuminuria. Lipid abnormalities, obesity, and other metabolic and hemodynamic stressors also contribute to DKD. Evidence suggests that early intervention against modifiable risk factors can significantly delay or prevent the onset of DKD. Preventive strategies should be implemented not only at the individual level but also at the community level and further by strengthening the healthcare networks and interdepartmental collaborations within the healthcare systems and services.

Keywords: Primary prevention, DKD, India, eGFR, microalbuminuria.

INTRODUCTION

Diabetic kidney disease (DKD) is considered a subset of chronic kidney disease (CKD), which comprises both physiological and structural pathological alterations. DKD, one of the complications of diabetes, is noted as one of the leading causes of CKD and an important cause of end-stage renal disease (ESRD). DKD accounts for more than half of the people affected with ESRD worldwide.[1] There were about 107 million people with chronic type 2 DKD globally in 2021, an 85% increase from 58 million in 1990. The projection for the global burden of DKD from 2020 to 2040 suggests a significant increase in these numbers.[2] A recent review showed that a total of 115 million people are living with CKD in India. It also suggests that the majority of the Asian countries reported a 100% increase or more in the overall burden of CKD from 2009 to 2019.[3] CKD due to type 2 diabetes (T2D) increased worldwide by about 74% between 1990 and 2017.[4] In addition, DKD is closely linked to a significant increase in cardiovascular morbidity and mortality.[5]

PATHOPHYSIOLOGY

The pathophysiology of DKD involves intricate mechanisms that result in renal injury and a gradual decline in kidney function. The main trigger of DKD's pathophysiology is chronic hyperglycemia, which leads to the accumulation of advanced glycation end products in the renal tissues.[6] Hyperglycemia-induced oxidative stress generates reactive oxygen species, which activate proinflammatory pathways such as the nuclear factor-kappa B (NF-κB) pathway and the mitogen-activated protein kinase pathway. These pathways stimulate the production of cytokines, chemokines, and adhesion molecules, recruiting inflammatory cells to the renal tissues and intensifying the inflammatory response.[7] Another crucial mechanism in the pathophysiology of DKD is the activation of the renin–angiotensin–aldosterone system (RAAS), leading to the production of angiotensin II, which induces vasoconstriction and oxidative stress in the kidneys. Angiotensin II also triggers the production of profibrotic factors, such as transforming growth factor-β (TGF-β), facilitating the accumulation of extracellular matrix proteins and the onset of kidney fibrosis.[8]

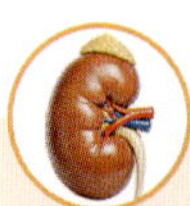

- *DKD, which is recognized as one of the complications of diabetes, is noted as the leading cause of CKD and an important reason for ESRD.*
- *The pathophysiology of DKD is quite complex and involves intricate mechanisms that result in renal injury and a gradual decline in kidney function.*

Existing Evidence on Prevention or Decreased Progression of Diabetic Kidney Disease

Diabetic kidney disease is quite a common outcome of long-term, uncontrolled diabetes in both type 1 diabetes (T1D) and T2D. Although DKD has a gradual onset, there are several risk factors and associated diseases that can exacerbate renal injury and DKD progression. A thorough preventive approach for DKD includes glycemic control, treatment of hypertension and hyperlipidemia comorbidities, and lifestyle modifications (diet, exercise, and cessation of smoking).

Hyperglycemia is a major determinant for the progression of DKD. In people with early DKD, management of glycemic control remains a key aspect of care and plays a vital role in minimizing microvascular kidney damage or reducing DKD progression. There is a strong association between insulin resistance and DKD in the Indian population with T2D.[9] Maintaining the blood glucose levels within the target range can prevent or decrease the progression of the disease. There are several landmark trials such as DCCT, UKPDS, ACCORD trial, and DIAS trial which show evidences on prevention or decreased progression of DKD which are elucidated in **Table 1**. DCCT (Diabetes Control and Complications Trial) in type1 diabetes highlighted that an intensive diabetes treatment reduces the incidence of microalbuminuria (36%) and was observed that individuals who followed strict glycemic control showed a long-lasting 40% risk reduction in developing microalbuminuria and hypertension even after 7–8 years at the end of DCCT trial.[10] It has also been well documented that hyperfiltration predicts progression to microalbuminuria and overt proteinuria, which is markedly decreased by improved glycemic control.[11] In the UKPDS study, it was observed that intensive blood glucose control over 12 years in people with newly diagnosed T2D led to a significant reduction in the risk of microvascular

TABLE 1: Landmark trials for prevention/decreased progression of DKD.

Risk factor	Diabetes type	Target level	Effect/Risk reduction	Study (year)
Hyperglycemia	T2D	Glycemic control (HbA1c <7%)	• 33% ↓ risk of microalbuminuria onset • 34% ↓ proteinuria • 74% ↓ risk of 2× ↑ in plasma creatinine	UKPDS 33[13] (1998)
	T1D	Good glycemic control (HbA1c <7%)	36% ↓ risk of incident microalbuminuria	DCCT-EDIC (2003)[11]
	T1D	Strict glycemic control (HbA1c <6.5%)	40% ↓ risk of incident microalbuminuria	DCCT-EDIC (2003)[11]
Hypertension	T2D	BP reduction by 10 mm Hg (e.g., from 154 to 144 mm Hg)	29% ↓ risk of microalbuminuria onset	UKPDS 38[22] (1998)
	T2D	BP <140/90 mm Hg or <130/80 mm Hg	↓ Progression of DKD	JNC 7 (2003)[24]
	T2D	Intensive BP control (<120 mm Hg systolic) vs. standard (<140 mm Hg)	↓Serum creatinine levels	ACCORD-BP Trial (2010)[23]
Hyperlipidemia	T2D	LDL <100 mg/dL (or <70 mg/dL in established CVD)	↓ Risk of progression from normoalbuminuria to microalbuminuria	DAIS (2005)[28]

(CVD: cardiovascular disease; DKD: diabetic kidney disease; HbA1c: glycated hemoglobin; LDL: low-density lipoprotein)

complications compared to conventional treatment. There was a risk reduction of 33% in the onset of microalbuminuria, 34% risk reduction in proteinuria, and 74% risk reduction in a twofold increase of plasma creatinine.[12] The ACCORD trial showed a significant reduction of estimated glomerular filtration rate (eGFR) and microalbuminuria in the intensive group compared to the standard group during the initial years. However, it was observed that the composite renal outcomes were similar at transition and at the end of the study period. In addition, it revealed that tight control of glucose resulted in increased hypoglycemia and deaths in high-risk individuals.[13] Therefore, strategies of primary prevention of DKD should be well focused on achieving intensive blood glucose

control with a recommendation of an A1c goal of <7.0% for adults with diabetes.[14] Kidney Disease: Improving Global Outcomes (KDIGO) guidelines recommended an A1c for people with DKD not treated with dialysis from <6.5 to <8% considering comorbid conditions, CKD stage, life expectancy, and hypoglycemic risk.[15]

Hypertension is also a strong risk factor for the development and progression of DKD,[16] which is more common among people with diabetes, even when renal involvement is not present. This risk factor adds another dimension to the prevention and progression of DKD, which has been proven to have an active role in the development of microvascular complications among people with diabetes.[17] Compared to the general population, people with diabetes are twice as likely to be hypertensive[18] and nearly one-third of people with hypertension develop diabetes in subsequent years.[18,19] Several placebo-controlled trials have analyzed the risks and benefits of intense blood pressure management among people with diabetes and hypertension. Several studies have shown that intensive control of blood pressure is associated with delayed albuminuria as well as decreased rates of serious extrarenal cardiac events.[20,21] The UKPDS study demonstrated that a reduction in systolic blood pressure (154–144 mm Hg) in T2D with newly diagnosed hypertension was associated with a 29% decrease in the onset of microalbuminuria.[22] Intensive BP control had a significant effect on serum creatinine levels as evident in the ACCORD BP trial.[23] BP control also plays a major role in the prevention of other comorbidities in terms of CVD risk factors. Hypertension optimal study highlighted that the risk of cardiovascular events was reduced by 50% for a reduction in DBP by 85–81 mm Hg and the targeted BP should be <130/80 mm Hg in people with diabetes.[24] Blood pressure levels <140/90 mm Hg are mandated to reduce the risk or slow the progression of DKD, with strong consideration of lower targets (<130/80 mm Hg) and further recommendations should be based on individualized assessment of treatment benefits and risks.[25] Hence, a strict control of blood pressure is a key aspect of diabetes care to prevent DKD. KDIGO guidelines recommend maintaining <120 mm Hg SBP to reduce the risk of DKD.[26]

Hyperlipidemia should be considered as another important comorbid condition in the development and progression of DKD, because of its strong association with the CVD risk and CVD-related deaths. Thus, treating hyperlipidemia is crucial for disease prognosis and to improve kidney function. The clinical recommendations by American Diabetes Association (ADA) suggest a target low-density lipoprotein (LDL) of <100 mg/dL for people with diabete or LDL <70 mg/dL for people with diabetes who have established cardiovascular disease.[27] In the Diabetes

Atherosclerosis Intervention Study, fenofibrate usage significantly reduced the rate of progression from normoalbuminuria to microalbuminuria in T2D.[28] The Heart Protection Study[29] highlighted the use of statins, and ACCORD lipid trial[30] investigated combination therapy to reduce the development of microalbuminuria in people with diabetes. To summarize, effective treatment for hyperlipidemia in people with diabetes is recommended as it also has a promising effect on decreasing cardiovascular events and mortality.

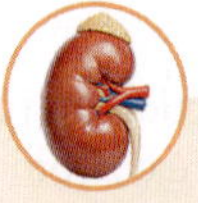

- *Management of hyperglycemia and hypertension in people with diabetes showed a significant improvement in kidney function.*
- *A lower occurrence of microalbuminuria and a significant decrease in serum creatinine levels were evident with intensive glycemic and BP control.*

LIFESTYLE MODIFICATION

Dietary protein requirement becomes essential for people with diabetes for systemic metabolic needs, but a high intake level can lead to albuminuria and renal injury. The low protein diet was associated with an overall slow rate of GFR decline in people with diabetes over time.[31] However, ADA recommends an optimal protein intake of 0.8 g/kg/day.[32] High dietary sodium is recognized as a silent killer responsible for millions of deaths worldwide, secondary to hypertension and its complications. Dietary sodium reduction is broadly recommended for people with DKD. A reduction in salt intake reduces systemic blood pressure and thus minimizes hypertension, stress, and injury to the kidneys.[33] Salt consumption of Indians was estimated to be higher than the recommended values due to their food habits and culture[34] and intake of sodium was an independent risk factor associated with systolic BP.[35] A study conducted by Vijay et al. indicated the consumption of high amounts of dietary salt and an inappropriate proportion of macronutrients in the South Indian population with diabetes and other comorbid conditions.[36] Practical suggestions would include decreased intake of salt and sodium, and reduced consumption of highly processed and packaged foods.

Exercise and physical activity should be included in patient care plans, including DKD treatment, due to their multisystem benefits in the whole body. There are few evidences which provide data on exercise therapy in DKD or CKD. Improved weight management, increased aerobic and cardiovascular capacity, and decreased inflammation and muscle atrophy may help in delaying CKD progression among people living with diabetes.[37] Other possible mechanisms by which physical activity can prevent the development of DKD are reduction of BP, improvement of the lipid profile, glycemic control, insulin sensitivity, and endothelial function. Incorporation of more research plans for exercise routine in DKD and CKD treatment may show promising benefits.

Smoking cessation should be identified as a part of the prevention approach for DKD and associated comorbidities. Persons with diabetes who smoke were at an increased risk for microalbuminuria.[38] There was an increased risk for the decline in GFR for smokers when compared to their counterparts, provided the risk for progression to ESRD was much higher in smokers.[39] The use of toxic chemicals like nicotine can trigger chronic vasoconstriction, leading to kidney fibrosis[40] and also significantly increases the risk and severity of cardiovascular events in people with diabetes.[41] Hence, smoking cessation should be considered for renal protection and prevention of DKD.

Our kidneys can be affected by the consumption of alcohol. Excessive alcohol intake, may worsen kidney function,[42] increasing the risk of DKD. Some studies have shown that moderate alcohol consumption was associated with decreased risk of DKD.[43] A recent cross-sectional study conducted in US adults showed daily alcohol consumption was associated with increased risk of DKD, whereas moderate consumption had reduced risk, which further highlighted the importance of drinking behavior in the progression and management of DKD.[44] Therefore, it becomes essential to be cautious about alcohol consumption and seek guidance from a healthcare professional, especially for people who are at high risk of developing DKD.

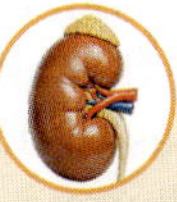

- *Lifestyle changes, including dietary habits (low sodium intake) and weight reduction, play a major role in improving kidney function.*
- *Cessation of smoking and quitting alcohol help maintain kidney health.*

SCREENING AND EARLY CLINICAL DIAGNOSIS FOR DIABETIC KIDNEY DISEASE

Diabetic kidney disease usually is an asymptomatic condition in the initial stages; guidelines from the ADA and KDIGO group recommend that kidney function and albuminuria should be measured at diagnosis and at least annually thereafter in people with T2D. While in T1D, it is recommended to start screening after 5 years of diagnosis.[45] In a South Indian study, persistent microalbuminuria was reported in 28.2% of T1D subjects, with prevalence increasing with longer disease duration and association with hypertension and retinopathy.[46] Albuminuria is assessed using the albumin-to-creatinine ratio (ACR) measured on spot urine samples (ideally early morning samples). 24 hours urine collections to measure albumin excretion are also appropriate, although they are less convenient and more prone to collection errors. Estimation of kidney function was based on serum creatinine-derived eGFR using the CKD-EPI equation, which offers greater accuracy than alternative equations, particularly within the 60–90 mL/min/1.73 m² range. Assessment of both eGFR and albuminuria is important to diagnose, assess the stage, and manage appropriate kidney health. The semiquantitative and quantitative methods for estimating urine albumin concentration are shown in **Figure 1**. The dipstick test identifies gross or overt proteinuria, mainly detecting albumin when its concentration exceeds about 300 mg/L. It is quick, inexpensive, and widely available, but not sensitive enough to detect early kidney damage. In contrast, the Micral test is an immunoassay that specifically detects small amounts of albumin in the range of 20–200 mg/L, allowing identification of microalbuminuria—an early marker of DKD. While the Micral test is more sensitive and useful for early detection, it is slightly more costly and requires careful handling. Thus, the dipstick test, a semiquantitative method, is suitable for screening overt proteinuria, whereas the Micral test is preferred for detecting early, subtle renal impairment in people with diabetes. This would initiate the first step toward the detection of incipient diabetic nephropathy in developing countries.[47] The cost efficiency and the high sensitivity and specificity of the urine dipstick test when compared to the Micral test will encourage its use among primary care physicians and private practitioners as a diagnostic tool to detect urine albumin concentration. A flowchart for the detection and quantification of microalbuminuria is shown in **Flowchart 1**. Early detection of

microalbuminuria[48] identifies patients at risk and allows for early treatment of the disease. Therapies that produce a lasting decrease in urine albumin may slow the progression of DKD.[49] A diagrammatic representation for the screening of microalbuminuria is depicted in **Flowchart 2**.

In T1D, a clinical diagnosis of DKD can be made when there is persistent moderate (A2) (30–300 mg/g) or severe (A3) (>300 mg/g) albuminuria or a persistent reduction in eGFR to <60 mL/min/1.73 m², occurring at least 5 years after onset of

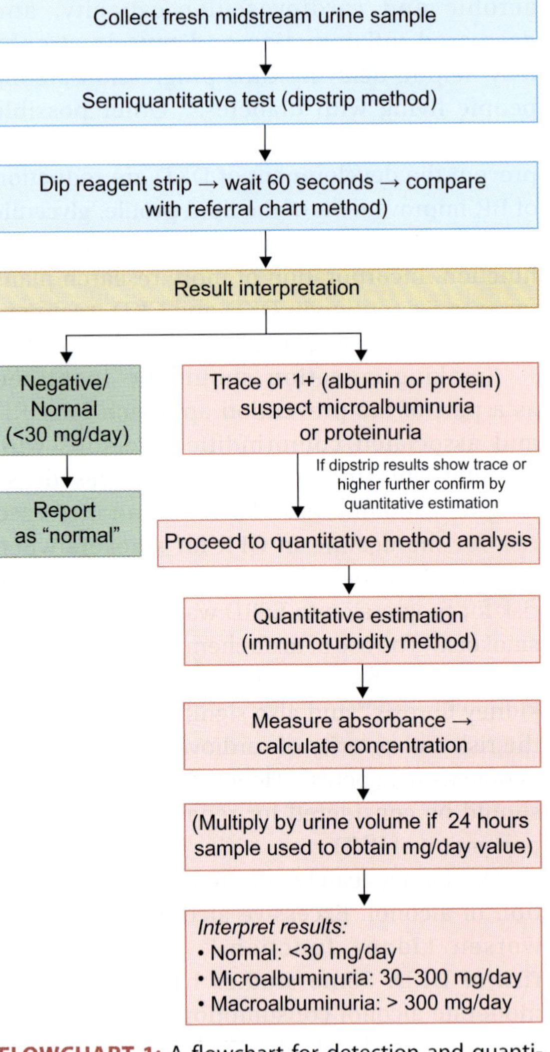

FLOWCHART 1: A flowchart for detection and quantification of microalbuminuria.

FIG. 1: Semiquantitative and quantitative method for urine albumin concentration.

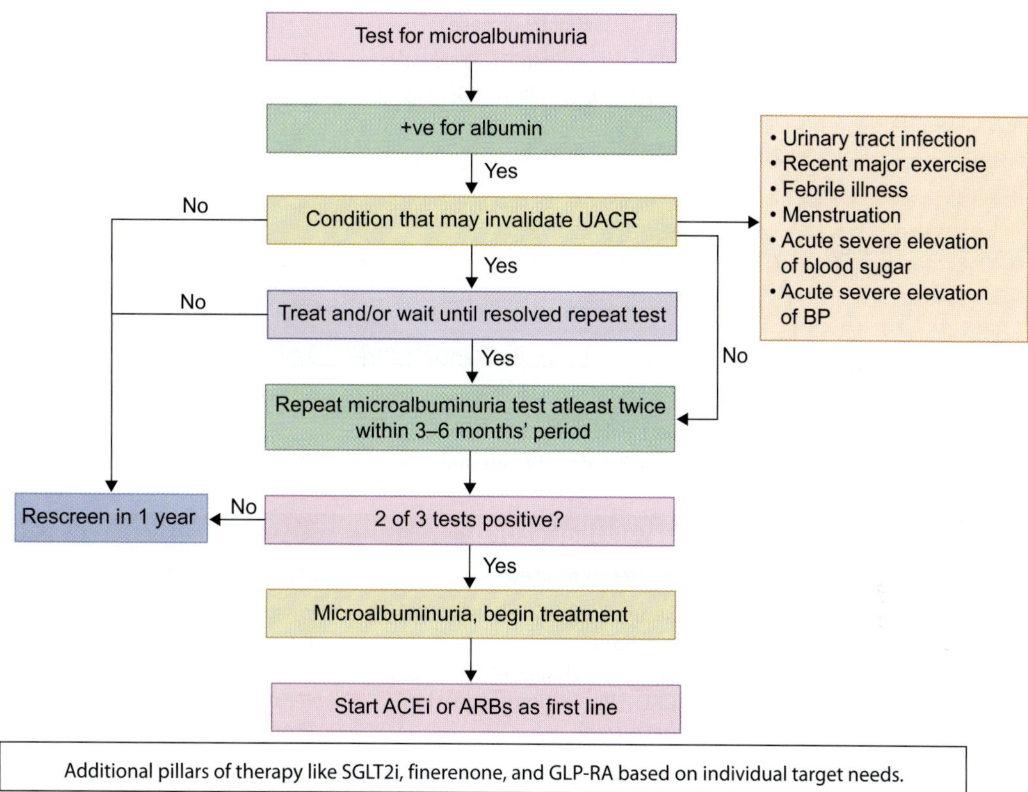

FLOWCHART 2: Algorithm for screening for microalbiminuria.[48]
(ACEi: angiotensin-converting enzyme inhibitors; ARBs: angiotensin receptor blockers; SGLT2i: sodium-glucose cotransporter-2 inhibitor)

diabetes. In over 95% of cases, diabetic retinopathy will also be present, and there should be no clinical suggestions of an alternative kidney disease. Persistent reduction in eGFR without albuminuria can indicate evaluation for nonalbuminuric DKDs. Similarly, the presence of albuminuria without diabetic retinopathy should raise consideration of alternative diagnoses such as hypertensive nephrosclerosis, primary glomerular disease, or other nondiabetic renal pathologies.

In T2D, the clinical diagnosis can be more challenging due to the increased heterogeneity of clinical presentation, although the same principles of persistent albuminuria or persistently reduced eGFR can be applied. A diagnosis of DKD can be made when eGFR is persistently below 60 mL/min/1.73 m^2, although this finding should also prompt assessment for other potential causes of kidney disease. The different stages of kidney disease using eGFR based on KDIGO guidelines are seen in **Figure 2**. Longer duration of diabetes and presence of retinopathy are important indicators toward the diagnosis when they are present, but neither a short duration of diabetes nor absence of retinopathy is useful to rule out DKD in T2D. Nevertheless, a clinical confirmation of DKD can be made if there is a persistent reduction in eGFR or an increase in albuminuria is detected, and reconfirmed on repeat testing over 3–6 months; a minimum of two elevated ACR levels more than 3 months apart are required before an individual is considered to have increased albuminuria. Similarly, two eGFR values below 60 mL/min/1.73 m^2 at least 90 days apart are required to make a diagnosis of CKD.[32] In addition, a random estimated protein excretion (EPE) can also be used to assess the renal function in poor resource settings. People with protein

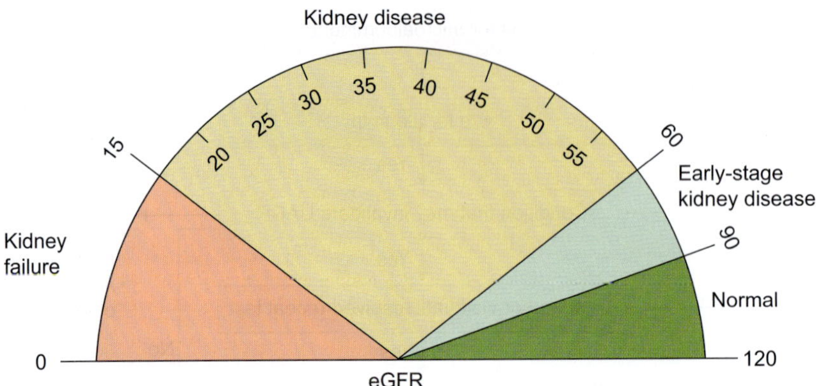

FIG. 2: The stages of kidney disease using eGFR based on KDIGO.

(eGFR: estimated glomerular filtration rate; KDIGO: Kidney Disease: Improving Global Outcomes)

TABLE 2: Quantitative or laboratory evaluation of DKD.[51-53]		
Test	*Measurement used*	*Diagnostic result*
Creatinine measurement and eGFR calculation	• Serum creatinine level (Jaffe's method) • eGFR calculated using the 2021 CKD-EPI creatinine equation (race-free)	*Early stage*: • Decline in eGFR • 60–90 mL/min/1.73 m^2 *Later stages*: • Progressive decline in eGFR indicating worsening renal function • eGFR <60 mL/min/1.73 m^2
Spot urine test (urinary albumin-creatinine ratio—UACR)	Albumin concentration (mg of albumin per g of creatinine)	• Normoalbuminuria: <30 mg/g • Microalbuminuria: 30–300 mg/g • Macroalbuminuria: >300 mg/g
Spot urine test for proteinuria (urinary protein and creatinine ratio—UPCR)	Protein concentration (mg of protein per g of creatinine)	• Normoalbuminuria: <0.2 • Macroalbuminuria: >0.2
24 hours urine test	Estimated protein excretion	• Normal protein excretion <150 mg/day • Abnormal >150 mg/day

(DKD: diabetic kidney disease; eGFR: estimated glomerular filtration rate)

excretion of <100 mg/dL were classified as normal, 100–500 mg/dL as mild proteinuria, and >500 mg/dL as persistent proteinuria.[50] The various tests evolved in the laboratory evaluation of DKD are tabulated in **Table 2**.

Screening for Normoalbuminuric Diabetic Kidney Disease

Nonalbuminuric DKD is a condition in which there is a decline in renal function in people with diabetes without proteinuria. Traditionally, DKD is characterized by the presence of albuminuria along with a progressive decline in renal function. However, studies have shown that in some people with diabetes, renal function decline can occur even before the onset of proteinuria. The reduction in eGFR without albuminuria, known as nonproteinuric DKD, has been increasingly recognized in individuals with T2D. It has a weaker association with diabetic retinopathy and is caused by vascular and tubulointerstitial abnormalities. There are many underlying possibilities that might explain the occurrence of nonproteinuric DKD, which include coexisting conditions of other vascular diseases, tubulointerstitial fibrosis, decline in eGFR due to previous episodes of AKI, and decreased albuminuria due to RAAS inhibitors.[54] The prevalence of nonproteinuric kidney disease in T2DM is estimated to be between 39 and 70%,[54-56] while in T1D, it is reported to be between 7 and 60%.[55,57,58] It has a better prognosis than DKD with proteinuria but is a significant risk factor for death and major cardiovascular disease.[59]

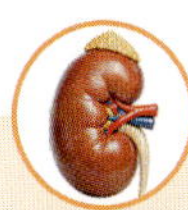

- *DKD can be assessed using UACR and also serum creatinine-based eGFR calculation (CKD-EPI equation).*
- *As a considerable proportion of people with diabetes experience nonalbuminuric DKD, there is a need to assess both eGFR and albuminuria.*

Importance of Patient Education and Support

Patient education is another important aspect of diabetes clinical care that must be incorporated into current DKD preventive strategies. Despite DKD being the most prevalent complication of diabetes, it is noted from the larger population studies that less than one-fourth of the people with DKD are aware of this condition.[49] It is always underscored that there is a major unmet need for improved screening and self-management education for people with diabetes, which suggests that the majority of people with DKD do not have access to education about diagnosis, inadequate intervention and poor therapy adherence. Currently, the ADA recommends that all people with T1D with a diagnosis ≥5 years and all those with T2D need to undergo annual urinary albumin and eGFR assessments.[45] Adhering to these guidelines is

essential to ensure that all patients at risk for DKD are identified early and timely interventions are implemented to prevent further renal damage. A study conducted by Vijay et al. showed that the direct cost of hospital admission for treating CKD was considerably greater than for those without complications,[60] and this emphasizes the need for early diagnosis and detection of risk factors to prevent diabetic nephropathy,[61] through appropriate intervention, education, care, and support. Educating people with newly diagnosed diabetes on the long-term sequelae of the disease and information provided at the time of diagnosis to promote self-care management and improve long-term health outcomes is the key to targeting people with diabetes before DKD develops. Empowering patients with self-driven preventive strategies will have many potential advantages, including better awareness of the disease, treatment adherence and ultimately, could contribute toward a reduction in DKD rates. A structured framework with an appropriate support system is important in primary healthcare services for the prevention of DKD.

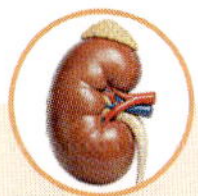

- *Low DKD awareness: Less than 25% of people with diabetes are aware of their condition.*
- *Early screening is the key: ADA recommends annual urinary albumin and eGFR tests for people at risk (type 1 ≥5 years, all type 2) to prevent renal damage.*
- *Empowering people with self-care education at diagnosis improves adherence, awareness, and long-term health outcomes.*

Primary Care Model for the Prevention of Diabetic Kidney Disease

A multifaceted approach is essential for any preventive health measure. To reduce the onset and progression of DKD, key strategies include providing self-management education to individuals with diabetes, promoting healthy lifestyle changes, ensuring appropriate pharmacological interventions, preventing comorbidities—particularly cardiovascular disease—and offering comprehensive psychosocial support. The main objectives of a primary care model are to decrease the onset and progression of DKD.

- To reduce the incidence of DKD
- To facilitate screening and effective management of early DKD to delay the progression further and reduce associated complications.[62] Indian evidence also emphasizes these two aspects.[63,64] Greater emphasis should be placed on primary care, as most diabetes management occurs at this level, where the majority of interactions between healthcare providers and people with diabetes take place. The model's key stakeholders are people with diabetes and their caregivers, primary and specialty care practitioners, community partners, health policymakers, and the health system as a whole. A prevention care model for DKD is given in **Figure 3**.[62] This model gives a comprehensive framework for DKD prevention at different levels—individual, family and community, and the health services system.

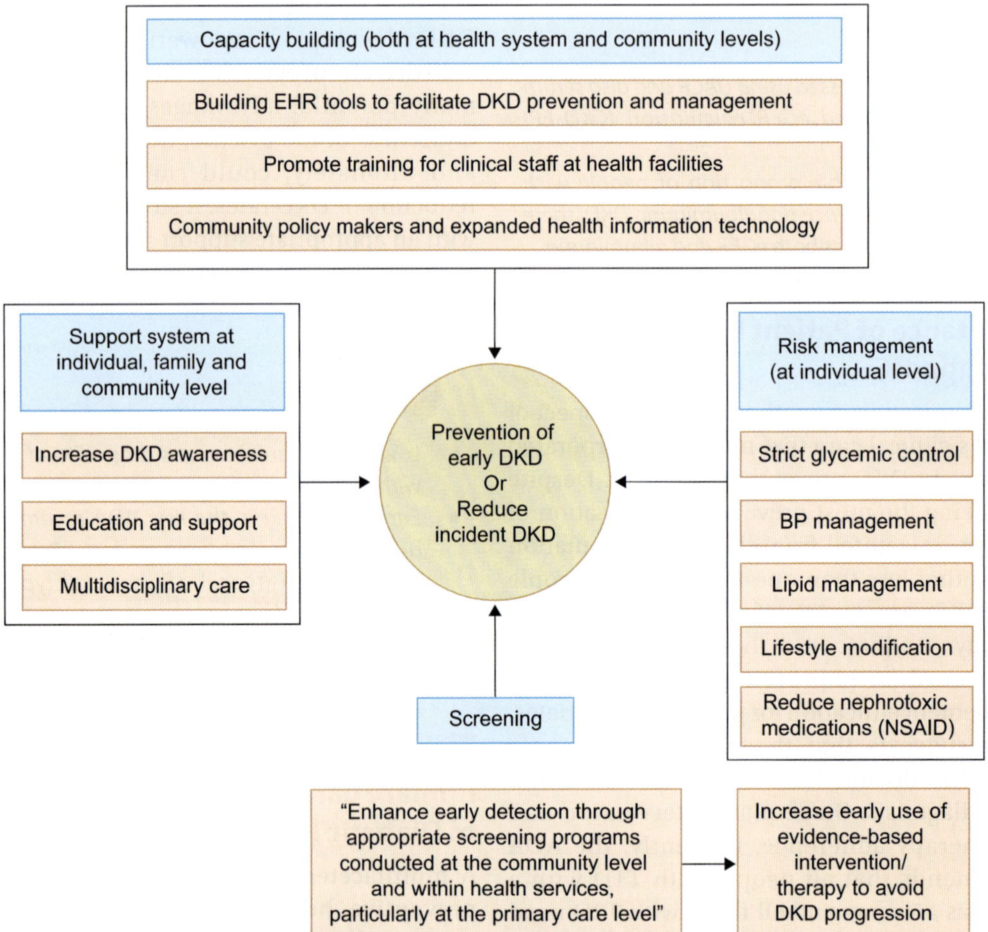

FIG. 3: Healthcare model for prevention of diabetic kidney disease (DKD).[62]

Individual Level

The individual level focuses on managing diabetes and related risk factors for people living with the condition. Therefore, individuals with diabetes must take proactive steps to manage the following aspects:

- *Glycemic control*: Regular monitoring and control of plasma glucose levels and HbA1c are essential. Aim to maintain fasting blood glucose below 100 mg/dL and HbA1c levels below 7%.
- *Hypertension control*: Managing blood pressure (target BP < 130/80 mm Hg) is crucial for preventing DKD. This can be achieved through a low-sodium diet, regular physical activity, and adherence to medications prescribed by healthcare providers.
- *Dyslipidemia management*: It is important to manage lipid levels in the body. This includes maintaining low LDL cholesterol (<70 mg/dL), high HDL cholesterol, and keeping triglyceride levels below 150 mg/dL.
- *Lifestyle modifications*: Key lifestyle changes to prevent DKD include adopting a balanced diet, increasing physical activity, reducing stress, and cessation of smoking/alcohol.
- *Minimizing nephrotoxic medications (NSAIDs) and over-the-counter drugs*: Nonsteroidal anti-inflammatory drugs (NSAIDs) are known to contribute to renal problems in people with diabetes. Their use should be minimized by opting for alternative medications or reducing dosages and durations. Additionally, it is important to avoid over-the-counter (OTC) drugs that may harm kidney function. Regular monitoring of renal function is essential to detect any adverse effects early.

Support System at Individual, Family, and Community Levels

This level mainly includes the availability of resources, accessibility, and interaction between individuals and healthcare providers and also the caregivers who are mostly the family members.

- *Increased DKD awareness*: Increased DKD awareness is crucial for early detection and management. Education and awareness at individual levels lead to early detection and the avoidance of progression of the disease.
- *Education and support*: Education and support for DKD are very important. It includes education on self-management of plasma glucose levels, counseling, and guidance on diet and lifestyle changes. These supports should be made available through appropriate healthcare professionals on online platforms, too.
- *Multidisciplinary care*: A multidisciplinary team for DKD at the primary care level includes a physician, nurse, diabetic educator/dietitian, and psychosocial counselors. Each team member should focus on specific aspects of care for preventing kidney damage and managing other complications in people with diabetes.

Screening and Early Intervention

- Increased screening and early detection of DKD at the individual and community levels are crucial to prevent DKD.
- Screening at healthcare services, mainly primary care, also helps in identifying people with DKD and will be of help in the prevention of progression of the disease.
- Early screening helps in early interventions, which include therapies such as glucose, BP, and lipid management.

Capacity Building (Both at Health Services and Community Levels)

Developing EHR tools for DKD prevention and management: Creating electronic health records (EHR) systems that integrate patient data to facilitate early screening, detection, and education for DKD prevention and management.

Training healthcare providers: It is crucial to enhance the capacity and skills of healthcare providers to screen and diagnose DKD. This can be achieved through tailored educational programs, including interactive webinars, workshops, case studies, and online modules that offer continuing education credits.

Engaging policymakers and expanding health information technology: Policymakers should prioritize health equity when developing policies to ensure all individuals with diabetes have equal access to care. Bridging the digital divide is essential to ensure that all communities have access to digital health tools, ultimately improving DKD prevention, early detection, and management.

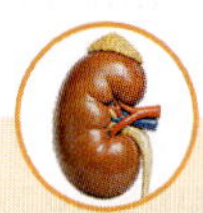

- *Use EHR systems for early DKD screening and education*
- *Educate healthcare providers on DKD screening and management*
- *Ensure equitable access to digital health tools for DKD prevention*

STRATEGIES FOR IMPLEMENTATION OF COMMUNITY-BASED PREVENTION PROGRAM

Implementation is the most challenging part of the DKD prevention program, more so in a large country like India. Other community-based programs that were implemented in low-populated smaller countries like Australia and Singapore[65,66] are not suitable in India because of the diversified and huge population size. A community-based prevention study of chronic renal failure conducted in India[67] looked quite encouraging, but is still far away and also needs to be accepted by healthcare policy makers. The most possible way and the best approach will be screening of DKD in the high-risk group, like the first-degree relatives of people with diabetes and hypertension and annual screening of people

with established diabetes and hypertension. Studies on insulin-dependent diabetes mellitus (IDDM) show that individuals with a family history of nephropathy face a 72% increased long-term risk of developing nephropathy, compared to just 25% in patients whose relatives do not have kidney disease.[68] This familial aggregation is notably significant, even in cases of nephropathy associated with hypertension.[69] Programs like the Kidney Early Evaluation Program (KEEP) and those focusing on family history of end-stage renal disease (ESRD) in the United States highlight the importance of familial screening within high-risk groups.[70,71] Additionally, large-scale screening camps at the community level play a crucial role in early detection and prevention in these high-risk population. Hence, the key points to be considered in framing and implementation of DKD prevention programs at community level are summarized in **Box 1**.

> **BOX 1: Key points in framing and implementing preventive DKD programs at the community level.**
>
> - Assessment of the burden of DKD at the national or regional level by conducting multicentric studies and framing targeted interventions for high-risk groups to minimize the DKD progression
> - Education and training programs on burden and prevention of DKD to healthcare providers and to conduct awareness programs through a multimedia approach to the general population
> - Proper planning and implementation of regular screening of DKD (dipstick for albuminuria and serum creatinine for eGFR) in people with diabetes and hypertension
> - Screening the first-degree relatives of people with DKD, as they are at high risk and identifying them for early detection of DKD
> - Referral of people diagnosed with DKD to an appropriate health facility and ensuring the use of evidence-based therapies, including pharmacological and lifestyle interventions to prevent or halt the progression of DKD
>
> (DKD: diabetic kidney disease)

CONCLUSION

Diabetic kidney disease affects nearly half of those with T2D and is a leading cause of ESRD. Preventive care, early screening, and targeted therapies are essential to slow its progression and improve outcomes. Preventing DKD progression involves lifestyle changes such as quitting smoking, reducing alcohol intake, including a weight loss program, exercises, and personalized dietary adjustments that include moderate protein and sodium intake. These strategies improve glycemic control, reduce hypertension, and slow kidney damage more effectively, in addition to the pharmacological treatment. Overall, good management of diabetes represents the best strategy for the prevention of DKD.

SUMMARY

Diabetic kidney disease is a common complication of long-term, poorly controlled diabetes in both people with T1D and T2D. Early diagnosis through the detection of microalbuminuria and a decline in eGFR is crucial for preventing the progression of DKD. Although DKD has a gradual onset, there are several risk factors and associated diseases that can exacerbate renal injury and DKD progression. Framing of a comprehensive preventive approach for DKD includes glycemic control, treatment of hypertension, and hyperlipidemia comorbidities, and lifestyle modifications (diet, exercise, and smoking cessation) are important. Patient education on DKD in the clinical setting with an interdisciplinary care team is equally important and highly encouraged. Since DKD is initially asymptomatic, early intervention through patient education is an essential step in the collective goal to reduce the future DKD and ESRD burden. Nonalbuminuric DKD generally has a better prognosis than albuminuric DKD, even when kidney function is severely impaired. However, it still presents a significant cardiovascular risk. Nonalbuminuric DKD has a better prognosis than albuminuric DKD when kidney function is severely decreased. Thus, early screening and diagnosis at the individual and community level, self-management of blood sugars, awareness and education on diabetes and its complications, along with other comorbid conditions, play a key role in prevention and management strategies to optimize beneficial outcomes in DKD. Capacity building of the healthcare team and regular efforts to frame appropriate policies and strategies are important to deal with chronic conditions like diabetes and the prevention of DKD.

TAKE HOME MESSAGES

- All people with diabetes should be screened for DKD, and should undergo regular screening for albuminuria and eGFR.
- The key objective in the management of DKD is to prevent the decline of GFR. This can be achieved by optimizing glycemic control (target HbA1c <7%), blood pressure control (target BP < 130/80 mm Hg), and optimal lipid profiles (LDL of <100 mg/dL).
- The prevention care model approach is highly recommended to prevent or delay the onset of DKD and can be achieved at the primary care level.

REFERENCES

1. Guo W, Song Y, Sun Y, Du H, Cai Y, You Q, et al. Systemic immune-inflammation index is associated with DKD in Type 2 diabetes mellitus patients: Evidence from NHANES 2011-2018. Front Endocrinol (Lausanne). 2022;13:1071465.

2. He Y, Wang X, Li L, Liu M, Wu Y, Chen R, et al. Global, Regional, and National Prevalence of Chronic Type 2 DKD From 1990 to 2021: A Trend and Health Inequality Analyses Based on the Global Burden of Disease Study 2021. J Diabetes. 2025;17(5):e70098.

3. Makmun A, Satirapoj B, Tuyen DG, Foo MWY, Danguilan R, Gulati S, et al. The burden of chronic kidney disease in Asia region: a review of the evidence, current challenges, and future directions. Kidney Res Clin Pract. 2025;44(3):411-33.

4. International Diabetes Federation. (2023). Diabetes and Kidney Disease. [online] Available from https://diabetesatlas.org/resources/idf-diabetes-atlas-reports/diabetes-and-kidney-disease/[Last accessed March, 2026].

5. American Diabetes Association. 11. Microvascular complications and foot care: Standards of medical care in diabetes-2020. Diabetes Care. 2020;43:S135-51.

6. Bierhaus A, Humpert PM, Morcos M, Wendt T, Chavakis T, Arnold B, et al. Understanding RAGE, the Receptor for Advanced Glycation End Products. J Mol Med. 2005;83:876-86.

7. Oda Y, Nishi H, Nangaku M. Role of Inflammation in Progression of Chronic Kidney Disease in Type 2 Diabetes Mellitus: Clinical Implications. Semin Nephrol. 2023;43(3):151431.

8. Lin YC, Chang YH, Yang SY, Wu KD, Chu TS. Update of pathophysiology and management of DKD. J Formos Med Assoc. 2018;117(8):662-75.

9. Viswanathan V, Tilak P, Meerza R, Kumpatla S. Insulin resistance at different stages of DKD in India. J Assoc Physicians India. 2010;58:612-5.

10. Writing Team for the Diabetes Control and Complications Trial/Epidemiology of Diabetes Interventions and Complications Research Group. Sustained effect of intensive treatment of type 1 diabetes mellitus on development and progression of diabetic nephropathy: The Epidemiology of Diabetes Interventions and Complications (EDIC) study. JAMA. 2003;290:2159-67.

11. Kalra OP. Preventive strategies for diabetic nephropathy. In: Singal RK (Ed). Medicine Update. The Association of Physicians of India. New Delhi: Jaypee Brothers Medical Publishers; 2007. pp. 261-72.

12. UK Prospective Diabetes Study Group. Intensive blood-glucose control with sulphonylureas or insulin compared with conventional treatment and risk of complications in patients with type 2 diabetes: UKPDS 33. Lancet. 1998;352:837-53.

13. Ismail-Beigi F, Craven T, Banerji MA, Basile J, Calles J, Cohen RM, et al.; ACCORD Trial Group. Effect of intensive treatment of hyperglycaemia on microvascular outcomes in type 2 diabetes: an analysis of the ACCORD randomised trial. Lancet. 2010;376(9739):419-30.

14. ElSayed NA, Aleppo G, Aroda VR, Bannuru RR, Brown FM, Bruemmer D, et al.; American Diabetes Association. 6-Glycemic targets: Standards of Care in Diabetes—2023. Diabetes Care. 2023;46(Suppl. 1):S97-S110.

15. Kidney Disease: Improving Global Outcomes Diabetes Work Group. KDIGO 2020 clinical practice guideline for diabetes management in chronic kidney disease. Kidney Int. 2020;98(Suppl.):S1-S115.

16. Leehey DJ, Zhang JH, Emanuele NV, Whaley-Connell A, Palevsky PM, Reilly RF, et al.; VA NEPHRON-D Study Group. BP and renal outcomes in DKD: the Veterans Affairs Nephropathy in Diabetes Trial. Clin J Am Soc Nephrol. 2015;10:2159-69.

17. Viswanathan V, Smina TP. Blood pressure control in diabetes-the Indian perspective. J Hum Hypertens. 2019;33(8):588-93.

18. Sahay BK. API-ICP guidelines on diabetes 2007. J Assoc Physicians India. 2007;55:1-50.

19. Hypertension in Diabetic Study (HDS). Prevalence of hypertension in newly presenting type 2 diabetic patients and the association with risk factors for cardiovascular and diabetic complications. J Hypertens. 1993;11:309-17.

20. Cushman WC, Evans GW, Byington RP, Goff DC Jr, Grimm RH Jr, Cutler JA, et al. Effects of intensive blood-pressure control in type 2 diabetes mellitus. N Engl J Med. 2010;362:1575-85.

21. Zac-Varghese S, Winocour P. Managing DKD. Br Med Bull. 2018;125:55-66.

22. UK Prospective Diabetes Study Group. Tight blood pressure control and risk of macrovascular and microvascular complications in type 2 diabetes: UKPDS 38. BMJ. 1998;317:703-13.

23. ACCORD Study Group. Effects of intensive blood-pressure control in type 2 diabetes mellitus. N Engl J Med. 2010;362(17):1575-85.

24. Chobanian AV, Bakris GL, Black HR, Cushman WC, Green LA, Izzo JL Jr, et al. The Seventh Report of the Joint National Committee on Prevention, Detection, Evaluation, and Treatment of High Blood Pressure: The JNC 7 report. JAMA. 2003;289:2560-72.

25. ElSayed NA, Aleppo G, Aroda VR, Bannuru RR, Brown FM, Bruemmer D, et al.; American Diabetes Association. 11. Chronic kidney disease and risk management: Standards of Care in Diabetes—2023. Diabetes Care. 2023;46(Suppl. 1):S191-S202.

26. Kidney Disease: Improving Global Outcomes (KDIGO) CKD Work Group. KDIGO 2024 Clinical Practice Guideline for the Evaluation and Management of Chronic Kidney Disease. Kidney Int. 2024;105(4S):S117-S314.

27. Tuttle KR, Bakris GL, Bilous RW, Chiang JL, de Boer IH, Goldstein-Fuchs J, et al. DKD: A report from an ADA Consensus Conference. Diabetes Care. 2014;37:2864-83.

28. Ansquer JC, Foucher C, Rattier S, Taskinen MR, Steiner G; DAIS Investigators. Fenofibrate reduces progression to microalbuminuria over 3 years in a placebo-controlled study in type 2 diabetes: results from the Diabetes Atherosclerosis Intervention Study (DAIS). Am J Kidney Dis. 2005;45:485-93.

29. Collins R, Armitage J, Parish S, Sleigh P, Peto R. MRC/BHF Heart Protection Study of cholesterol lowering with simvastatin in 5963 people with diabetes: A randomized placebo-controlled trial. Lancet. 2003;361:2005-16.

30. Elam M, Lovato L, Ginsberg H. The ACCORD-Lipid study: implications for treatment of dyslipidemia in Type 2 diabetes mellitus. Clin Lipidol. 2011;6(1): 9-20.

31. Pan Y, Guo LL, Jin HM. Low-protein diet for diabetic nephropathy: A meta-analysis of randomized controlled trials. Am J Clin Nutr. 2008;88:660-6.

32. Association AD. Microvascular Complications and Foot Care: Standards of Medical Care in Diabetes-2020. Diabetes Care. 2020;43:S135-51.

33. Sulaiman MK. Diabetic nephropathy: Recent advances in pathophysiology and challenges in dietary management. Diabetol Metab Syndr. 2019;11:7.

34. Dhemla S, Varma K. Salt intake in India-an alarming situation. JFAV. 2015;5(1):1-10.

35. Ravi S, Bermudez OI, Harivanzan V, Kenneth Chui KH, Vasudevan P, Must A, et al. Sodium Intake, Blood Pressure, and Dietary Sources of Sodium in an Adult South Indian Population. Ann Glob Health. 2016;82(2):234-42.

36. Smina TP, Kumpatla S, Viswanathan V. Higher dietary salt and inappropriate proportion of macronutrients consumption among people with diabetes and other co morbid conditions in South India: Estimation of salt intake with a formula. Diabetes Metab Syndr. 2019;13(5):2863-8.

37. Qiu Z, Zheng K, Zhang H, Feng J, Wang L, Zhou H. Physical Exercise and Patients with Chronic Renal Failure: A Meta-Analysis. Biomed Res Int. 2017;2017:7191826.

38. Remuzzi G. Cigarette smoking and renal function impairment. Am J Kidney Dis. 1994;33:807-13.

39. Orth SR, Stockmann A, Conradt C, Ritz E, Ferro M, Kreusser W, et al. Smoking as a risk factor for end stage renal failure in men with primary renal disease. Kidney Int. 1998;54:9.

40. Liao D, Ma L, Liu J, Fu P. Cigarette smoking as a risk factor for diabetic nephropathy: A systematic review and meta-analysis of prospective cohort studies. PLoS One. 2019;14:e0210213.

41. Onyenwenyi C, Ricardo AC. Impact of Lifestyle Modification on DKD. Curr Diab Rep. 2015;15:60.

42. Shibata M, Sato KK, Koh H, Shibata I, Okamura K, Takeuchi Y, et al. The Relationship of Alcohol Consumption and Drinking Pattern to the Risk of Glomerular Hyperfiltration in Middle-aged Japanese Men: The Kansai Healthcare Study. J Epidemiol. 2024;34(3):137-43.

43. Roy S, Schweiker-Kahn O, Jafry B, Masel-Miller R, Raju RS, O'Neill LMO, et al. Risk Factors and Comorbidities associated with DKD. J Prim Care Comm Health. 2021;12:21501327211048556.

44. Yang X. Association between drinking patterns and DKD in United States adults: a cross-sectional study based on data from NHANES 1999-2016. Ren Fail. 2025;47(1):2454970.

45. de Boer IH, Khunti K, Sadusky T, Tuttle KR, Neumiller JJ, Rhee CM, et al. Diabetes Management in Chronic Kidney Disease: A Consensus Report by the American Diabetes Association (ADA) and Kidney Disease: Improving Global Outcomes (KDIGO). Diabetes Care. 2022;45(12):3075-90.

46. Viswanathan V, Snehalatha C, Shina K, Ramachandran A. Persistent microalbuminuria in type 1 diabetic subjects in South India. Diabetes Res Clin Pract. 2003;59(3):127-31.

47. Viswanathan V, Nalr MB, Suresh S, Chamukuttan S, Ambady R. An Inexpensive Method to Diagnose Incipient Diabetic Nephropathy in Developing Countries. Diabetes Care. 2005;28(5):1259-60.

48. Centers for Disease Control and Prevention. (2023). Chronic kidney disease in the United States, 2023. [online] Available from https://www.cdc.gov/kidney-disease/php/data-research/index.html [Last accessed March, 2026]

49. American Diabetes Association. 11. Microvascular complications and foot care: standards of medical care in diabetes—2019. Diabetes Care. 2019;42(suppl 1):S124-S138.

50. Viswanathan V, Chamukuttan S, Kuniyil S, Ambady R. Evaluation of a simple, random urine test for prospective analysis of proteinuria in type 2 diabetes: a six year follow-up study. Diabetes Res Clin Pract. 2000;49(2-3):143-7.

51. Reidy K, Kang HM, Hostetter T, Susztak K. Molecular mechanisms of DKD. J Clin Invest. 2014;124(6):2333-40.

52. KDOQI. Clinical practice guidelines and clinical practice recommendations for diabetes and chronic kidney disease. Am J Kidney Dis. 2007;49(2 suppl 2):S12-S154.

53. Deem M, Rice J, Valentine K, Zavertnik JE, Lakra M. Screening for DKD in primary care: A quality improvement initiative. Nurse Pract. 2020;45(4):34-41.

54. MacIsaac RJ, Tsalamandris C, Panagiotopoulos S, Smith TJ, McNeil KJ, Jerums G. Nonalbuminuric

renal insufficiency in type 2 diabetes. Diabetes Care. 2004;27(1):195-200.

55. Samsu N. Diabetic nephropathy: Challenges in pathogenesis, diagnosis, and treatment. Biomed Res Int. 2021;2021:1497449.

56. Shi S, Ni L, Gao L, Wu X. Comparison of nonalbuminuric and albuminuric DKD among patients with type 2 diabetes: A systematic review and meta-analysis. Front Endocrinol (Lausanne). 2022;13:871272.

57. Penno G, Solini A, Bonora E, Fondelli C, Orsi E, Zerbini G, et al. Clinical significance of nonalbuminuric renal impairment in type 2 diabetes. J Hypertens. 2011;29:1802-9.

58. Thorn LM, Gordin D, Harjutsalo V, Hägg S, Masar R, Saraheimo M, et al. The presence and consequence of nonalbuminuric chronic kidney disease in patients with type 1 diabetes. Diabetes Care. 2015;38:2128-33.

59. Selby NM, Taal MW. An updated overview of diabetic nephropathy: Diagnosis, prognosis, treatment goals and latest guidelines. Diabetes Obes Metab. 2020;22 Suppl 1:3-15.

60. Satyavani K, Kothandan H, Jayaraman M, Viswanathan V. Direct costs associated with chronic kidney disease among type 2 diabetic patients in India. Indian J Nephrol. 2014;24(3):141-7.

61. Viswanathan V. Prevention of diabetic nephropathy: a diabetologist's perspective. Indian J Nephrol. 2004;14:157-62.

62. ElSayed NA, Bannuru RR, Bakris G, Bardsley J, de Boer IH, Gabbay RA, et al. DKD Prevention Care Model Development. Clin Diabetes. 2024;42(2):274-94.

63. Agarwal SK. Chronic kidney disease and its prevention in India. Kidney Int Suppl. 2005;(98):S41-5.

64. Ghotekar LH, Yadav M. Current Strategies for Preventing DKD. Int J Adv Med Health Res. 2025;12(1):4-11.

65. Hoy W, Wang Z, Baker PRA, Kelly AM. Reduction in natural death and renal failure from a systematic screening and treatment program in an Australian Aboriginal community. Kidney Int. 2003;63(Suppl 83):S66-S73.

66. Ramirez SBP, Hsu SIH, Mcclellan W. Taking the public health approach to the prevention of end stage renal disease: The NKF Singapore program. Kidney Int. 2003;63(Suppl 83):S61-5.

67. Mani MK. Prevention of chronic renal failure at the community level. Kidney Int. 2003;63(Suppl 83):S86-9.

68. Quinn M, Angelico MC, Warram JH, Krolewski AS. Familial factors determine the development of diabetic nephropathy in patients with IDDM. Diabetologia. 1996;39:940-5.

69. Freedman BI, Tuttle AB, Spray BJ. Familial predisposition to nephropathy in African-Americans with non–insulin-dependent diabetes mellitus. Am J Kidney Dis. 1995;25:710-3.

70. Brown WW, Peters RM, Ohmit SE, Keane WF, Collins A, Chen SC, et al. Early detection of kidney disease in community setting. The Kidney Early Evaluation Program (KEEP). Am J Kidney Dis. 2003;42:22-35.

71. Freedman BI, Soucie JM, Mcclellan WM. Family history of end stage renal disease among incident dialysis patients. J Am Soc Nephrol. 1997;8:1942-5.

Key Research Takeaway

LETTERS

An Inexpensive Method to Diagnose Incipient Diabetic Nephropathy in Developing Countries

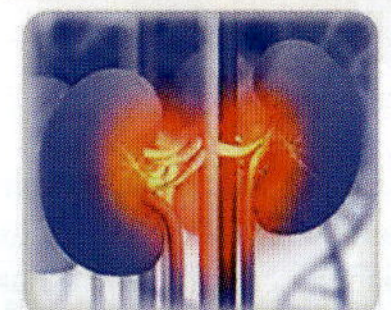

Diabetic patients with microalbuminuria are at a high risk for developing overt nephropathy and cardiovascular complications (1). Constantmonitoring is mandatory to prevent vascular complications. Due to socioeconomic reasons, many patients in developing countries cannot afford to regularly test their blood glucose. In such a scenario, the test of urine albumin-tocreatinine ratio or albumin excretion rate to diagnose diabetic albuminuria is beyond the reach of many patients. In addition, only a few speciality centers provide facilities for doing these tests. Urine protein dipstick testing is, however, easily available to most patients. We aimed to evaluate whether a dipstick test showing "trace" for urinary protein reliably indicated the presence of microalbuminuria. Urine dipstick for protein was done in 500 consecutive random urine samples of type 2 diabetic subjects, using Uristik (Bayer Diagnostics India). The results were read visually as "negative" or as "positive," indicated as trace, 1, 2, or greater, representing a protein concentration of 0.15, 0.15– 0.30, 0.30, or 1 g/l, respectively. Three trained technicians tested all samples, and the interobserver variations were 5%, measured statistically. Urine microscopy was done on all samples, and samples with significant presence of white blood cells and other cell types were excluded. Among the 500 urine samples, 360 were negative for dipstick, 99 were trace, and 41 were 1or greater. In the subjects without clinical proteinuria (n 459), albumin-to-creatinine ratio was determined. The results were ranked as normoalbuminuria (men 2.5, women 3.5 mg/mmol [n 356]) and microalbuminuria(men 2.525, women 3.5–35 mg/mmol; n 103). Quantification of urine creatinine (mg/dl) was by the Jaffe method, urine albumin by immunoturbidimetry, and urine protein by the biuret method using a Hitachi 912 analyzer (Roche, Mannheim, Germany). The data of 459 urine samples were used to determine the sensitivity and specificity of the dipstick to detect a negative or a positive test. The sensitivity, specificity, positive predictive value, and negative predictive value of trace to detect microalbuminuria were 68, 98, 92, and 88%, respectively; the accuracy was 89%. This study showed that the dipstick test with a reading of trace = was highly specific and fairly sensitive in determining the presence of microalbuminuria. Micral-test II was found to be an effective screening tool in various Caucasian studies (2). However, even micral-test II is an expensive screening tool in develop-ing countries. In a study by Baskar et al. (3), Combur 5 test D strips (Roche Diagnostics, Vilvoorde, Belgium) were found to have little or no benefit in repeat testing outside the low microalbuminuric range. In our study, we found that the positive test had 98% sensitivity and 100% specificity to determine proteinuria. In developing countries like India, the cost of doing an albumin-to-creatinine ratio in a random sample is $5.60 U.S. (INR 250), while 100 patients can be screened for albuminuria by a dipstick at the cost of $9.80 U.S. (INR 439). A repeat test is, however, essential in positive cases to ascertain the presence of microalbuminuria or proteinuria. The cost efficiency and the high sensitivity and specificity of the urine dipstick test will =encourage its use among primary care physicians and private practitioners as a diagnostic tool for microalbuminuria and proteinuria. This would initiate the first step toward detection of incipient diabetic nephropathy in developing countries.

Vijay Viswanathan, Md, Phd

Mamtha B. Nair, Msc

Sheethal Suresh, Msc

Snehalatha Chamukuttan, Msc, Dsc

Ramachandran Ambady, Md, Phd, Dsc, Frcp

Diabetes Care, volume 28, number 5, May 2005

Evaluation of a simple, random urine test for prospective analysis of proteinuria in Type 2 diabetes: a six year follow-up study

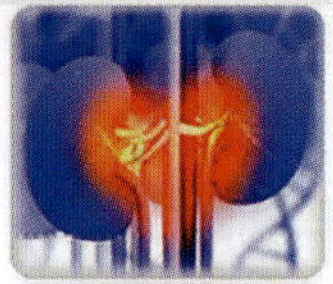

Vijay Viswanathan *, Snehalatha Chamukuttan, Shina Kuniyil, Ramachandran Ambady

Diabetes Research Centre, No. 4, Main Road, Royapuram, Madras 600 013, India

Received 13 September 1999; received in revised form 26 January 2000; accepted 12 February 2000

Abstract

Aim: To assess the usefulness of an estimated proteinuria (EPE) using the protein to creatinine ratio (P:C ratio) in a random urine sample for follow-up evaluation of kidney function in diabetic patients. Research designs and methods: 410 newly registered Type 2 diabetic patients had annual follow-up for 6 years (M:F 263:147). EPE was calculated by estimation of P:C ratio in random urine sample. Based on the EPE they were divided into those with normal protein excretion (B100 mg:dl), mild proteinuria (100 to B500 mg:dl) and nephropathy (persistent proteinuria \500mg:dl) cases. The study subjects were divided into 4 groups based on the proteinuria status at follow-up. Anthropometry, measurement of blood pressure and retinopathy were carried out for all study subjects.

Results: at the baseline, 342 (83.4%) had normal protein excretion, 53 (12.9%) had mild proteinuria and 15 (3.7%) had nephropathy. At the follow-up the respective numbers were 276 (67.3%), 64 (15.6%) and 70(17%). During the study period nephropathy developed in 55 (13.4%) and mild proteinuria in 11 (2.7%). Nephropathy developed in 32 (6.7%) subjects in the non-proteinuria group and in 23 (43.4%) of the mild proteinuric subjects. Conversion to nephropathy was greater in the latter group (x241.6, PB0.0001). Nephropathy cases had higher duration of diabetes at the baseline (8.896.4 years) and at follow-up (7.196.0 years) and higher prevalence of hypertension when compared with non-proteinuric group (60 and 43.5% compared with 11.1%, PB0.01). New cases of hypertension were detected in 32.8% of proteinuric and 0.7% of normal protein excretion subjects (x232.24, P0.0001). During the follow-up 55 of the 70 nephropathy subjects (78.6%) developed retinopathy compared with ten out of the 276 subjects with normal protein excretion (3.6%) (x2200.6, P0.0001).

Conclusion: EPE is useful in serial evaluation of kidney function. The risk conferred by hypertension, mild proteinuria and duration of diabetes in producing nephropathy are also highlighted. EPE could be used in developing countries to assess the renal function on a follow-up basis.

Persistent Microalbuminuria in Type 1 Diabetic Subjects in South India.

V Viswanathan, C Snehalatha, K Shina, A Ramachandran

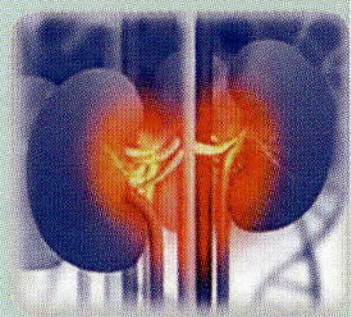

Aim : There are only a few reports on the prevalence Of microalbuminuria (MAU) in type I diabetic subjects in India. This study was done to assess the prevalence of MAU in South Indian diabetic subjects.

Material and Methods : MAU was estimated by measuring albumin/creatinine ratio in an early morning urine sample on three occasions using immunoturbidimetry (> 30 pg albumin/mg creatinine) in South Indian patients. Kidney function tests were done in 95 type I DM, (M:F, 56:39). Persistent proteinuria was detected in 17 (17.9%) and they were excluded from the study. Further details were taken only in the remaining 78 subjects. Persistent MAU was seen in 22 (28.2%) and other 56 subjects had normoalbuminuria (NAU) (71.8%).

Results : There was no significant difference in the age, duration of DM and the average HbAlc between MAU and NAU. MAU developed at the age of 2 20 years, even in subjects with onset of diabetes at a younger age. Diabetic retinopathy was present in 3 (13.6%) and ECG abnormalities were seen in one patient with MAU. None of the subjects in NAU group had these abnormalities. Prevalence of MAU increased with increasing duration of diabetes, MAU was present in 3 patients (10.3%) with duration of diabetes S 5 years, in five patients (23.8%) with duration of diabetes > 5 to S 10 years and in 14 (50%) patients with duration of diabetes > 10 years. Hypertension was present in 5 (22.7%) of MAU and only in one subject with NAG.

Conclusion : It is observed that MAU occurs in type I diabetes after the age of 20 years and it is present in a large proportion of the study subjects.

J Assoc Physicians India 2022;50:1259-1261

Indian J Nephrol 2004;14: 157–162

Prevention of diabetic nephropathy: A diabetologist's perspective

V Viswanathan
Diabetes Research Centre, [WHO Collaborating Centre for Research, Education and Training in Diabetes], Chennai

Abstract

Diabetes mellitus causes considerable morbidity and mortality due to micro and macro vascular complications. One such complication is diabetic nephropathy which causes chronic renal failure in 30% of diabetic patients in India. Early diagnosis and detection of risk factors for diabetic nephropathy is important step for prevention of diabetic nephropathy.

Diabetes mellitus is a major health problem1 and causes considerable morbidity and mortality primarily due to micro and macro vascular complications. The prevalence of diabetes is increasing globally and the maximum increase is expected to be in developing countries like India. By the year 2010, it is estimated that nearly 220 million people worldwide will have diabetes. India is facing a major health care burden due to the high prevalence of type 2 diabetes and there are indications that this would increase further in the next few decades. Diabetes is preventable and so are its complications. One such microvascular complication of diabetes is diabetic nephropathy. Nearly 30% of chronic renal failures in India are due to diabetic nephropathy2. Nonetheless attention towards diabetic nephropathy is not directed until the patient has progressed towards the stage of renal failure. Nephropathy due to diabetes can be diagnosed very easily and can be prevented. This review article aims at describing diabetic nephropathy, its prevalence and pathogenesis and management. Diabetic nephropathy is clinically defined by the presence of persistent proteinuria of > 500 mg/day in a diabetic patient who has concomitant diabetic retinopathy and hypertension and in the absence of clinical or laboratory evidence of other kidney or renal tract disease3.

Increased prevalence of diabetic nephropathy in South Asians

Racial differences in the prevalence of diabetic renal disease have been reported. Asian subjects have significantly (p < 0.01) higher prevalence (52.6%) of diabetic end stage renal disease (ESRD) when compared with the Caucasians (36.2%)4. Migrant Asian Indians had 40 times greater risk of developing ESRD when compared with the Caucasians5. The prevalence of diabetic nephropathy in type 2 diabetic subjects is reported to be 5-9% from various Indian studies6,7,8. Patients with diabetic nephropathy, especially with type 2 diabetes, have a high cardiovascular risk. The risk for cardiovascular disease (CVD) was 3 fold higher in South Indian NIDDM subjects with nephropathy when compared with their non-nephropathic counterparts9. Thus, in type 2 diabetes, many patients may not reach end stage renal disease due to premature death from CVD.

Pathophysiology

The pathogenesis of diabetic nephropathy is multifactorial and genetic susceptibility has been proposed to be an important factor in the development and progression of diabetic nephropathy. Two major causative factors have been implicated in the development of diabetic nephropathy: metabolic and hemodynamic. Three major histologic changes occur in the glomeruli in diabetic nephropathy (1) mesangial expansion is directly induced by hyperglycemia, perhaps via increased matrix production or glycosylation of matrix proteins, (2) glomerular basement membrane thickening occurs, (3) glomerular sclerosis is caused by

11

Diabetic Foot Ulcers and Renal Dysfunction: A Complex Interplay

Manisha Jadaun, Rajeshwar Singh Jadaun, Sivashankari Selva Elavarasan

- ➤ Risk factors and development of renal dysfunction in people with diabetes
- ➤ Pathophysiological links between diabetic foot ulcer (DFU) and chronic kidney disease (CKD)
- ➤ Acute kidney injury (AKI) due to DFUs
- ➤ Impact of AKI on diabetic foot wound healing
- ➤ Impact of CKD on DFU progression and wound healing
- ➤ End-stage renal disease and AKI (acute-on-chronic injury)
- ➤ Management of diabetic foot disease (DFD) with renal dysfunction

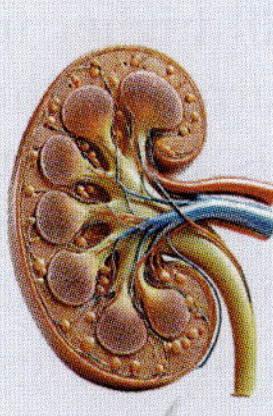

Abstract

A varying degree of renal dysfunction occurs as a serious complication of diabetes mellitus, from a combination of the associated triad of peripheral sensorimotor neuropathy, ischemia, and infection-related foot ulcers. Multiple pathophysiological links exist between renal impairment and foot ulcers, suggestive of a bidirectional relationship, as chronic kidney disease (CKD) may be found in up to 40% of patients with long-standing diabetes and significantly worsened prognosis with 75% 2-year mortality postamputation is found in patients with diabetic foot ulcers with concomitant end-stage renal disease (ESRD) with ongoing dialysis.

Nephropathy may progress to ESRD in the presence of risk factors such as elevated glycosylated hemoglobin (HbA1c), hypertension, microalbuminuria, or gross proteinuria. High mortality has been reported in cases of diabetes with chronic renal disease/ESRD and poorly perfused lower limbs with low ankle brachial index (ABI). Advanced cases of CKD with associated uremic nephropathy adversely affect the immune system and perfusion of the lower limbs. In cases of moderate to severe diabetic foot infections, acute kidney injury (AKI) may be precipitated due to sepsis and nephrotoxic drug use. The spot urine-protein-creatinine ratio provides a good estimate of total protein excretion per day from the kidneys. Screening of diabetes patients for diabetic kidney disease (DKD) to focus on elevated serum creatinine, proteinuria, assessment of peripheral circulation, and foot at regular intervals and good glycemic control (HbA1c near target values) to improve wound healing.

Keywords: Diabetic foot ulcer, acute kidney injury, chronic kidney disease, diabetic kidney disease, end-stage renal disease.

INTRODUCTION

Diabetes related renal dysfunction is a very significant and serious complication of diabetes mellitus, which is a global health challenge arising from a complex group of pathologies or from a combination of peripheral neuropathy, ischemia, and infection-related ulcers in the foot. Multiple pathophysiologic links between renal impairment and diabetic foot ulcers (DFU) as they frequently coexist with other diabetic microvascular complications such as retinopathy, vasculopathy, neuropathy, nephropathy, chronic renal failure, or end-stage renal disease (ESRD).[1] Diabetes is a strong risk factor with a bidirectional relationship for chronic kidney disease (CKD), as patients with DFUs usually have evidence of diabetic kidney disease (DKD), e.g., proteinuria or reduced glomerular filtration rate (GFR). Coexisting with DKD, hypertension, and atherosclerotic cardiovascular disease (CVD) are leading causes of morbidity and mortality in diabetics. The last decade witnessed a lot of work being done to prove the association between these two pathologies to prevent the health cost burden.

DEFINITIONS OF AKI, DKD, CKD, ESRD, AND RENAL FOOT

In the presence of severe foot infections and in the course of their treatment, acute damage to the kidneys (e.g., via sepsis or nephrotoxic antibiotics) may precipitate acute kidney injury (AKI). There is a sudden decline in renal function (e.g., rise in serum creatinine by ≥ 0.3 mg/dL within 48 hours) due to prerenal, intrinsic, or postrenal causes.

In people with diabetes, chronic involvement of the kidney is termed DKD. When renal dysfunction exists for a duration of 3 months along with kidney damage markers such as albuminuria or other electrolyte imbalances and a GFR below 60 mL/min/1.73 m^2, it is described by the term CKD. ESRD is defined as the progression of CKD or AKI characterized by a fall in GFR to below 15 mL/min/1.73 m^2. The new term "renal foot" encompasses people living with diabetes with CKD stage 4 or 5 [renal replacement therapy (RRT)], along with infected or uninfected DFU, PAD (with or without gangrene), and/or Charcot osteoarthropathy of the foot.[2]

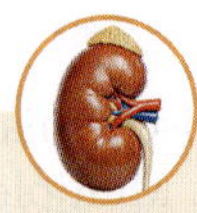

Diabetes is a strong risk factor with a bidirectional relationship for CKD, as patients with DFUs usually have evidence of DKD (e.g., proteinuria or reduced

EPIDEMIOLOGY AND RISK FACTORS

With an estimated lifetime risk of ulceration in feet of 19–34% of people with diabetes, the prevalence of diabetic foot disease (DFD) in CKD patients may be higher than that of CKD patients without diabetes and still higher in those with diabetes and ESRD. Currently, the total number of patients with CKD is more than 800 million (10% of the world's population) as per the suggestion from global prevalence, and further rise is expected in patients with diabetes, hypertension, and in the elderly age group. The prevalence of DFU in CKD patients may range from 5–10% and 15–25% depending on high to low-income countries respectively. The prevalence of DFU may rise to 22% in ESRD and in patients.

Reflecting the systemic nature of long-standing diabetes, CKD is present in up to 40% of diabetic patients, and its presence significantly worsens outcomes in DFU, particularly when on dialysis (ESRD) as per a published report; worse prognosis than many cancers with almost 70%, 5-year mortality postamputation.[3]

Initially, due to hypertension and DKD, there is microalbuminuria or gross proteinuria, nephropathy, which may progress to ESRD in the background of uncontrolled hyperglycemia.

Under the influence of risk factors other than diabetes, such as elevated systolic and diastolic blood pressures, microalbuminuria, or gross proteinuria, nephropathy occurs, which may progress to ESRD in presence of uncontrolled glycemic status or elevated glycosylated hemoglobin (HbA1c).[4] Microalbuminuria in the range of 30–300 mg/dL is a risk biomarker for CVD but does not represent renal injury. A quick, noninvasive and rapidly performed test, namely the spot urine protein/creatinine ratio, provides a good estimation of total protein excretion per day from the kidney. When microalbuminuria exceeds 300 mg albumin per day (gross proteinuria), then spot urine protein estimation is helpful. In addition to this, HbA1c values must be near target values and glycemic control must be optimal to improve wound healing, prevent diabetic foot complications, and worsening of kidney functions **(Flowchart 1)**.[5]

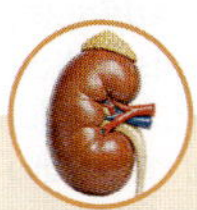

The prevalence of DFU in CKD patients may range from 5 to 10% and 15 to 25% depending on high- to low-income countries, respectively. Microalbuminuria in the range of 30–300 mg/dL is a risk biomarker for CVD but does not represent renal injury. A quick, noninvasive and rapidly performed test, namely the spot urine protein/creatinine ratio, provides a good estimation of total protein excretion per day from the kidney. When microalbuminuria exceeds 300 mg albumin per day (gross proteinuria), then spot urine protein estimation is helpful.

Multiple research trials have found a low ankle brachial index (ABI) of <0.9 to be a predictor and risk factor for coronary artery disease and peripheral vascular disease. Low ABI and poor blood supply to the feet with high mortality have been reported in cases of diabetes with chronic renal dysfunction on dialysis. It is essential to perform screening for diabetes complications, including hypertension, dyslipidemia, nephropathy, DKD, assessment of peripheral circulation, and foot at regular intervals and to focus on elevated serum creatinine, proteinuria, and renal failure.[6]

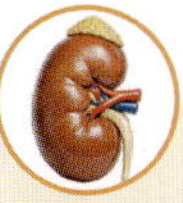

*Advanced CKD exacerbates neuropathy via uremic neuropathy and also accelerates peripheral arterial disease (PAD), compounding ischemia in the diabetic limb. In addition, immune dysfunction in uremia increases infection risk in foot wounds **(Flowchart 2)**.*

In study by Anitha Rani et al., from a tertiary diabetes center in South India it was concluded

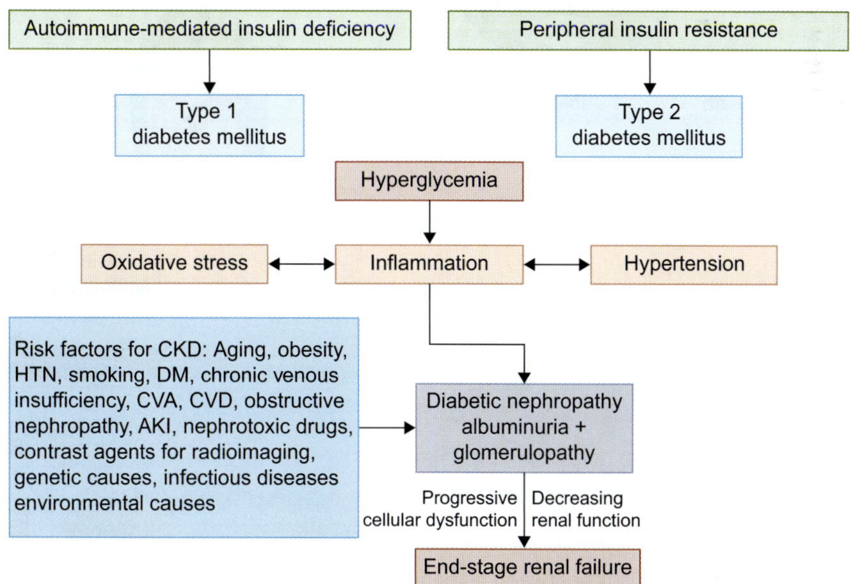

FLOWCHART 1: Risk factors and development of renal dysfunction in diabetes patients.

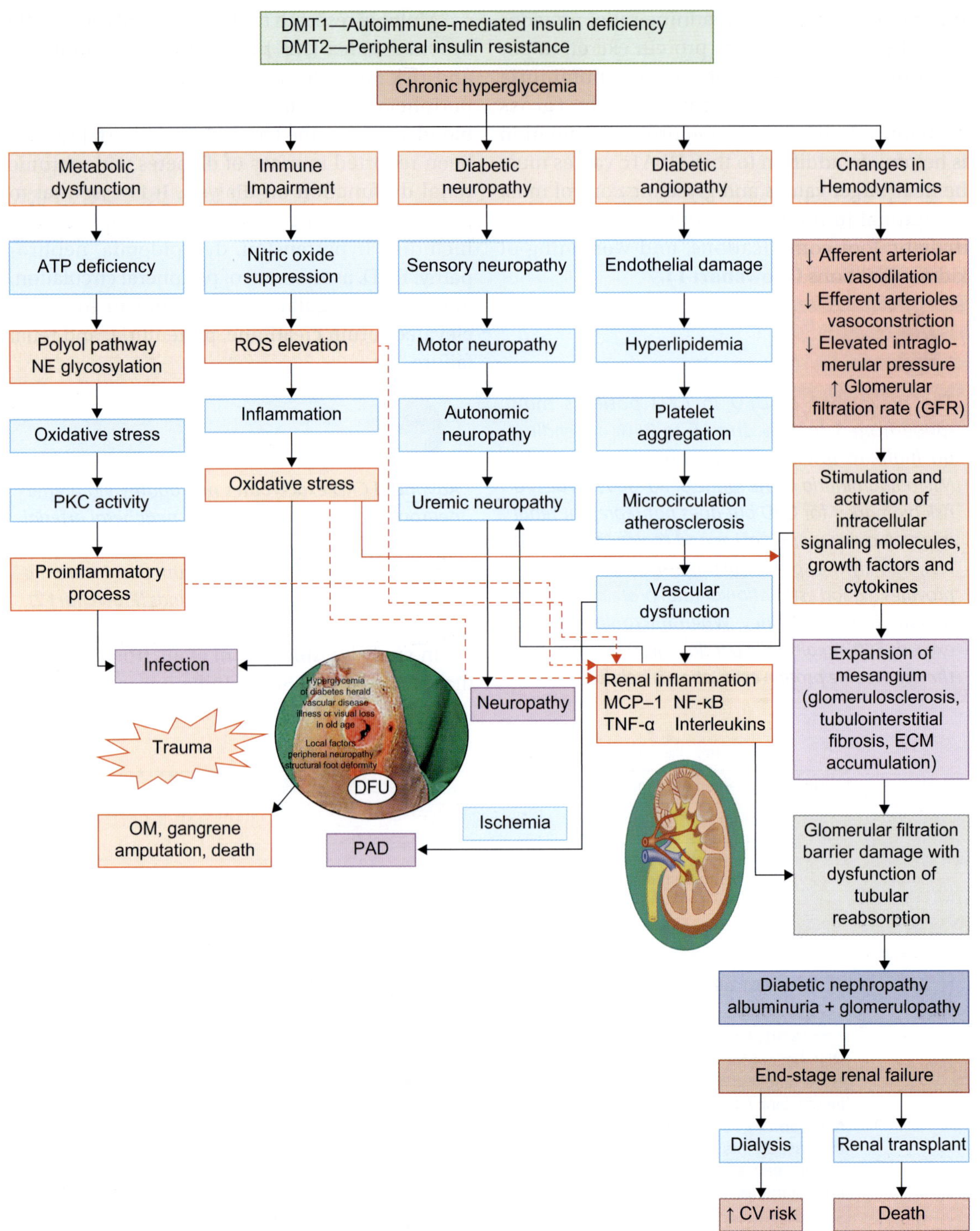

FLOWCHART 2: Pathophysiological links between diabetic foot ulcer (DFU) and chronic kidney disease (CKD) and shared mechanisms driven by diabetes and its complications [endothelial dysfunction, ischemia (peripheral arterial disease or PAD), neuropathy, infection, and impaired immunology].

that there is a significant reduction in eGFR among CKD patients with DFI and DFI patients without CKD. Hence development of DFI may cause decline in renal function irrespective of CKD status and preventive steps to prevent a DFI is mandatory in all T2DM.[7]

In another study by Smina TP et al. from South India, a gradual and uniform reduction of eGFR was observed throughout the study period in the participants affected with either CKD or DFU alone. Whereas in participants with both CKD and DFU, there was a sharp decline in the eGFR during the 6 months prior to the baseline.[8]

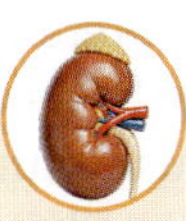

In this chapter, we shall discuss the effect of AKI on DFU healing, ESRD contributing to AKI risk (acute-on-chronic kidney injury), and how CKD/ESRD influences neuropathy, vascular insufficiency, and infection in the context of DFD.

ACUTE KIDNEY INJURY DUE TO DIABETIC FOOT ULCERS

Acute kidney injury is defined as a sudden decline in renal function (e.g., a rise in serum creatinine by ≥0.3 mg/dL within 48 hours) due to prerenal, intrinsic, or postrenal causes. Most commonly affecting hospitalized or critically ill patients as part of multiorgan dysfunction, the development of AKI is a known marker of poor prognosis. Additional risk factors for AKI are increasing age, CKD, systemic hypertension, previous history of AKI, and congestive cardiac failure. The combination of type 2 diabetes with congestive cardiac failure or systemic hypertension further increases the risk of AKI. Preexisting proteinuria, hypertension, and diabetes mellitus were all independent AKI risk factors.[9]

Proteinuria and Decreased eGFR

Research studies by Prabhu et al., Moseu et al., and other cohort studies have proven that a correlation exists between AKI incidence and lower baseline eGFR, and higher proteinuria.[10]

Hypoglycemic Agents

Diabetic patients taking oral hypoglycemic agents and posted for surgery had a 30% higher chance of developing acute renal failure in the operative period compared to those taking insulin, who had a 70% higher risk.

Drugs

Around 20% of cases are prone to develop drug-induced AKI, and the pathophysiological mechanism depends on the type of drug used, such as nephrotoxic drugs or contrast agents. Risk of AKI is considerably higher in diabetics with CKD. In diabetic foot infection cases (moderate to severe IDSA grade) with preexisting nephropathy, patients who are receiving drugs for treatment are predisposed to a high risk of acute renal injury. The angiotensin-converting enzyme inhibitor (ACEi)/angiotensin receptor blocker (ARB) is the main cause of AKI, contributing to 35% of cases due to their increased use in diabetic patients. The risk was even higher in patients with congestive heart failure, volume depletion, diuretics, hydrochlorothiazide, nonsteroidal anti-inflammatory drugs (NSAIDs), and bilateral renal artery stenosis. Drugs responsible for AKI are aminoglycosides (gentamicin) and NSAIDs, followed by statins, antitubercular agents (rifampicin), and ifosfamide, with an even higher risk with the combination of these drugs. Nonsteroidal anti-inflammatory drugs reduce GFR and renal blood flow by suppression of prostaglandin production.[11]

Contrast Agent-induced Injury

In people with diabetes and associated DN (CI-AKI), the conditions are mutually causative, causing kidney function to deteriorate further. Renal hypoxia, apoptosis, immunological changes, generation of reactive oxygen species (ROS), and increased oxidative stress in diabetic patients lead to vascular constriction due to vasoactive substances. Impaired nitrovasodilation, increased endothelin synthesis, and hyperresponsivity to adenosine-related vasoconstriction, along with an effect on peritubular blood flow. Research data show that the incidence of contrast-induced AKI ranges from 5.7 to 29.4% in diabetes patients.[12]

Dehydration

Extracellular volume depletion due to glycosuria, because of uncontrolled diabetes, especially in pediatric patients, leads to prerenal AKI. The combined effect of uncontrolled diabetes along with prerenal AKI may cause intrinsic renal AKI, characterized by renal parenchymal damage and tubular necrosis.[13]

Sepsis

Along with dysfunctional immune systems, both humoral and cell-mediated, increased neutrophil dysfunction also contributes to an increased risk of sepsis. A higher eGFR declines secondary to sepsis-related AKI compared to other etiologies. Diabetes mellitus has been demonstrated to be an independent risk factor.[14]

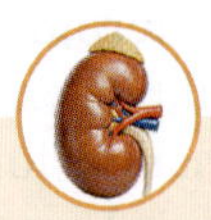

Proteinuria and decreased eGFR, hypoglycemic agents, drugs such as ACEi/ARB, aminoglycosides, NSAIDs, statins, antitubercular agents and ifosfamide, contrast agent-induced injury, dehydration and sepsis were recognized as the contributing risk factors for AKI in people with DFUs.

PATHOPHYSIOLOGY OF ACUTE KIDNEY INJURY IN PEOPLE WITH DIABETES

Multifactorial pathophysiologic mechanisms are described in causing diabetes-related kidney damage. Probably structural and functional alterations in the renal vasculature and the tubular epithelial cells increase the generation of cytokines and chemokines, which produce inflammation, ischemia, and isolated proximal tubulopathy. There is endothelial cellular dysfunction due to distorted nitric oxide (NO) metabolism in people with diabetes, and the renal vasculature is more vulnerable to stimuli that cause vasoconstriction, which leads to glomerular hyperfiltration. There is intraglomerular hypertension due to glomerular hyperfiltration that contributes to glomerulosclerosis, causing DKD with progressive decline in kidney function. A dysregulation in normal renal vascular tone or increased renal vascular resistance in the prerenal cause may exacerbate the kidney damage by renal hypoperfusion. Hyperuricemia can cause acute or chronic renal damage by crystal-mediated and crystal-independent nephropathy, glomerular injury, and tubulo-interstitial involvement, signifying dehydration. Uncontrolled blood sugars lead to increased risk of AKI, which results in CKD and ESRD via another pathophysiologic pathway. It may also lead to apoptosis of endothelial cells, vascular rarefaction and hypoxia, mitochondrial dysfunction, proximal tubular disorder, podocyte disorder, podocyte apoptosis, and autophagy.[15]

Impact of Acute Kidney Injury on Diabetic Foot Wound Healing

Effect of Acute Hyperuremia

The uremic and inflammatory milieu of AKI can significantly impair wound healing in DFUs. Renal impairment (even acute) leads to accumulation of uremic toxins and fluid/electrolyte disturbances that disrupt normal tissue repair. Uremia causes endothelial dysfunction, characterized by altered basement membranes, increased vascular permeability, and prothrombotic changes. This endothelial dysfunction reduces perfusion and oxygen delivery to the wound, delaying healing. AKI often brings fluid overload and edema as well, which can increase tissue pressure and reduce microcirculatory flow in the ulcer bed, further hampering oxygenation and nutrient delivery for healing. Additionally, acute uremia adversely affects the function of fibroblasts and keratinocytes by reducing fibroblast proliferation, collagen synthesis, and keratinocyte growth. Even short-term renal failure can thus stall the normal phases of wound repair (granulation and re-epithelialization) and lead to persistent ulcers.[16]

Metabolic and Immune Effects

Acute Kidney Injury is a highly catabolic state. Toxin accumulation (e.g., guanidines and reactive nitrogen species) and metabolic acidosis in AKI disrupt cellular metabolism and enzyme function needed for tissue regeneration. AKI-related hyperkalemia and acidosis can impair cardiac output and tissue perfusion, compounding ischemia in the extremities.[17] Moreover, acute renal failure causes immune dysfunction similar to chronic uremia—neutrophil and lymphocyte functions are blunted, and there is a proinflammatory yet immunosuppressed state. Clinically, this means an acute kidney insult can render a DFU patient less prone to fight infection, facilitating the spread of infection or sepsis. Indeed, one study noted that hyperuremia in AKI can worsen preexisting peripheral neuropathy and "promote infection" in diabetic foot wounds. The need for urgent dialysis in AKI may also remove nutrients and trace elements (such as zinc and selenium) vital for wound healing. All these factors—hemodynamic instability, toxin buildup, malnutrition, and immune impairment—converge to delay ulcer healing and can even precipitate wound deterioration or wet gangrene in a diabetic limb.[18]

Clinical Correlation

The presence of AKI in a patient with a DFU usually signifies severe illness and is associated with worse outcomes. In ICU trauma, patients with major wounds, early AKI is common (~18% incidence) and correlates with extremely high mortality (50–70%). Similarly, in diabetic foot infections, AKI often develops in the context of sepsis **(Figs. 1A and B)** or nephrotoxic antibiotic use. A study in diabetic foot patients found that GFR significantly declined after antibiotic therapy, especially with nephrotoxic regimens.[19]

This acute loss of kidney function can force clinicians to hold or dose-reduce essential antibiotics, potentially compromising infection control. It can also necessitate dialysis, which may temporarily improve uremia but poses risks of hypotension and reduced tissue perfusion during treatments. In short, AKI can complicate a DFU which in turn triggers a vicious cycle: the foot infection can cause AKI (via sepsis or drugs), and the AKI in turn impairs wound healing and infection clearance, raising the risk of amputations or death. Aggressive supportive

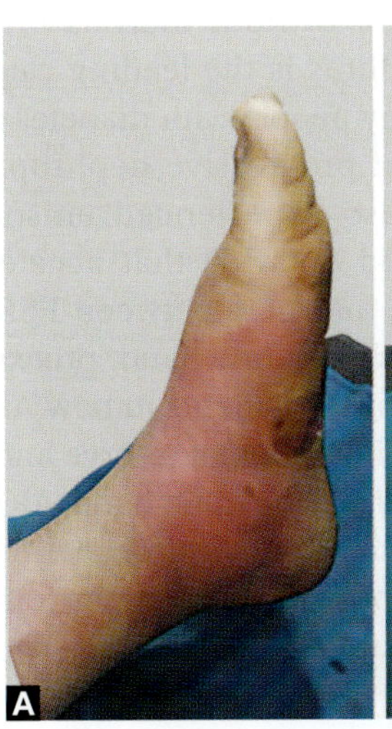
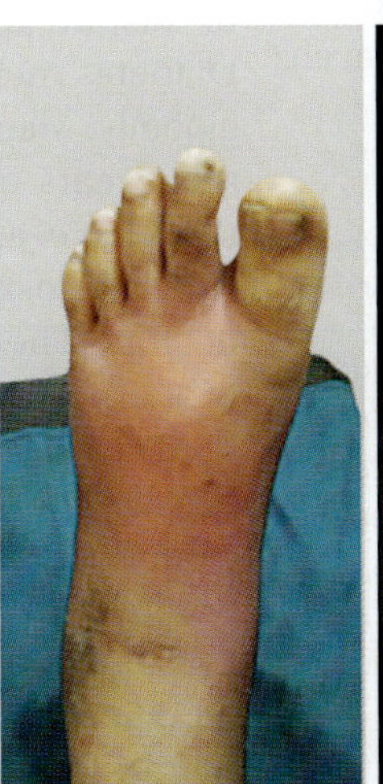
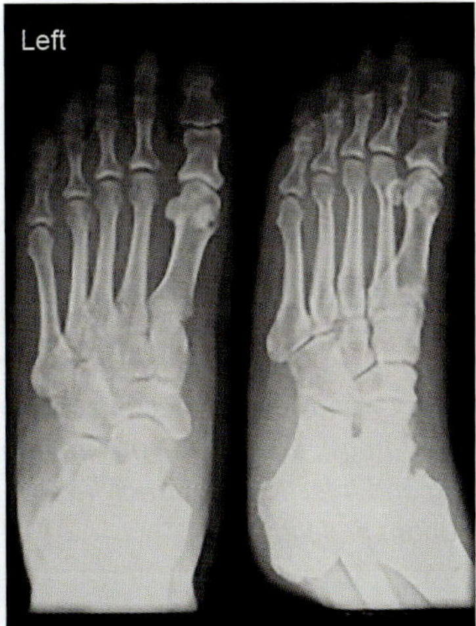

FIGS. 1A AND B: *(Continued)*

Continued

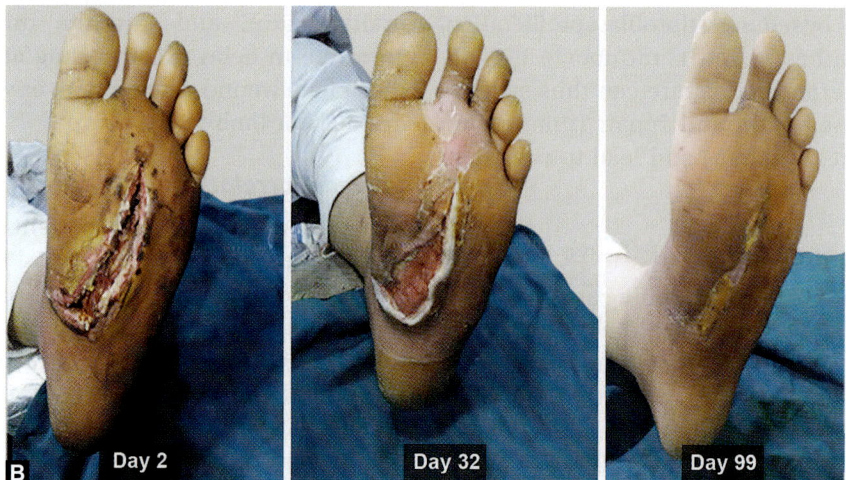

FIGS. 1A AND B: (A) Photographs of a clinical case of a 52-year-old shopkeeper with neuropathy, uncontrolled diabetes, and fever with history of trauma to sole while walking barefoot. ABI 0.9, WBC >14,000, serum creatinine—3 mg/dL, UACR—>300 mg/g. (B) Postdebridement and drainage, thick pus was evacuated but later wound appeared pale and dusky with slough. Worsening of wound, renal and liver functions with pallor were noted and AKI was diagnosed. Delayed wound healing was noted.

care—optimizing hemodynamics, timely RRT, and adjusting medications—is required to break this cycle. Encouragingly, if patients survive the acute illness and renal function recovers, the previously stalled ulcers may resume healing. Notably, one review observed that when adequately treated, DFUs in patients who had AKI or CKD can heal at rates comparable to those in patients with normal renal function and the importance of not giving up on limb salvage even in patients with declining kidney function.[20]

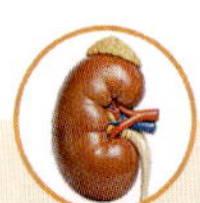

The presence of AKI in a patient with a DFU usually signifies severe illness and is associated with worse outcomes. AKI can complicate a DFU which in turn triggers a vicious cycle: The foot infection can cause AKI (via sepsis or drugs), and the AKI in turn impairs wound healing and infection clearance, raising the risk of amputations or death.

END-STAGE RENAL DISEASE AND ACUTE KIDNEY INJURY (ACUTE-ON-CHRONIC INJURY)

Background

End-stage renal disease refers to the most advanced stage of CKD (usually stage 5, GFR <15 mL/min), where kidney function is insufficient to sustain life without dialysis or transplant. Diabetes mellitus is the leading cause of ESRD globally. Many people with diabetes reach ESRD after years of progressive nephropathy; often, they have also experienced episodes of AKI superimposed on CKD that accelerated their decline. The interplay between ESRD and AKI is bidirectional. On one hand, preexisting CKD/ESRD predisposes patients to new AKI episodes, because of minimal renal reserve and associated comorbidities. On the other hand, AKI can hasten progression to ESRD in those with underlying CKD, a phenomenon sometimes termed "acute-on-chronic" kidney injury.[21]

End-stage Renal Disease as a Risk Factor for Acute Kidney Injury

Patients with ESRD on dialysis have virtually no remaining renal function, yet they remain vulnerable to acute hemodynamic and metabolic insults. For example, an ESRD patient with a residual urine output can lose that residual function if they develop hypotension or sepsis—an AKI on top of ESRD (often meaning acute injury to a transplanted kidney or acute damage superimposed on any remaining nephrons). In practice, any acute illness in an ESRD patient can be viewed as AKI, in that it often requires more intensive dialysis support and may cause further organ dysfunction. Hemodialysis itself can contribute to intradialytic hypotension episodes, which may cause ischemic injury to any residual renal tissue and other organs. If a person with diabetes and ESRD receives a kidney transplant, that transplanted kidney is at high risk for AKI from causes such as rejection, calcineurin-inhibitor toxicity, or infections. Thus, ESRD patients must be monitored closely for acute changes in kidney function or graft function.[22]

Moreover, the likelihood and severity of AKI are inversely related to baseline renal function. A minor nephrotoxic insult (e.g., contrast dye and NSAIDs) that a person with normal kidneys might tolerate could precipitate severe AKI in someone with advanced CKD **(Figs. 2A and B).**

Nephropathy is far more frequent in people with diabetes and CKD. In diabetic foot care, this is pertinent: Imaging studies for limb ischemia (arteriography) or repeated IV antibiotics may pose increased AKI risk in patients with CKD/ESRD. Clinical data support this heightened susceptibility: One study found that CKD patients who developed an AKI had 41-fold higher odds of progressing to ESRD compared to those without CKD. Even having CKD alone raised ESRD risk ~8-fold relative to non-CKD, but AKI *superimposed* on CKD boosted the risk further (approximately fourfold higher than CKD without AKI). Thus, ESRD is often the result of cumulative injuries—each episode of AKI pushes residual kidney function closer to zero.[23]

Acute Kidney Injury Worsening in End-stage Renal Disease

When an ESRD patient (especially one on dialysis) sustains an acute insult, the consequences can be dire. Without any renal reserve, toxins and fluid accumulate quickly until the next dialysis. For instance, consider a diabetic dialysis patient who develops a severe foot infection with sepsis: The combination of sepsis-related hypotension and nephrotoxic antibiotics can cause whatever little kidney function remains to acutely deteriorate (if they have a transplant or residual function). The patient may become anuric, volume overloaded,

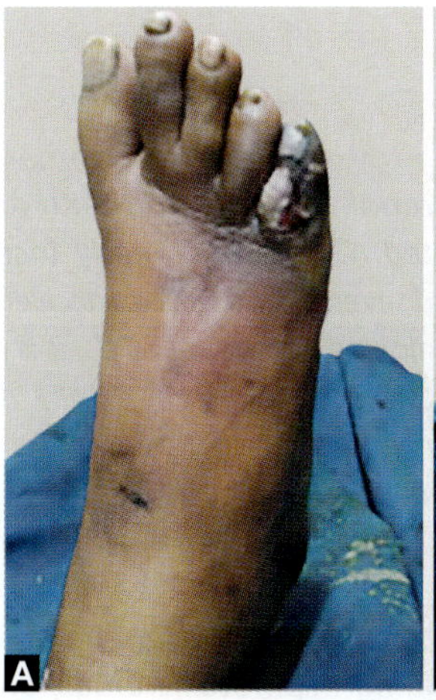
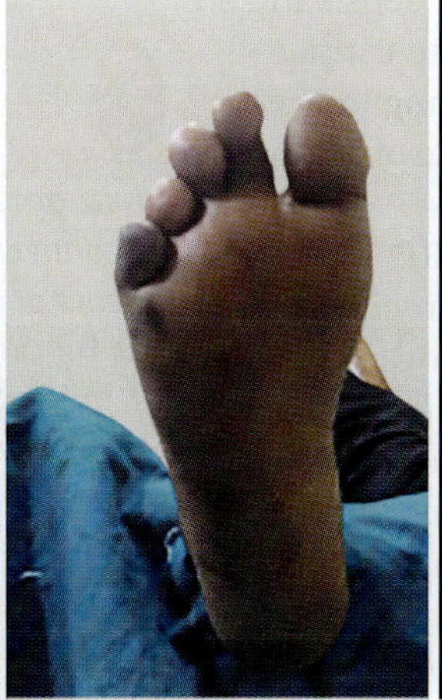
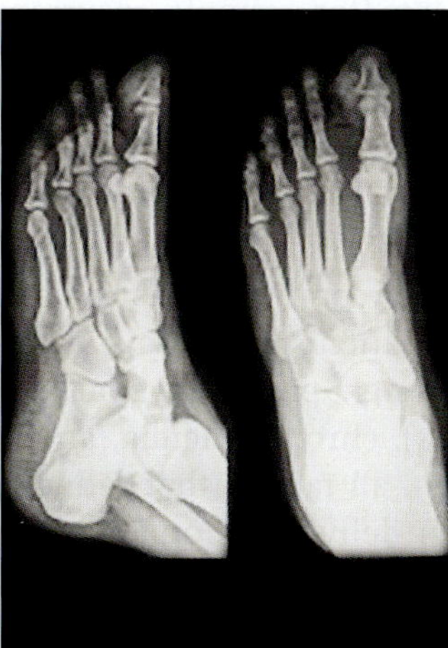

FIGS. 2A AND B: *(Continued)*

Continued

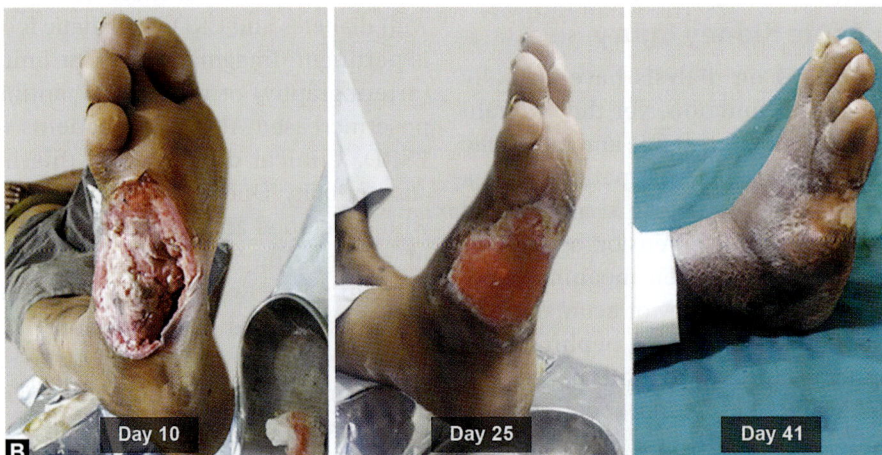

FIGS. 2A AND B: (A) Photographs of a clinical case of a 61-year-old lawyer with DMT2, HTN, and mild pulmonary veno-occlusive disease (POVD), nephropathy, uncontrolled sugars presented with severe pain and swelling right foot and fifth toe gangrene with foul smell. ABI 0.8, Wagner grade 4 ulcer. WBC count >11,000/mm^3, blood urea 63 mg/dL, and serum creatinine 2.9 mg/dL. (B) Wound debridement, 5th toe disarticulation, 5th metatarsal head resection.

hyperkalemic, and acidotic within hours—essentially an AKI on top of chronic failure. This scenario often mandates urgent extra dialysis sessions. Unfortunately, such acute episodes in ESRD carry high mortality. Studies in both elderly and ICU populations show that AKI in CKD/ESRD exponentially increases the risk of death and progression to permanent ESRD. In-hospital mortality is significantly higher when dialysis patients get "acute" multiorgan failure. Additionally, repeated AKI insults in ESRD patients (for example, recurrent sepsis in a DFU) can injure other systems—acute cardiac strain (cardiorenal syndrome), acute lung injury (pulmonary edema), etc., creating a cycle of organ crosstalk failure.[24]

From another perspective, ESRD itself contributes to conditions that may precipitate AKI. ESRD patients often have cardiovascular instability (e.g., prone to heart failure and arrhythmias), chronic anemia, and autonomic neuropathy—all factors that reduce perfusion and oxygen delivery to organs during stress. ESRD also entails chronic inflammation and oxidative stress, which can "prime" the kidneys for injury. For example, an ESRD patient has an elevated baseline level of inflammatory cytokines and endothelial activation; an acute second hit (like infection) on this background triggers disproportionate damage (so-called "two-hit" model). Also, certain ESRD-related medications or treatments can cause acute insults: Improper dosing of anticoagulation or antibiotics (due to altered pharmacokinetics in ESRD) may lead to toxic accumulation; or dialysis catheter-related bloodstream infections can cause sepsis and AKI in a transplanted kidney.[25]

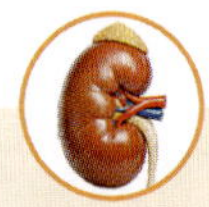

End-stage renal disease and AKI are tightly interconnected. CKD/ESRD greatly increases AKI incidence and severity, and AKI can accelerate CKD to ESRD. For clinicians managing DFUs, it is imperative that patients with advanced kidney disease be treated as very high risk and that small deteriorations in kidney function should be addressed immediately, as well as nephrotoxic exposures minimized. Conversely, aggressive measures to prevent AKI (such as adequate hydration before contrast studies, avoiding nephrotoxic drugs, and prompt

infection control) can slow progression to ESRD and improve overall outcomes, including limb outcomes. Multidisciplinary care (nephrologist, diabetologist, and foot surgeon) is essential in such patients to balance renoprotective strategies with effective foot ulcer management.

Strategies for Acute Kidney Injury Prevention

Universal therapy for AKI does not exist. The primary goal of treatment is to address underlying causes, such as dehydration, avoiding nephrotoxic drugs, and resorting to electrolyte management along with RRT. Obese patients have glomerulomegaly, increased renal blood flow, hyperfiltration, and higher albuminuria in the absence of hypertension. Sleep apnea in obese patients leads to hypoxic episodes, contributing to renal impairment. Maintaining body weight is an important preventive aspect for decreasing renal injury.

Chronic Kidney Disease

Overview

Progressive kidney function loss, which necessitates the need for RRT in the form of dialysis or transplantation, is termed CKD or renal failure.

Compared with the urine protein-to-creatinine ratio, the urine albumin creatinine ratio is a more sensitive marker of glomerular pathology.[26]

This condition can be classified based on GFR and albuminuria **(Boxes 1 and 2)**.

BOX 1: Categories of CKD based on GFR.

- *G1:* GFR 90 mL/min/1.73 m^2 and above
- *G2:* GFR 60–89 mL/min/1.73 m^2
- *G3a:* GFR 45–59 mL/min/1.73 m^2
- *G3b:* GFR 30–44 mL/min/1.73 m^2
- *G4:* GFR 15–29 mL/min/1.73 m^2
- *G5:* GFR less than 15 mL/min/1.73 m^2 or treatment by dialysis.[1]

BOX 2: Categories of CKD based on albuminuria.

- *A1* (urine ACR < 30 mg/g)
- *A2* (30–300 mg/g)
- *A3* (>300 mg/g)

IMPACT OF CKD ON DFU PROGRESSION AND WOUND HEALING

The physiopathological link suggests the role of diabetes, arterial disease, uremic neuropathy, and nutritional deficiencies in between CKD and diabetic foot. However, these foot ulcers may also present in nondiabetic individuals with renal failure along with vasculopathy and neuropathy **(Flowchart 3)**.

Effect of Hypoalbuminemia on Wound Healing in Diabetic Foot with CKD

Proteinuria, malnutrition, poor hepatic synthesis, increased protein catabolism, and oxidative stress in CKD patients lead to poor immune function, vulnerability to infections, and compromised wound healing.[27] Low albumin levels affect proliferative and regenerative (angiogenesis, collagen laying down, and cellular synthesis) phases of wound healing as well as cause zinc deficiency. Pedal edema due to hypoalbuminemia causes tissue hypoperfusion and also prevents wound contraction, leading to stalled wounds. Immune dysfunction associated with poor neutrophil response promotes severe deep limb and life-threatening infections by virulent bacteria. In cases of advanced CKD, low albumin levels are a predictor of amputation and related mortality.[28,29]

Effects of Uremic Neuropathy on Diabetic Foot Ulcer Healing

Diabetic peripheral neuropathy (DPN) is typically a distal symmetric polyneuropathy due to chronic hyperglycemia, causing nerve ischemia and demyelination. It leads to loss of protective sensation, motor denervation of small foot muscles with intrinsic minus foot and

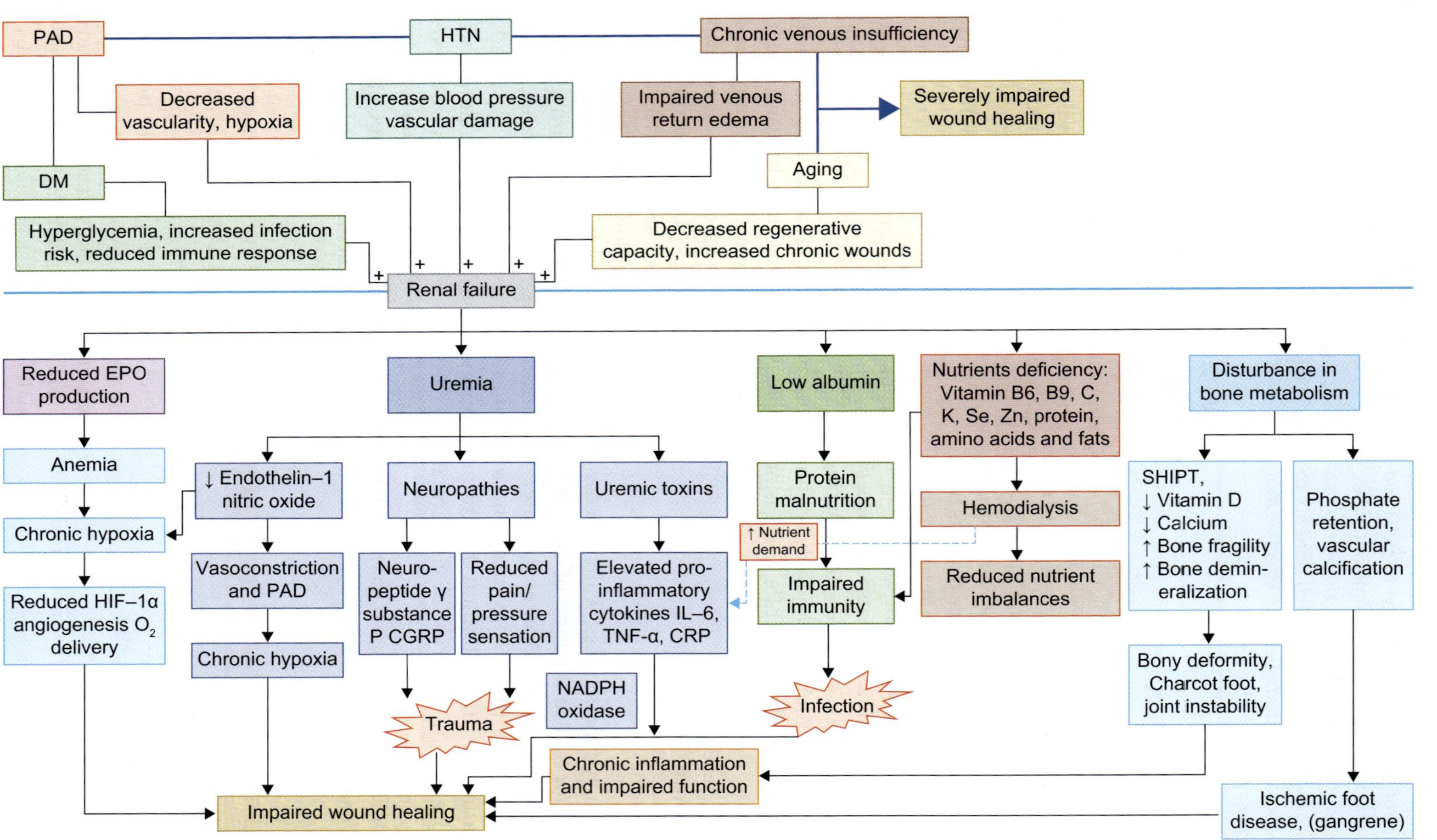

FLOWCHART 3: A complex interplay of aberrant wound healing, diabetes kidney disease (DKD), and other comorbidities.

related foot or toes deformities, gait disturbances, frequent chances of injuries due to falls, and autonomic dysfunction related to dry skin and plantar fissures. These changes of sensorimotor neuropathy pave the way for the development of foot ulceration, infection, and limb loss.

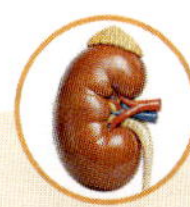

Chronic kidney disease has a systemic impact that profoundly affects the development and course of diabetic foot complications. Beyond its contribution to AKI risk, CKD alters the neurologic, vascular, and immune landscape in ways that worsen peripheral neuropathy, impair circulation, and heighten infection susceptibility.

People with diabetes and nephropathy therefore face a "triple threat" to foot health: More severe neuropathy (from both diabetes and uremia), accelerated atherosclerosis/PAD, and immune dysfunction with proneness for infections.[30]

A distal sensorimotor neuropathic process known as *uremic neuropathy*, caused by the accumulation of uremic toxins, is seen in advanced renal failure. Uremic neuropathy is considered to exist independently in ESRD (being present in more than half of renal patients on dialysis) and its severity correlates with the level of renal dysfunction. It predominantly affects large fibers, resulting in numbness, tingling, and reduced reflexes with notable worsening of preexisting neuropathy as CKD sets in. Hyperuremia of advanced CKD is an "aggravating factor" on top of hyperglycemia-induced nerve damage; hence, patients with combined diabetic and uremic neuropathy had profound sensory loss and muscle weakness than those with diabetes alone.[31] Uremic toxins such as guanidino compounds and parathyroid hormone fragments. In addition, vitamin B6 and folate deficiencies cause impairment of axonal function and disrupt dorsal root ganglia metabolism. Diabetic

nephropathy patients suffer from treatment-resistant neuropathy, and even dialysis is unable to reverse uremic neuropathy

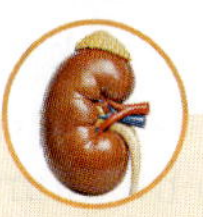

The combined neuropathy from diabetes and CKD greatly heightens foot ulcer risk. Loss of pain sensation is more complete, so patients fail to notice ulcers or tissue breakdown. Motor neuropathy leads to greater foot deformities (claw toes and Charcot joints) that concentrate pressure on certain areas, precipitating ulcers. Autonomic neuropathy (from both diabetes and uremia) causes dry, fissured skin and impaired sweat/oil glands, breaking the protective skin barrier. Peripheral neuropathy is the primary driver of foot ulceration in renal failure patients. All these neuropathic changes occur earlier and more aggressively if CKD is present. In summary, CKD "potentiates" diabetic neuropathy, creating profound insensitivity of the feet and making ulcer prevention and healing far more challenging.

Effect of Uremic Vasculopathy

Accumulation of uremic toxins in ESRD is a well-known risk factor for worsened cardiovascular outcomes. It can contribute to calcification and stiffening of peripheral arteries, in turn predisposing patients to calciphylaxis and leading to overall impaired wound healing. Uremia induces differentiation of vascular smooth muscle cells into an osteogenic phenotype which, in combination with excess calcium and phosphate, accelerates calcification of vessel walls. This then leads to inflammation and oxidative stress via activation of NADPH oxidase, impairing endothelial cell function as outlined in **Flowchart 3**. Uremic toxins can also induce vasoconstriction by modulating the expression of endothelin-1 and downregulating the production of nitric oxide. Altogether, these effects of uremia result in narrow and stiff vessels, resulting in impaired oxygenation to wound sites.

Effect of Uremia on Calcium and Phosphate Balance

Hyperparathyroidism in combination with uremia causes hypercalcemia that increases the risk for calciphylaxis caused by circumferentially layered deposits of calcium apatite in small- to medium-sized vessels. Proposed mechanisms include increased expression of osteogenic markers, ectopic expression of bone morphogenic protein at wound sites and a chronic inflammatory state leading to increased activation of nuclear factor kappa B (NFkB) and overexpression of receptor activator of NFkB ligand (RANK-L).

Phosphate retention as a result of compromised renal function in CKD patients stimulates fibroblast growth factor 23 (FGF23) and PTH secretion. Elevated FGF23 contributes to deficiency of vitamin D and secondary hyperparathyroidism. Sustained hyperphosphatemia enhances calcification of vessels of the lower limbs, promotes inflammation, and delays wound healing. Medial arterial sclerosis of vessels due to calcification causes thickening and stiffening of vessels with reduced foot perfusion and critical limb-threatening ischemia. This results in foot ulcers, impaired wound healing, infection, and gangrene may cause loss of limb.

In normally functioning kidneys, about 60% of filtered magnesium is reabsorbed, compared to CKD, where mechanisms involving the calcium-sensing receptor may lead to increased magnesium excretion, causing impairment of several enzymatic processes and protein synthesis involved in wound healing.

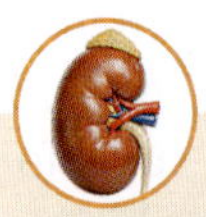

Uremic toxins can also induce vasoconstriction by modulating the expression of endothelin-1 and downregulating the production of nitric oxide. Sustained hyperphosphatemia enhances calcification of vessels of the lower limbs, promotes inflammation and delays wound healing. Medial arterial sclerosis of vessels due to calcification causes

thickening and stiffening of vessels with reduced foot perfusion and critical limb-threatening ischemia. This results in foot ulcers, impaired wound healing, infection, and gangrene may cause loss of limb.

Effect of Nutritional Deficiency on Wound Healing in Diabetic Foot with CKD

Renal failure patients often have deficiencies in vitamins B6, B9, and C, selenium, and zinc. Chronic inflammatory state results in a reduction of proteins, amino acids, and fats, which makes the patients malnourished and prone to develop chronic wounds along with impaired wound healing. Deficiency of vitamin C and arginine, which play a vital role in collagen formation, causes delayed wound healing. Vitamin B6 is essential for collagen formation, and vitamin B9 is essential to fibroblast proliferation.

Zinc is a cofactor in the enzymatic activity of matrix metalloproteinases (MMPs), which play a role throughout the stages of wound healing, including inflammation, angiogenesis, re-epithelialization and tissue remodeling.[32] Zinc also independently plays a role in differentiating proinflammatory (M1) and anti-inflammatory (M2) macrophages, which is essential to the transition from proinflammatory to anti-inflammatory states of wound healing.[33] Finally, it has been shown to accelerate hemostasis, although the exact mechanism is not well understood.[34] Although zinc supplementation has been shown to improve immune response and stabilize hemoglobin levels in patients with CKD, its role in enhancing wound healing is not well studied.[35]

During hemodialysis, vitamin K deficiency may occur due to warfarin therapy or use of vitamin K antagonists or reduced intake of foods rich in vitamin K. Reduced concentration of circulating calcification inhibitors due to vitamin K deficiency is seen in patients on hemodialysis. Vitamin K plays a role in the gamma-carboxylation of matrix GLA protein and protects from vessel wall calcification.

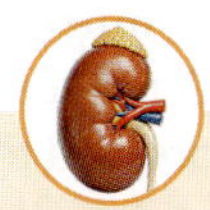

Chronic inflammatory state results in a reduction of proteins, amino acids, and fats, which makes the patients malnourished and prone to develop chronic wounds along with impaired wound healing.

Effect of Anemia on Wound Healing in Diabetic Foot with CKD

The various important causes of anemia in CKD include chronic inflammatory state associated with DFU, blood loss during repeated debridement, use of blood thinners, which cause more bleeding during surgery or bedside debridements, hypothyroidism, severe sepsis, malnutrition, and vitamin B12 deficiency. Erythropoietin gene (EPO) activation occurs by HIF-1α in a hypoxic background. In chronic renal impairment, there is an inadequate response to hypoxia and erythropoietin production is reduced, which, coupled with chronic inflammation and iron deficiency, leads to anemia, thus hampering oxygen delivery to wound sites. Target hemoglobin levels to be attained with anemia correction as per guidelines are between 10 g/dL and 11.5 g/dL (risk associated with erythropoietin-stimulating agents). When anemia is due to CKD in DFD, intravenous iron infusion is a good option to achieve hemoglobin levels >10 g/dL, but it is important to keep transferrin saturation levels >30% and serum ferritin levels > 500 ng/dL with dosage adjustment for ESAs.

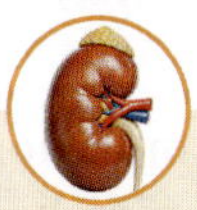

In chronic renal impairment, there is an inadequate response to hypoxia and erythropoietin production is reduced, which, coupled with chronic inflammation and iron deficiency, leads to anemia, thus hampering oxygen delivery to wound sites.

Effect of PAD on Wound Healing in Diabetic Foot with Chronic Kidney Disease

Atherosclerosis in Chronic Kidney Disease

Chronic kidney disease is recognized as a major risk factor for atherosclerosis and PAD. With the progression of CKD, a "dose-dependent dysfunction of most organ systems occurs, called the uremic syndrome," which includes vascular pathology.[36] Patients with CKD have high rates of dyslipidemia, endothelial dysfunction, vascular calcification, and arterial stiffness. Secondary hyperparathyroidism in ESRD leads to calcium-phosphate deposition in vessel walls, causing media calcification (Monckeberg's sclerosis) that particularly affects lower extremity arteries. Consequently, the prevalence of PAD is markedly elevated (24–37%) in CKD, which rises above 30% in those with stage 5 CKD. Together as a powerful combination, diabetes predisposes to large and small artery disease, whereas CKD accelerates and amplifies this process via inflammation and mineral bone disorder.

Vascular Insufficiency/Peripheral Arterial Disease in Chronic Kidney Disease

A significantly higher prevalence of mortality related to CVD is seen in patients with renal failure. A 38% increase in the risk of CVD in patients with a GFR of 15–59 mL/min/1.73 per 1.73 m^2 at baseline due to endothelial dysfunction, compared with an estimated GFR of 90–150 mL/min/1.73 m^2, was found by the Atherosclerosis Risk in Communities Study. Endothelial cells malfunction in CKD, contributing to reduced nitric oxide (NO) production. NO is essential for vasodilation, so with reduced NO production, there is vasoconstriction and increased blood pressure.[37] Due to deficiencies in l-arginine in CKD, there is limited NO production and worsening endothelial dysfunction. Elevated ROS levels in CKD also damage endothelial cells and impair their function. Dysfunction occurs in the peripheral vasculature of patients with both moderate and severe stages of the disease.[38]

Peripheral arterial disease reduces blood flow to the legs and feet, contributing to ischemic ulcers and poor wound healing. In diabetes, PAD tends to be segmental and shows predilection for below knee arteries (tibioperoneal arteries). CKD-related PAD often presents with a more diffuse pattern, characterized by calcified arteries that are difficult to revascularize and have poor collateral formation. Large vessel calcification and calciphylaxis of medium and small vessels of the foot promote ischemic symptoms in the foot along with gangrenous skin changes, progressive necrosis and nonhealing foot ulcers. Together, CKD and DFU "share several pathophysiologic elements, the first of which is peripheral arterial disease (PAD)". This implies that much of the excess risk of foot complications in CKD can be attributed to worsened ischemia. Clinically, diabetic patients with nephropathy are more likely to have critical limb ischemia (rest pain and gangrene) than diabetics with normal renal function. In fact, nephropathy is an independent predictor of peripheral vascular disease in diabetic foot patients. Wolf et al. (2009) found a strong inverse relationship between GFR and diabetic foot severity such that lower GFR correlated with higher Wagner ulcer grade and higher amputation rates. Simply put, poorer kidney function implies poorer limb perfusion and outcomes.[39]

Pathophysiologically, CKD causes endothelial dysfunction (due to uremic toxins and nitric oxide imbalance) and promotes arterial stiffening. Uremic toxins such as asymmetric dimethylarginine (ADMA) inhibit endothelial nitric oxide, reducing vasodilatory capacity. CKD also induces a proinflammatory state with elevated cytokines and oxidative stress that damage vessels. High levels of sPTH and phosphate in ESRD trigger vascular smooth muscle to undergo osteogenic change, depositing calcium in arterial walls (vascular calcification). These calcified, noncompliant arteries in ESRD patients (sometimes detected as "medial artery

calcification" on X-ray) can lead to falsely elevated ankle-brachial indices and a special form of ischemia with stiff vessels and poor muscle perfusion. Furthermore, anemia of CKD reduces oxygen delivery to tissues. All these factors lead to impaired wound healing: Even if a DFU is primarily neuropathic in origin, superimposed CKD/PAD will slow granulation and re-epithelialization due to lack of blood supply.[40]

This is why DFUs in CKD often become chronic and may require vascular interventions. Unfortunately, CKD patients also have a higher perioperative risk for such interventions, making management difficult. In summary, CKD aggravates diabetic foot ischemia through high PAD burden, making foot ulcers more likely to develop and less likely to heal without revascularization.[41]

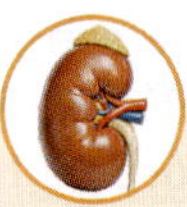

Diabetes is considered an independent risk factor for large and small artery disease, whereas CKD accelerates and amplifies this process via inflammation and mineral bone disorder. Elevated ROS levels in CKD also damage endothelial cells and impair their function. In diabetes, PAD tends to involve below-knee arteries (tibial vessels), which, combined with neuropathy, leads to the classic neuroischemic foot ulcer. CKD-related PAD often presents with a more diffuse pattern, characterized by calcified arteries that are difficult to revascularize and have poor collateral formation.

Effect of Immunodysfunction on Wound Healing in Diabetic Foot with Chronic Kidney Disease

Chronic renal failure leads to accumulation of uremic toxins, which leads to diminished immune defense, contributing to the high rate of infections.[42] Derangement of neutrophil function includes impaired chemotaxis, phagocytosis, dysfunctional macrophages/monocytes, reduced lymphocyte proliferation, and the complement pathway is less effective. Factors driving this immune dysfunction apart from accumulated toxins also include chronic inflammation, malnutrition, anemia, and vitamin D deficiency. Vitamin D deficiency and hyperparathyroidism in CKD also negatively affect innate immunity due to premature aging of the immune system.[43] High risk of both polymicrobial and opportunistic infections is liable to affect the healing of foot ulcers with increased chances of systemic spread if not managed appropriately.

Effect of Infection/Sepsis on Wound Healing in Diabetic Foot with Chronic Kidney Disease

The presence of CKD in itself is an independent risk factor for methicillin-resistant *Staphylococcus aureus* (MRSA) infection in DFUs. More severe foot infection (higher Wagner grade) with resistant organisms in developing countries increases the likelihood of amputation.[44] Poor glycemic control, immune dysfunction, hyperglycemia due to uremia-induced insulin resistance, and gluconeogenesis in CKD with DFD patients may predispose to further spread of infection. In advanced CKD, there is reduced insulin clearance, which causes a sudden fall in blood sugar levels or unpredictable glycemic swings. Suboptimal diabetes control predisposes to hyperglycemia a well-known promoter of infection, by impairing leukocyte function. Thus, CKD patients with diabetes may experience more frequent and recalcitrant foot infections.

Deficient cellular immunity due to uremia also leads to reduced bactericidal activity. In addition, many antibiotics require dose adjustments or are less effective in poorly perfused tissue. Aminoglycosides pose toxicity risks, such as gentamicin, which can cause acute tubular necrosis, and prolonged use (>14 days) carries up to 50% risk of nephrotoxicity.[45] Furthermore, protein energy malnutrition is common in advanced CKD, leading to poor wound healing and weaker immune responses. Deficiencies of zinc and selenium (due to renal losses or dietary restrictions) impair immune cell function and wound collagen synthesis. Anemia in CKD reduces tissue oxygenation needed for bacterial killing and tissue repair.[46]

As the spread of infection is faster and host defenses are compromised, hospitalization is a must for limb and life-threatening infections. Early surgical intervention (debridement or minor amputation) may be warranted to control infection in certain cases, necessitating a high index of suspicion, early diagnosis and rapid referral to a foot specialist. Guidelines by IDSA/IWGDF in 2023 highlight that diabetic patients with nephropathy should be considered "high-risk foot" patients necessitating more frequent foot inspections and aggressive management of even minor wounds to prevent infection. Preventive foot care is critical, as emphasized by an observation that neglecting podiatric care in dialysis patients led to a drastic increase in hospitalizations and amputations.

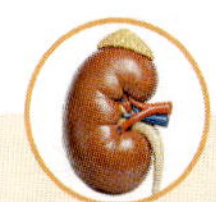

Chronic kidney disease/ESRD amplifies infection risk in the diabetic foot through uremic immune dysfunction, malnutrition, and treatment dilemmas. This manifests as more frequent infections, unusual or resistant organisms (MDRs) such as MRSA, Klebsiella pneumonia, Pseudomonas aeruginosa, and E. coli, as well as propensity for minor wounds to become limb threatening. Bacterial overgrowth due to gut microbiome dysbiosis allows endotoxins to trigger systemic inflammation with further cellular immune dysfunction. To add to this weakening of skin integrity also makes foot ulcers vulnerable to infection.

Effect of Chronic Inflammation and Oxidative Stress on Wound Healing in Diabetic Foot with CKD

Patients of CKD and ESRD suffer from a state of chronic inflammation due to underlying uremic toxins, oxidative stress, hyperglycemic state of diabetes, and CVD, which triggers the elevation of proinflammatory cytokines [interleukins IL–6, tumor necrosis factor-alpha, and C-reactive protein (CRP)]. Inflammatory response is further exacerbated by oxidative stress in renal dysfunction due to the damaging influence of excess ROS on cellular components. Persistent oxidative stress causes endothelial dysfunction, poor angiogenesis, and tissue reparative responses. Despite elevated inflammatory cytokines due to immune exhaustion, the infection fails to be controlled.

The hypoxia inducible factor-1 alpha promotes angiogenesis via vascular endothelial growth factor in a low oxygen level environment, but in renal dysfunction, it may not remain stable and its activity is compromised, thereby causing impaired wound healing.

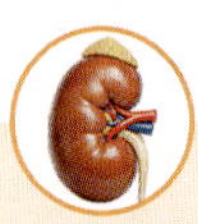

A combination of neuropathy, ischemia, immunopathy, and DKD faces a "perfect storm" for foot ulceration with a high risk of cardiovascular complications. In addition, this sustained inflammatory state leads to excessive tissue damage and fibrosis with delayed wound healing.

Effect of Chronic Kidney Disease, with Impaired Bone Health, on Wound Healing

Excessive bone resorption coupled with poor bone formation due to renal osteodystrophy and secondary hyperparathyroidism in DKD leads to increased risk of stress fractures of metatarsals and tarsals, poor union, deformities, and Charcot feet. Underlying factors for renal dystrophy include secondary hyperparathyroidism, vitamin D deficiency-induced hypocalcemia causing poor bone mineralization, hyperphosphatemia-induced vascular calcification, chronic inflammation, medial sclerosis of lower extremity vessels with resultant ischemia, and compromised wound healing. Chronic systemically elevated proinflammatory markers also promote poor bone formation and impaired fracture healing.

Effect of Diabetes Mellitus and Glycemic Fluctuations on Wound Healing

Diabetes mellitus is one of the most common renal failure comorbidities. Poor glycemic control with fluctuations or peaks in blood sugar levels induces accelerated vascular calcification, causing tissue hypoxia, renal damage, increased predisposition to PAD and also has adverse diabetic foot outcomes. Unstable glycemic control exacerbates neuropathy, triggers the renin angiotensin aldosterone system, nitric oxide (NO reduction, which induces glomerular damage with persistent albuminuria, causing increased risk of infection, deficient collagen laying down, poor wound response, and increased chances of limb loss.

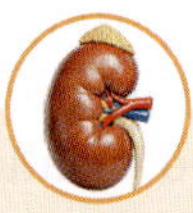

Diabetes mellitus is one of the most common renal failure comorbidities. Excessive bone resorption coupled with poor bone formation due to renal osteodystrophy and secondary hyperparathyroidism in DKD leads to increased risk of stress fractures of metatarsals and tarsals, poor union, deformities, and Charcot feet. Poor glycemic control with fluctuations or peaks in blood sugar levels induces accelerated vascular calcification, causing tissue hypoxia, renal damage, increased predisposition to PAD and also has adverse diabetic foot outcomes.

MANAGEMENT OF DIABETIC FOOT DISEASE WITH RENAL DYSFUNCTION

Comprehensive Preventive Foot Care in Diabetic Foot Disease with Renal Dysfunction

Challenges in managing patients with DFUs and renal dysfunction mainly target factors and comorbidities that impair wound healing.

Wound Care, Ideal Dressings, and Adjuvant Therapies

These wounds need standard of care practices such as debridement, infection control, restoration of blood flow, moist wound dressings, and offloading.

An ideal wound dressing for DKD foot wounds has not been researched. Topical esmolol 14% dressings have been researched to promote wound healing in hypoalbuminemia and anemia due to CKD. The efficacy of other adjuvant healing agents, such as topical oxygen, ozone therapy, or hyperbaric oxygen therapy, has not been researched in CKD patients in particular. Sucrose octasulfate dressings, which target metallo-matrix proteases, may be used.

Infection Control

Aggressive infection control is a must in patients with CKD with DFUs to prevent limb loss and related mortality, as they are at four times higher risk. The polymicrobial flora in these wounds is mostly severe and multidrug-resistant, such as MRSA, vancomycin-resistant strains, etc. Fungal infections may be more prevalent and need antifungal therapy with fluconazole, terbinafine, etc. and for anaerobic coverage, metronidazole or clindamycin may be added. Nephrotoxic drugs such as aminoglycosides should be better avoided, and the dosage schedule is titrated accordingly.

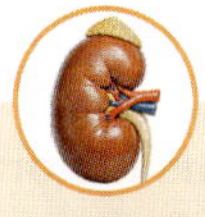

Challenges in managing patients with DFUs and renal dysfunction mainly target factors and comorbidities that impair wound healing. Aggressive wound care and infection control is necessary in patients with CKD and DFUs to prevent limb loss and related mortality.

Managing Hypoalbuminemia in Diabetic Foot Disease with Chronic Kidney Disease

Albumin has an essential role in maintaining immunity and wound healing. Hypoalbuminemia as a result of proteinuria of renal dysfunction leads to impaired wound healing by deficient angiogenesis, collagen laying down and inefficient clearing of infection. To expedite wound closure and prevent limb loss, it is important to reinforce protein intake (0.8 g/kg body weight/day for those without dialysis and 1.0–1.2 g/kg/day for those on dialysis) within the permissibility of renal diet. Allaying the underlying cause is important for relief for a longer duration, and albumin infusions are reserved only for severe cases.[47]

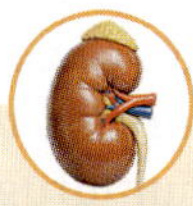

Hypoalbuminemia as a result of proteinuria of renal dysfunction leads to impaired wound healing by deficient angiogenesis, collagen laying down and inefficient clearing of infection.

Managing Anemia in Diabetic Foot Disease with Chronic Kidney Disease

Reduced erythropoietin levels, along with iron deficiency, are two major causes of anemia and consequently poor wound outcomes in CKD patients. Erythropoietin-stimulating agents/ESA (epoetin alfa, darbepoetin alfa, and glycol-epoetin beta) improve oxygen perfusion and must be considered in those without iron deficiency but with hemoglobin levels <g/dL and caution must be exercised due to the risk of thrombosis or hypertension.

Iron infusion with ferric carboxymaltose or iron sucrose is considered for those not on ESA, with no active infection, but transferrin saturation must be <30%, ferritin levels <500 ng/mL, and Hb <10 g/dL.[48]

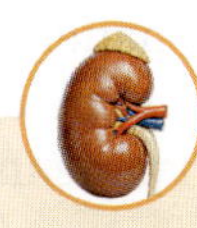

Reduced erythropoietin levels, along with iron deficiency, are two major causes of anemia and consequently poor wound outcomes in CKD patients.

Managing Infection/Sepsis in Diabetic Foot Disease with Chronic Kidney Disease

Chronic renal disease alters immune response, causes extensive vascular calcification leading to ischemic foot disease, disturbed bone metabolism with demineralization causing increased fragility of foot bones, chronic systemic inflammation, and glycemic fluctuations. As a result, the DFUs develop more severe, aggressive, deep infections involving bones and are difficult to heal with prolonged hospitalization periods. Presence of uremic toxins, low albumin levels, iron deficiency anemia contribute further to impaired wound healing, along with multidrug-resistant organisms, increased susceptibility to polymicrobial flora such as MRSA, vancomycin-resistant enterococci, anaerobic pathogens such as *Bacteroides fragilis*, and *Candida* species fungus infections.[49]

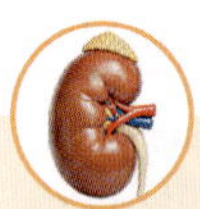

In patients undergoing dialysis, the course of healing may be protracted further with increased propensity to limb loss. The choice and dosage schedule of antibiotics needs to be altered to avoid nephrotoxicity. Poor limb outcomes with morbidity due to amputations, poor quality of life, higher mortality rates due to cardiovascular risks, chronic inflammation, and fulminant sepsis are the hallmark of DFD with CKD.

Managing Ischemia/PAD in Diabetic Foot Disease with Chronic Kidney Disease

A combined medical treatment and surgical revascularization is needed in patients of CKD with PAD, as ischemia is very common patients of CKD. Presence of vascular calcification in tibial and peroneal arteries is very common in patients with DKD.

Medical management—Statins are most commonly used whereas ARBs may be used caution due to risk of hyperkalemia. Antiplatelet therapy (aspirin/clopidogrel) with oral anticoagulants (rivaroxaban) may be used considering safety profile due to increased risk of bleeding.[50]

Surgical management—endovascular intervention may be rendered difficult in cases of advanced CKD due to extensive tunica media calcification which may have adverse outcomes.[51]

Managing Charcot Foot in Diabetic Foot Disease with Chronic Kidney Disease

Total contact casting is the gold standard in managing the active phase of Charcot foot. Denosumab, a new drug, has shown a promising role in inducing remission in active cases and acts by inhibiting the RANKL pathway-induced osteoclast activation.[52]

Managing CKD Progression in DFD with CKD

It is of paramount importance to reduce the speed of progression of CKD as it impairs DFU healing as well as worsening of neuropathy, PAD, and immune status. These drugs also have an indirect beneficial effect of stabilizing blood sugar levels and improving vascularity.[53]

Managing DFD with CKD/ESRD in Patients on Dialysis Therapy

Those dialysis patients with a previous history of foot ulcers or amputation, DPN, or macrovascular disease are at reasonably high risk of developing DFU or suffering amputation.[54,55] Further, dialysis patients are often bedridden and are prone to develop bed sores or pressure ulcers and additionally lack dexterity to practice self-foot care behavior or inspect for new and recent ulcers. High incidence of DFU and amputation was found after initiating dialysis therapy in a retrospective study, which concluded that dialysis acts as a driving force. These negative effects and postdialysis findings were further corroborated in another multicentric study.[56] One research study established that major amputation rates in diabetic patients on hemodialysis were markedly increased irrespective of revascularization and had worse prognosis.[57] A proactive approach to podiatrist care for vigilant preventive foot care, as well as DFU cases with or without sepsis at dialysis centers, is an essential practice to reduce major amputation rates **(Figs. 3A to D)**.[58]

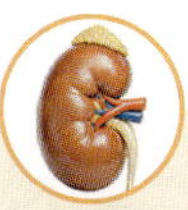

Diabetes mellitus is considered to be a major risk factor for lower extremity amputation in patients undergoing hemodialysis. Sepsis or infection is the major triggering factor in DFU progression, as well as amputation and postamputation mortality, particularly in patients with worsening renal function and those on dialysis, as they demonstrate vulnerability to infection.

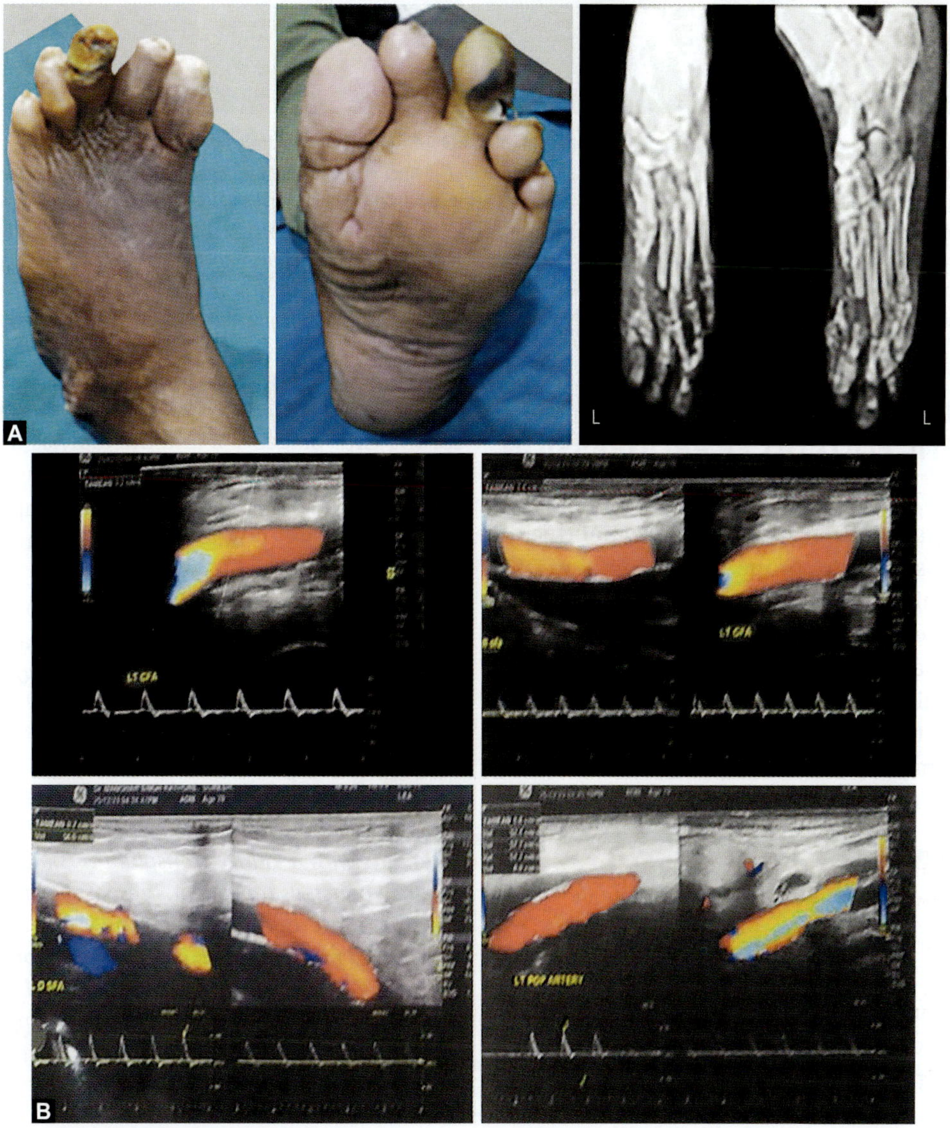

FIGS. 3A TO D: *(Continued)*

Continued

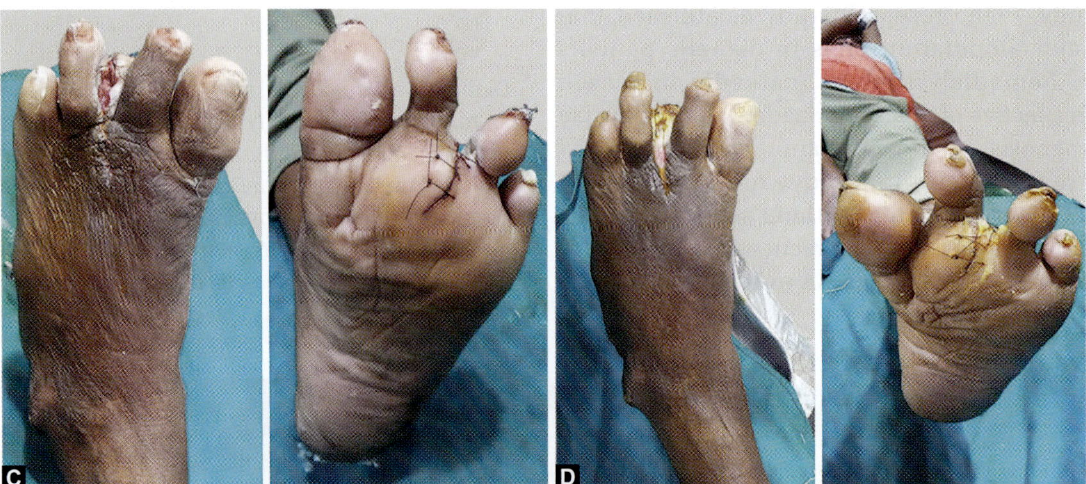

FIGS. 3A TO D: (A) A patient with type 2 diabetes, HTN, CAD, ESRD, on hemodialysis mild POVD, ABI 0.8, gangrene second toe with painful foul smelling ulcer. X-ray left Foot (AP and oblique view). Areas of bony erosion are noted in 1st and 2nd metatarsal with overlying soft tissue swelling—like postinfective. Distal phalynx of 3rd toe is not visualized. Accessory navicular bone was noted. Visualized joints are grossly normal in space, articular surfaces, and articulation. (B) A color arterial Doppler study—left lower limb findings are suggested of peripheral arterial disease with below knee significant gradually increase luminal narrowing in tibial arteries up to DPA. (C) Third toe excision with removal of metatarsal head. Postoperatively topical oxygen was given. (D) Healed wound on 28th day.

RENAL TRANSPLANTATION AND DIABETIC FOOT ULCER PROGRESSION

Patients with a kidney transplant or simultaneous kidney-pancreas transplant, irrespective of glycemic status, are prone to develop new DFU or worsening of the progression of existing ones, as peripheral vascular disease is quite common in these patients. Opportunistic infections due to compromised immune system in these patients, as a result of immunosuppression therapy they receive, may necessitate hospitalization as well as increased major amputation rates.[59]

Amputation Rates and Survival after Amputation

Several studies have demonstrated increased mortality and risk of amputation among those with chronic wounds and renal disease. Renal failure increases the likelihood of amputation surgery. In a research analysis, Otte et al. found a significantly higher risk of major amputation for the CKD stages 4–5 and the dialysis treatment groups when compared to the CKD 3 group. Another study on transmetatarsal amputations showed that ESRD was a significant predictor of failure to heal at the amputation site. However, the study also demonstrated that none of the comorbid conditions, such as coronary artery disease, hypertension, and diabetes, proved to be statistically significant for nonhealing.[60]

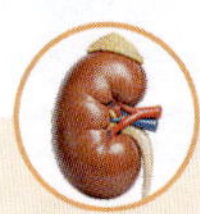

Patients with a kidney transplant or simultaneous kidney-pancreas transplant, irrespective of glycemic status, are prone to develop new DFU. There is increased mortality and risk of amputation among those with chronic wounds and renal disease. Renal failure increases the likelihood of amputation surgery.

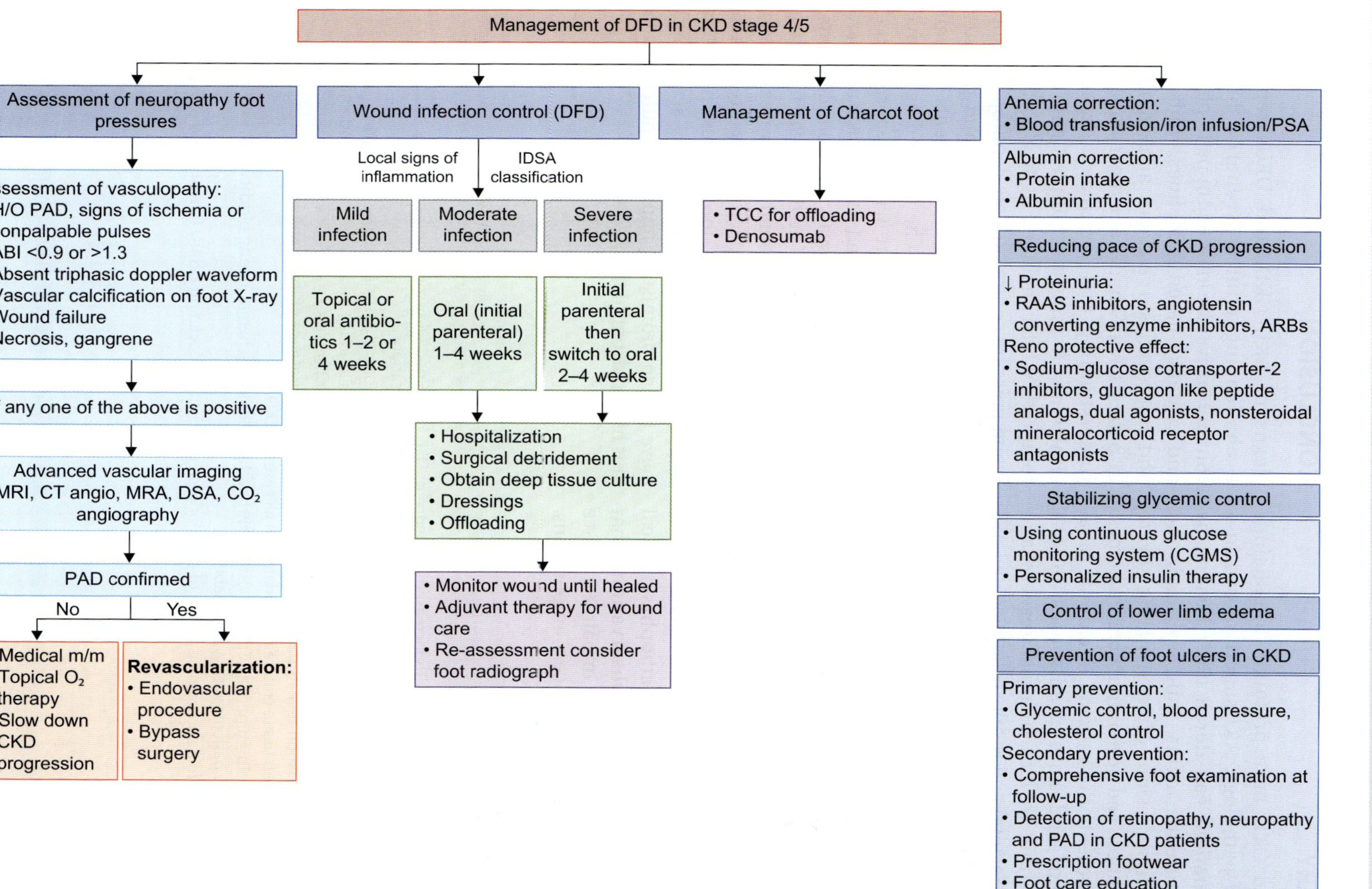

FLOWCHART 4: A flowchart for the management of diabetic foot ulcer in chronic kidney disease (CKD) patients.

SUMMARY

Acute and CKD have profound interactions with DFU pathology. AKI superimposed in a diabetic patient can derail ulcer healing by inducing uremic toxins, fluid overload, and immune suppression, often signaling severe systemic illness and portending poor outcomes. ESRD represents the extreme of chronic renal impairment and both predisposes to AKI episodes (due to lack of renal reserve and comorbid factors) and results from repeated AKI hits, forming a vicious cycle that worsens patient survival and complicates foot ulcer management. CKD, including diabetic nephropathy, exacerbates the key pathways leading to DFUs: It aggravates peripheral neuropathy (via uremic neuropathy) causing insensate, injury-prone feet; it accelerates peripheral vascular insufficiency (via diffuse atherosclerosis and calcification) causing ischemic, poorly healing ulcers; and it induces immune dysfunction (via uremia and malnutrition) leading to higher infection risk and severity. These interwoven pathophysiological links explain the clinical observations that diabetic patients with kidney impairment have markedly higher rates of foot ulcers, amputations, and mortality **(Flowchart 4)**.

CONCLUSION

Nexus of AKI, CKD, and DFUs represents a challenging clinical scenario, but with comprehensive care informed by pathophysiology and evidence-based guidelines, limb salvage and improved survival are achievable even in patients with significant renal impairment. Understanding this interplay is crucial for clinicians. A multidisciplinary approach is required, which includes tight glycemic and blood pressure control to slow nephropathy and neuropathy, routine foot exams, and podiatry care, especially in CKD/ESRD patients, prompt revascularization for ischemia, and aggressive infection management with renal-adjusted therapies. Prevention and early intervention are key to preventing microvascular complications, and "putting feet first" with regular foot care in patients with nephropathy. As research and guidelines indicate, specific measures (such as specialized dialysis-foot clinics, nutrition supplementation, and neuropathy screening) have shown promise in improving outcomes in this high-risk population.

TAKE HOME MESSAGES

- Presence of DKD is correlated with increased incidence of DFU combined with compromised wound healing and increased susceptibility for infection leading to lower extremity amputations.
- Early identification of patients with AKI and CKD promises better limb outcomes and reduced mortality.
- Assessment of neuropathy and vasculopathy is essential. Toe brachial index and duplex ultrasound should be considered as ABI may not be reliable in these cases with calcification of vessels.
- Local wound examination reveals paucity of signs of infection with presence of foul smell and prominent wound pallor. Obtaining deep tissue culture is mandatory in all cases of CKD.
- Correction of hypoalbuminemia, Charcot osteoarthropathy, anemia, ischemia needs biochemical and cardiac evaluation in all CKD patients with type 2 diabetes.
- Avoiding hypoglycemia and administration of antibiotics in people with declining kidney function and DFD is very important.

REFERENCES

1. Bonnet JB, Sultan A. Narrative Review of the Relationship Between CKD and Diabetic Foot Ulcer. Kidney Int Rep. 2021;7(3):381-8.

2. KDIGO. 2012 Clinical Practice Guideline for the Evaluation and Management of Chronic Kidney Disease. Elsevier; 2013.

3. Gök Ü, Selek Ö, Selek A, Güdük A, Güner MÇ. Survival evaluation of the patients with diabetic major lower-extremity amputations. Musculoskelet Surg. 2016;100:145-8.

4. American Diabetes Association. Cardiovascular disease and risk management. Diabetes Care. 2016;40:S75-87.

5. Aziz KMA. Correlation of urine biomarkers: microalbuminuria and spot urine protein among diabetic patients. application of spot urine protein in diabetic kidney disease, nephropathy, proteinuria estimation, diagnosing and monitoring. Recent Pat Endocr Metab Immune Drug Discov. 2015;9(2):121-33.

6. Ix JH, Katz R, De Boer IH, Kestenbaum BR, Allison MA, Siscovick DS, et al. Newman AB, Sarnak MJ, Shlipak MG, Criqui MH. Association of chronic kidney disease with the spectrum of ankle brachial index: the CHS (Cardiovascular Health Study). J Am Coll Cardiol. 2009;54(13):1176-84.

7. Anitha Rani A, Viswanathan V. Diabetic Foot Infection and Worsening Kidney Function: Implication for Health Care in the Developing World. Int J Diabetol Vasc Dis Res. 2017;5(5):208-13.

8. Smina TP, Rabeka M, Viswanathan V. Diabetic Foot Ulcer as a Cause of Significant Decline in the Renal Function Among South Indian Population with Type 2 Diabetes: Role of TGF-β1 and CCN Family Proteins. Int J Low Extrem Wounds. 2019;18(4):354-61.

9. Hsu CY, Ordoñez JD, Chertow GM, Fan D, McCulloch CE, Go AS. The risk of acute renal failure in patients with chronic kidney disease. Kidney Int. 2008;74:101-7.

10. Prabhu RA, Shenoy SV, Nagaraju SP, Rangaswamy D, Rao IR, Bhojaraja MV, et al. Acute kidney injury and progressive diabetic kidney disease: an epidemiological perspective. Int J Nephrol Renovasc Dis. 2021;14:23-31.

11. Harzallah A, Kaaroud H, Hajji M, Hamida F, Khiari K, Gorsane I, et al. Drug-induced acute kidney injury in diabetes mellitus. Open J Nephrol. 2016;6:176-87.

12. Li Y, Ren K. The mechanism of contrast-induced acute kidney injury and its association with diabetes mellitus. Contrast Media Mol Imag. 2020;2020:3295176.

13. Hursh BE, Ronsley R, Islam N, Mammen C, Panagiotopoulos C. Acute kidney injury in children with type 1 diabetes hospitalized for diabetic ketoacidosis. JAMA Pediatr. 2017;171:e170020.

14. Liu J, Xie H, Ye Z, Li F, Wang L. Rates, predictors, and mortality of sepsis-associated acute kidney injury: a systematic review and meta-analysis. BMC Nephrol. 2020;21:318.

15. Yu SM, Bonventre JV. Acute kidney injury and progression of diabetic kidney disease. Adv Chronic Kidney Dis. 2018;25:166-80.

16. Basu RK. Acute kidney injury in hospitalized pediatric patients. Pediatr Ann. 2018;47:e286-91.

17. Lech M, Grobmayr R, Ryu M, Lorenz G, Hartter I, Mulay SR, et al. Macrophage phenotype controls long-term AKI outcomes—kidney regeneration versus atrophy. J Am Soc Nephrol. 2014;25:292-304.

18. Cohen G, Hörl WH. Immune dysfunction in uremia—an update. Toxins (Basel). 2012;4(11):962-90.

19. Akbari R, Javaniyan M, Fahimi A, Sadeghi M. Renal function in patients with diabetic foot infection; does antibiotherapy affect it? J Renal Inj Prev. 2016;6(2):117-21.

20. Deery HG 2nd, Sangeorzan JA. Saving the diabetic foot with special reference to the patient with chronic renal failure. Infect Dis Clin North Am. 2001;15(3):953-81.

21. Singbartl K, Kellum JA. AKI in the ICU: definition, epidemiology, risk stratification, and outcomes. Kidney Int. 2012;81:819-25.

22. Fiorentino M, Bagagli F, Deleonardis A, Stasi A, Franzin R, Conserva F, et al. Acute Kidney Injury in Kidney Transplant Patients in Intensive Care Unit: From Pathogenesis to Clinical Management. Biomedicines. 2023;11(5):1474.

23. Ishani A, Xue JL, Himmelfarb J, Eggers PW, Kimmel PL, Molitoris BA, et al. Acute kidney injury increases the risk of ESRD among elderly. J Am Soc Nephrol. 2009;20:223-8.

24. Bedford M, Farmer C, Levin A, Ali T, Stevens P. Acute kidney injury and CKD: chicken or egg? Am J Kidney Dis. 2012;59:485-91.

25. Ishani A, Xue JL, Himmelfarb J, Eggers PW, Kimmel PL, Molitoris BA, et al. Acute kidney injury increases risk of ESRD among elderly. J Am Soc Nephrol. 2009;20(1):223-8.

26. Rampoldi L, Scolari F, Amoroso A, Ghiggeri G, Devuyst O. The Rediscovery of Uromodulin (Tamm- Horsfall Protein): From Tubulointerstitial Nephropathy to Chronic Kidney Disease. Kidney Int. 2011;80(4):338-47.

27. Russell L. The importance of patients' nutritional status in wound healing. Br J Nurs. 2001;10(Suppl 6):S42:S44-9.

28. Otte J, van Netten JJ, Woittiez AJ. The association of chronic kidney disease and dialysis treatment with foot ulceration and major amputation. J Vasc Surg. 2015;62(2):406-11.

29. Chahrour MA, Kharroubi H, Al Tannir AH, Assi S, Habib JR, Hoballah JJ. Hypoalbuminemia is associated with mortality in patients undergoing lower extremity amputation. Ann Vasc Surg. 2021;77:138-45.

30. Kaminski MR, Raspovic A, McMahon LP, Lambert KA, Erbas B, Mount PF, et al. Factors associated with foot ulceration and amputation in adults on dialysis: a cross-sectional observational study. BMC Nephrol. 2017;18:293.

31. Pop-Busui R, Roberts L, Pennathur S, Kretzler M, Brosius FC, Feldman EL. The management of diabetic neuropathy in CKD. Am J Kidney Dis. 2010;55(2):365-85.

32. Momen-Heravi M, Barahimi E, Razzaghi R, Bahmani F, Gilasi HR, Asemi Z. The effects of zinc supplementation on wound healing and metabolic status in patients with diabetic foot ulcer: A randomized, double-blind, placebo-controlled trial. Wound Repair Regen. 2017;25:512-20.

33. Yarahmadi A, Saeed Modaghegh MH, Mostafavi-Pour Z, Azarpira N, Mousavian A, Bonakdaran S, et al. The effect of platelet-rich plasma-fibrin glue dressing in combination with oral vitamin E and C for treatment of non-healing diabetic foot ulcers: a randomized, double-blind, parallel-group, clinical trial. Expert Opin Biol Ther. 2021;21:687-96.

34. Shofler D, Rai V, Mansager S, Cramer K, Agrawal DK. Impact of resolvin mediators in the immunopathology of diabetes and wound healing. Expert Rev Clin Immunol. 2021;17:681-90.

35. Da Porto A, Miranda C, Brosolo G, Zanette G, Michelli A, Ros RD. Nutritional supplementation on wound healing in diabetic foot: What is known and what is new? World J Diabetes. 2022;13(11):940-8.

36. Arinze NV, Gregory A, Francis JM, Farber A, Chitalia VC. Unique aspects of peripheral artery disease in patients with chronic kidney disease. Vasc Med. 2019;24(3):251-60.

37. Chen J, Mohler ER 3rd, Xie D, Shlipak MG, Townsend RR, Appel LJ, et al. Risk factors for peripheral arterial disease among patients with chronic kidney disease. Am J Cardiol. 2012;110(1):136-41.

38. Garimella PS, Hirsch AT. Peripheral artery disease and chronic kidney disease: clinical synergy to improve outcomes. Adv Chronic Kidney Dis. 2014;21(6):460-71.

39. Wolf G, Müller N, Busch M, Eidner G, Kloos C, Hunger-Battefeld W, et al. Diabetic foot syndrome and renal function in type 1 and 2 diabetes mellitus show close association. Nephrol Dial Transplant. 2009;24(6):1896-901.

40. Harlacher E, Wollenhaupt J, Baaten CC, Noels H. Impact of uremic toxins on endothelial dysfunction in chronic kidney disease: A systematic review. Int J Mol Sci. 2022;23:531.

41. Sandepudi K, Shah KV, Melnick BA, Li RA, Ho K, O'Connor MJ, et al. Pathophysiology of Wound Development and Chronicity in Renal Disease: A Narrative Review. Int Wound J. 2025;22(7):e70713.

42. Cohen G, Hörl WH. Immune dysfunction in uremia—an update. Toxins (Basel). 2012;4(11):962-90.

43. Syed-Ahmed M, Narayanan M. Immune Dysfunction and Risk of Infection in Chronic Kidney Disease. Adv Chronic Kidney Dis. 2019;26(1):8-15.

44. Yates C, May K, Hale T, Allard B, Rowlings N, Freeman A, et al. Wound chronicity, inpatient care, and chronic kidney disease predispose to MRSA infection in diabetic foot ulcers. Diabetes Care. 2009;32(10):1907-9.

45. Campbell RE, Chen CH, Edelstein CL. Overview of Antibiotic-Induced Nephrotoxicity. Kidney Int Rep. 2023;8(11):2211-25.

46. Ashmi MF, Shaikh H, Rout P. Anemia of Chronic Kidney Disease. In: StatPearls. Treasure Island (FL): StatPearls Publishing; 2025.

47. Otte J, van Netten JJ, Woittiez AJ. The association of chronic kidney disease and dialysis treatment with foot ulceration and major amputation. J Vasc Surg. 2015;62(2):406-11.

48. Giangreco F, Iacopi E, Malquori V, Pieruzzi L, Goretti C, Piaggesi A. In Blood We Trust: Anemia as a Negative Healing Prognostic Factor in Diabetic Foot Patients. Acta Diabetologica. 2024;61(2):245-51.

49. Ross EA. Evolution of Treatment Strategies for Calciphylaxis. Am J Nephrol. 2011;34(5):460-7.

50. Rastogi A, Gupta R, Ghosh J, Jude EB. Renal Foot in Diabetes: Implications for Wound Healing and Solutions. Adv Wound Care (New Rochelle). 2025. doi: 10.1089/wound.2025.0074.

51. Greco T, Mascio A, Comisi C, Polichetti C, Caravelli S, Mosca M, et al. RANKL-RANK OPG pathway in charcot diabetic foot: Pathophysi ology and clinical-therapeutic implications. Int J Mol Sci. 2023;24(3):3014.

52. Rastogi A, Singh R, Ghosh J, Gupta R. Anti-RANKL antibody for active charcot foot neuro-osteoarthropathy in patients with diabetes and chronic kidney disease. Foot Ankle Int. 2024;45(10):1122-30.

53. Li Y, Hu Y, Huyan X, Chen K, Li B, Gu W, et al. Comparison of efficacy and safety of three novel hypoglycemic agents in patients with severe diabetic kidney disease: A systematic review and network meta-analysis of randomized controlled trials. Front Endocrinol (Lausanne). 2022;13:1003263.

54. Lavery LA, Hunt NA, Lafontaine J, Baxter CL, Ndip A, Boulton AJ. Diabetic foot prevention: A neglected

opportunity in high risk patients. Diabet Care. 2010;33(7):1460-2.

55. Speckman RA, Frankenfield DL, Roman SH, Eggers PW, Bedinger MR, Rocco MV, et al. Diabetes is the strongest risk factor for lower-extremity amputation in new hemodialysis patients. Diabetes Care. 2004;27:2198-203.

56. Allison GM, Flanagin E. How ESKD complicates the management of diabetic foot ulcers: The vital role of the dialysis team in prevention, early detection, and support of multidisciplinary treatment to reduce lower extremity amputations. Semin Dial. 2020;33(3):245-53.

57. Miyajima S, Shirai A, Yamamoto S, Okada N, Matsushita T. Risk factors for major limb amputations in diabetic foot gangrene patients. Diabet Res Clin Pract. 2006;71:272-9.

58. Hambleton IR, Jonnalagadda R, Davis CR, Fraser HS, Chaturvedi N, Hennis AJ. All-cause mortality after diabetes-related amputation in Barbados: A prospective case-control study. Diabetes Care. 2009;32:306-7.

59. Sharma A, Vas P, Cohen S, Patel T, Thomas S, Fountoulakis N, et al. Clinical features and burden of new onset diabetic foot ulcers post simultaneous pancreas kidney transplantation and kidney only transplantation. J Diabetes Complications. 2019;33(9):662-7.

60. Lavery LA, Hunt NA, Ndip A, Lavery DC, Van Houtum W, Boulton AJ. Impact of chronic kidney disease on survival after amputation in individuals with diabetes. Diabetes Care. 2010;33(11):2365-9.

Key Research Takeaway

OPEN ACCESS

http://scidoc.org/IJDVR.php

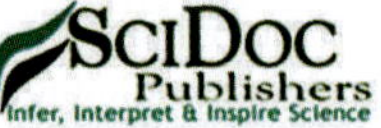

Diabetic Foot Infection and Worsening Kidney Function: Implication for Health Care in the Developing World

Anitha Rani A[1], Viswanathan V[2]

1 Post Doctoral Research Fellow, Prof. M. Viswanathan Diabetes Research Centre, Royapuram, Chennai, Tamil Nadu, India.
2 Head & Chief Diabetologist, M.V. Hospital for Diabetes and President, Prof. M.Viswanathan Diabetes Research Centre, West Madha Church Street, Royapuram, Chennai, Tamil Nadu, India.

Abstract

Background: Diabetic foot infection (DFI) and Chronic Kidney Disease (CKD) are two health care issues causing considerable burden in the developing world. The current study was aimed to examine the effect of DFI in declining renal function among patients with Type 2 Diabetes Mellitus (T2DM).

Methods: A total of 412 patients have been included in a prospective 12 months follow-up study. The study patients were categorized into Group I: T2DM with CKD and DFI, Group II: T2DM with CKD, Group III: T2DM with DFI and without CKD and Group IV- T2DM without any complications. Demographic, anthropometric and clinical parameters were recorded accordingly.

Results: Significant fall in eGFR was observed within group I at 6th month (p<0.0001) and 12th month (p<0.0001). In group II fall in eGFR was noticed in 3rd month (p<0.004); 6th month and (p<0.004); 12th months (p<0.0001) and in group III significant fall in eGFR was observed in 3rd month (p<0.0001), 6th month (p<0.004) and 12 months (p<0.004). No significant fall in eGFR was observed in group IV. The mean differences of eGFR from 0 to 12 months were 11.01, 8.36, 3.52, and 1.2 in all the groups respectively.

Conclusions: There was a significant reduction in eGFR among CKD patients with DFI and DFI patients without CKD. Therefore development of DFI may cause decline in renal function irrespective of CKD status and preventive steps to prevent a DFI is mandatory in all T2DM.

nt J Diabetol Vasc Dis Res,. 2017;5(5):208-213.

ORIGINAL ARTICLE

Diabetic Foot Ulcer as a Cause of Significant Decline in the Renal Function Among South Indian Population With Type 2 Diabetes: Role of TGF-β1 and CCN Family Proteins

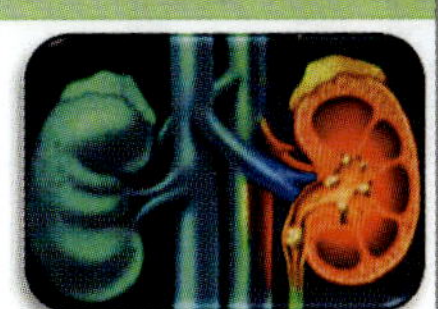

T. P. Smina, PhD[1], M. Rabeka, MSc[1], and Vijay Viswanathan, MD, PhD, FRCP[1]

Abstract

In the present study, a total of 428 South Indian subjects were divided into four different groups, consisting of individuals with type 2 diabetes without any other complications (T2DM), T2DM subjects with stage 2 and 3 diabetic kidney disease (CKD), T2DM subjects with grade 2 or 3 diabetic foot ulcer (DFU) and T2DM subjects having both diabetic kidney disease and diabetic foot ulcer (CKDDFU). The study was conducted ambispectively by comparing the changes in renal function among two consecutive periods, i.e., the period prior to the development of grade 2 and 3 diabetic foot ulcer (retrospectively) and after the development of DFU (prospectively). A gradual and uniform reduction of eGFR was observed throughout the study period in the subjects affected with either CKD or DFU alone. Whereas in subjects with both CKD and DFU, there was a sharp decline in the eGFR during the six months prior to the baseline, i.e., the period in which the development of ulcer and its progression to grade 2 or 3 happened. Remarkable elevations in the levels of TGF-β1 and CCN2 (CTGF), as well as a significant reduction in the level of CCN3 (NOV), were observed in the serum of CKDDFU group subjects, compared to the other groups. Increased production of TGF-β1 in response to the inflammatory stimulus from multiple sites in CKDDFU subjects caused a subsequent down regulation of CCN3, followed by the activation of a large quantity of CCN2.

The International Journal of Lower Extremity Wounds
1–8
© The Author(s) 2019
Article reuse guidelines:
sagepub.com/journals-permissions
DOI: 10.1177/1534734619862704
journals.sagepub.com/home/ijl

SAGE

¹M.V. Hospital for Diabetes and Prof. M. Viswanathan Diabetes Research Centre, Chennai, India

Corresponding Author: Vijay Viswanathan, M.V. Hospital for Diabetes and Prof. M. Viswanathan Diabetes Research Centre, No. 4, West Madha Church Street, Royapuram, Chennai 600013, India. Email: drvijay@mvdiabetes.com

12

When to Refer to Nephrologist and for Renal Replacement Therapy

T Navaneethan

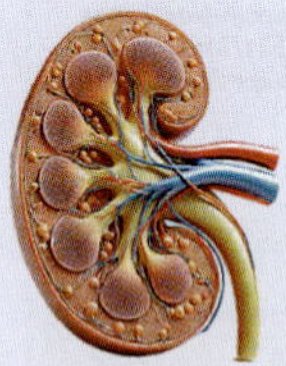

- ➤ Need for referral to a nephrologist
- ➤ Late and early referral
- ➤ How to decide the timing of referral?
- ➤ When to refer to a nephrologist?
- ➤ Referral for RRT
- ➤ Strategies for prevention of referral

Abstract

Diabetic kidney disease (DKD) is the most common cause of chronic kidney disease (CKD) in India; therefore, prompt referral of DKD patients to a nephrologist plays a major role in delaying the progression of CKD, designing the management of the patient through the stages of CKD, discussing the options of renal replacement therapy (RRT)—dialysis and transplantation, planning access for dialysis and appropriate initiation of RRT, and the management of its associated complications. Late referral results in increased overall morbidity and mortality and increased initiation of unplanned dialysis, which results in increased incidence of infection, whereas early referral reduced morbidity and mortality and hospitalization, better uptake of peritoneal dialysis as RRT option, and earlier placement of arteriovenous fistula (AVF). Referral to a nephrologist is decided by laboratory parameters, namely, albuminuria and estimated glomerular filtration rate (eGFR) and risk assessment equation named kidney failure risk equation (KFRE). The eGFR and the severity of albuminuria are the two important criteria that decide the frequency of assessment. Patient should be referred to a nephrologist when a nondiabetic kidney disease is suspected, faster progression of DKD is present, there are presence of comorbidities that would affect glomerular filtration rate (GFR), and there is presence of CKD complications. RRT may be required in patients on initial visit or irregularly followed-up patients or in the event of acute kidney injury (AKI). Primary care physician should be well aware of indications for RRT (severe uremic symptoms) for timely referral to a nephrologist.

Keywords: Renal replacement therapy, diabetic kidney disease, patient, nephrologist, referral.

INTRODUCTION

Diabetic kidney disease (DKD) being the most common cause of chronic kidney disease (CKD) (24.9%)[1] in India, prompt referral of DKD patients to a nephrologist plays a major role in delaying the progression of CKD, designing the management of the patient through the stages of CKD, discussing the options of renal replacement therapy (RRT)—dialysis and transplantation, planning access for dialysis and timely initiation of RRT, management of RRT complications, if any, and for palliative care if the patient and attenders do not choose RRT as treatment option or patient too sick to start on chronic maintenance hemodialysis (mHD). Timing of referral is important as it will decide the progress of disease. This chapter highlights the important indications for referral to a nephrologist, the benefits of early referral, and also clinical implications of late referral.

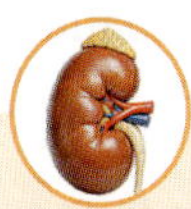

In India, prompt referral of DKD patients to a nephrologist plays a major role in delaying the progression of CKD, designing the management of the patient through the stages of CKD, and discussing the options of RRT.

LATE REFERRAL

Late referral means that the time interval between the first nephrology visit and initiation of RRT is <1–6 months. We will discuss the reasons and implications of late referral.

Reasons

The reasons for late referral could be both patient-related and primary-care physician-related. Patient-related factors include unawareness of the morbidity and mortality that CKD–end-stage renal disease (ESRD) would cause if not followed-up regularly and cost and time spent in visiting a nephrologist. Primary-care physician factors include failure to screen for albuminuria and estimated glomerular filtration rate (eGFR) during diagnosis of type-2 diabetes mellitus (T2DM) and biannually thereafter, after 5 years from the diagnosis of type-1 diabetes mellitus (T1DM), less knowledge about indications for referral, and unawareness of benefits of early referral.

Implications

Late referral leads to:
- Overall increased patient mortality and morbidity
- Commencement of unplanned dialysis with temporary catheter, which in turn increase the incidence of central-line-associated bloodstream infection (CLABSI) due to frequent manipulation
- Less acceptance of continuous ambulatory peritoneal dialysis (CAPD) as option of RRT
- Reduced likelihood of orientation to renal transplant program
- Increased cost and treatment burden to the patient
- Increased duration of hospital stay

Evidence

Chan et al. performed a meta-analysis of the English language literature from the year 1980 to 2005. 22 studies yielded a total of 12,749 patients. The duration of follow-up was from 0.8 to 4.9 years. Late referral was associated with increased overall mortality [risk ratio (RR) 1.99; 95% confidence interval (CI) 1.66–2.39]. The mortality was 29% at the end of first year in the late referral group and 13% in the early referral group respectively (RR 2.08; 95% CI 1.31–3.31). The duration of hospitalization at the initiation of dialysis was increased by 12 days in the late referral group (95% CI 8.0–16.1).[2]

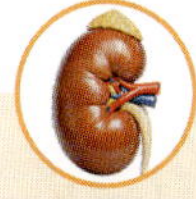

Late referral results in increased overall morbidity and mortality and increased initiation of unplanned dialysis, which results in increased incidence of infection.

EARLY REFERRAL

Early referral is defined as referral to nephrologist 6 months prior to initiation of RRT. The benefits of early referral should be explained clearly to the patient so that he/she accepts the need and also decision of referral. The benefits of early referral are discussed as follows.

Benefits

Early referral results in:

- Overall reduction in patient morbidity and mortality
- Preservation of residual renal function
- Better patient involvement in diabetic control
- Better insight to disease
- Better management of comorbidities (hypertension)
- Time spent with peer group of patients for better understanding of progress of disease and its complications
- Better management of CKD complications such as anemia and mineral bone disease.
- Increased rate of acceptance of RRT initiation and continuation
- Timely arteriovenous fistula (AVF) creation (3–6 months prior to the initiation of hemodialysis)
- Acceptance of CAPD as option for RRT continuation
- Better orientation to renal transplant program
- Guidance to palliation in patients who did not choose to continue RRT or unfit to continue RRT in view of multiple comorbidities
- Establishment of better rapport between patient and treating nephrologist, which is to be continued for patient's lifetime

Evidence

A Cochrane analysis of 40 longitudinal cohort studies provided data on 63,887 participants among which 43,209 (68%) were referred early and 20,678 (32%) were referred late. In this analysis, the patients who were referred early were less likely to receive temporary vascular access (RR 0.47; 95% 0.45–0.50; I^2 = 97%) when compared to those who were referred late. Patients referred early were more likely to receive permanent vascular access (RR 3.22; 95% CI 2.92–3.55; I^2 = 97%). Systolic blood pressure (BP) was significantly lower in early versus late referrals [mean difference (MD) –3.09 mm Hg; 95% CI –5.23 to –0.95; I^2 = 85%]; diastolic BP was significantly lower in early versus late referrals (MD –1.64 mm Hg; 95% CI –2.77 to –0.51; I^2 = 82%). Erythropoietin (EPO) use was significantly higher in those referred early (RR 2.92; 95% CI 2.42–3.52; I^2 = 0%). Inability to walk was less prevalent in early referrals (RR 0.66; 95% CI 0.51–0.86). It was concluded that early referral resulted in reduced mortality and hospitalization, as well as an enhanced uptake of peritoneal dialysis and earlier placement of AVF for patients with CKD.[3]

Importance of Continuous Ambulatory Peritoneal Dialysis in People with Diabetes

Arteriovenous fistula is the lifeline for chronic mHD. But creation, maturation, and maintenance of AVF is difficult in diabetic patients. There are many studies revealing that diabetes mellitus may be associated with AVF failure. A meta-analysis showed a higher rate of AVF failure in people with diabetes when compared to people without diabetes was also statistically significant.[4]

Possible mechanisms include high risk of platelet aggregation and increased release of von Willebrand factor, which promotes the platelet aggregation and results in damage to endothelial cells in blood vessels.[5] On account of atherosclerosis exists more often and severe in diabetes patients—there is a wide range of vascular lesions, making it difficult to establish a vascular access.[6] Diabetic patients are more prone for lipid deposition, especially in vascular wall near anastomotic stoma, causing blood clots of postoperative fistula more easily.[4] Hence, due to the difficulties in creating and maintaining AVF in some diabetic patients, CAPD plays the major role for such patients as option of RRT. Hence, early referral is important to get adequate time for preoperative assessment for AVF creation and allowing adequate time for AVF maturation. Early referral resulted in an increased acceptance of CAPD as a feasible option.

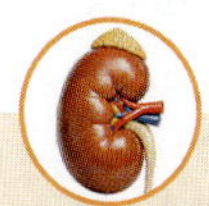

Early referral resulted in reduced mortality and hospitalization, as well as an enhanced uptake of peritoneal dialysis and earlier placement of AVFs for patients with CKD3 due to diabetes.

HOW TO DECIDE TIMING OF REFERRAL?

Referral to a nephrologist is decided by:
- Laboratory parameters
- Risk assessment equation

Laboratory Parameters

Decision for referral is made with the help of two laboratory parameters, namely, *albuminuria* and *eGFR*.

Albuminuria can be measured by either urine spot albumin-to-creatinine ratio (UACR) or 24-hour urine protein. 24-hour urine protein is cumbersome to collect resulting in fallacies in report. UACR is easy to collect, ideally early morning sample to be collected but can be done with sample collected during any time of the day. UACR shall be measured using CLINITEK microalbumin reagent strip test or Multistix PRO reagent strips, which measure both albumin and creatinine semiquantitatively. They detect albuminuria as low as 1.5–2 mg/dL and 2–4 mg/dL, respectively.[7] Due to the high biological variability of >20% between measurements in urinary albumin excretion, it is considered that two of three specimens of UACR collected within 3–6 months period should be abnormal to consider an individual to have moderately (30–299 mg/g) or severely elevated albuminuria (≥ 300 mg/g).[8]

The eGFR can be calculated using serum creatinine as filtration marker using the Chronic Kidney Disease Epidemiology Collaboration (CKD-EPI) equation, 2009 and 2021 [Kidney Disease: Improving Global Outcomes (KDIGO) recommended]. The 2009 equation used race as one of the variables but 2021 equation does not include race. The 2009 CKD-EPI equation is more accurate than 2021 equation for nonblack individuals. Additionally, using cystatin C as filtration marker, eGFRcys can be measured using CKD-EPI 2012 equation. However, eGFR calculated from the combination of creatinine and cystatin C (eGFRcr–cys) from CKD-EPI 2021 equation gives more accurate clinical decision.[8] eGFR can be calculated from eGFR calculators available online. Measured glomerular filtration rate (GFR) is the gold standard for GFR evaluation but more expensive, invasive, and more time consuming. Ideally it is done using urinary or plasma clearance of exogenous markers namely iohexol, iothalamate, Chromium-51-labeled ethylenediaminetetraacetic acid (^{51}Cr-EDTA scan), and Technetium-99m diethylene-triamine-pentaacetate (^{99m}Tc-DTPA). In a resource-limited setting like India, the CKD-EPI equation using serum creatinine is practically feasible and is also widely used among practitioners.

The frequency of assessment is important to decide on referral and it is based on severity of albuminuria and eGFR in the initial assessment and during further visit. The frequency of assessment that is recommended by KDIGO is depicted in **Table 1**.

Risk Assessment for Progression of Chronic Kidney Disease

In people with CKD G3–G5, KDIGO recommends using an externally validated risk equation to estimate the absolute risk of kidney failure (requirement of dialysis or renal transplantation). The KDIGO recommends three validated models for the risk assessment for the progression of CKD, namely, (1) the Kidney Failure Risk Equation (KFRE), (2) the Veterans Affairs model, and (3) the Z6 Score model.[8]

Among which KFRE is maximally used. The KFRE was developed and initially validated in 8,391 adults from 2 Canadian provinces and

TABLE 1: Risk of CKD progression, frequency of visits and referral according to GFR and albuminuria.[8]

			Albuminuria categories description and range		
	CKD is classified based on: • Cause (C) • GFR (G) • Albuminuria (A)		**A1** **Normal to mildly increased** <30 mg/g <3 mg/mmol	**A2** **Moderately increased** 30–299 mg/g 3–29 mg/mmol	**A3** **Severely increased** ≥300 mg/g ≥30 mg/mmol
GFR categories (mL/min/1.73 m²) description and range	G1	Normal or high ≥90	Screen (1)	Treat (1)	Treat and refer (3)
	G2	Mildly decreased 60–89	Screen (1)	Treat (1)	Treat and refer (3)
	G3a	Mildly to moderately decreased 45–59	Treat (1)	Treat (2)	Treat and refer (3)
	G3b	Moderately to severely decreased 30–44	Treat (2)	Treat and refer (3)	Treat and refer (3)
	G4	Severely decreased 15–29	Treat and refer* (3)	Treat and refer* (3)	Treat and refer (4+)
	G5	Kidney failure <15	Treat and refer (4+)	Treat and refer (4+)	Treat and refer (4+)

■ Low risk— if no other markers of kidney disease, no CKD   ■ High risk

■ Moderately increased risk   ■■ Very high risk

* Treat and refer to a nephrologist.

Note: This table shows staging of CKD according to GFR and albuminuria. The numbers in the brackets indicate the frequency of screening per year. The risk indicates risk of progression of CKD to ESRD and eventually RRT.[8]

(CKD: chronic kidney disease; ESRD: end-stage renal disease; GFR: glomerular filtration rate; RRT: renal replacement therapy)

subsequently validated in 721,357 individuals from more than 30 countries spanning 4 continents. KFRE depends upon four variables, namely: (1) age, (2) sex, (3) UACR, and (4) eGFR. More accurate information is provided by addition of four more parameters, namely: (1) serum albumin, (2) calcium, (3) phosphorus, and (4) bicarbonate. It provides 2- and 5-year probability of treating kidney failure (dialysis or transplantation) for a potential patient with CKD stage 3–5.[8] It also provides percentage reduction of progression of disease on addition of renoprotective drugs namely angiotensin-converting enzyme (ACE) inhibitors, angiotensin receptor blockers (ARBs), sodium-glucose cotransporter-2 (SGLT2) inhibitors, and non-steroidal mineralocorticoid receptor antagonist (finerenone). KFRE can be assessed in www.kidneyfailurerisk.com.

Interpretation of KFRE:

- A 5-year kidney failure risk of 3–5% needs nephrology referral.
- A 2-year kidney failure risk of >10% indicatse need for nephrology referral.
- A 2-year kidney failure risk threshold of >40% can be used to determine modality education and timing of preparation for RRT.

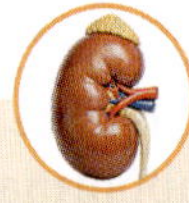

Referral is decided by two laboratory parameters, namely, albuminuria and eGFR and one risk assessment equation—KFRE equation.

WHEN TO REFER TO NEPHROLOGIST?

Appropriate and timely referral of patients with DKD to nephrologist plays a major role in outcome as discussed earlier. Hence the guidelines for referral are given by major organizations around the globe. The summary of the guidelines is enlisted as follows:

Kidney Disease: Improving Global Outcomes Recommendations[9]

Nephrology referral would require following situations:

- A fall in eGFR of >20% during follow up (frequency of testing indicated in **Table 1**)
- Among people with CKD who are initiated on hemodynamically active therapies (ACE inhibitor/ARB) and the GFR reductions of >30%
- A doubling of the ACR on a subsequent test (frequency of testing indicated in **Table 1**)
- A 5-year kidney failure risk of 3–5% (assessed by KFRE equation)
- A 2-year kidney failure risk of >10% (assessed by KFRE equation)

National Institute for Health and Care Excellence Guidelines[10]

Refer adults with DKD to nephrologist (taking into account their wishes and comorbidities) if they have any of the following:

- A 5-year risk of requiring RRT of greater than 5% (measured using the 4-variable KFRE).
- An albumin-to-creatinine ratio (ACR) of 300 mg/mmol or more and already treated with maximum tolerated dose of ACE/ARB and SGLT2 inhibitors
- An ACR of >30 mg/mmol (ACR category A3), along with hematuria (both micro and macrohematuria),
- A sustained decrease in eGFR of 25% or more and a change in eGFR category within 12 months
- A sustained decrease in eGFR of 15 mL/min/1.73 m^2 or more per year
- Poorly controlled hypertension
- Known or suspected rare or genetic causes of CKD
- Suspected renal artery stenosis

American Diabetes Association Recommendations[11]

Health-care professionals should consider referral to a nephrologist if the individual with diabetes has:

- Continuously rising UACR levels and/or continuously declining eGFR
- If there is uncertainty about the etiology of kidney disease
- For difficult management issues (anemia, secondary hyperparathyroidism, significant increases in albuminuria despite good blood pressure management, metabolic bone disease, resistant hypertension, or electrolyte disturbances)
- When there is advanced kidney disease (eGFR <30 mL/min/1.73 m^2) requiring discussion of renal replacement therapy for ESRD

What do Indian Guidelines Say?

The Indian Council of Medical Research (ICMR) 2018 guidelines recommend referral of DKD patients to a nephrologist if there is severe/resistant hypertension, serum potassium greater than 5.5 mEq/L, nephrotic range proteinuria, proteinuria in the absence of retinopathy, serum creatinine greater than 1.5 mg%, pregestational diabetes or gestational diabetes mellitus with proteinuria, and fluid overload.[12]

The Research Society for Study of Diabetes in India (RSSDI) (2017) guidelines for management of T2DM lay down four indications for referral of DKD to a nephrologist: (1) eGFR <30 mL/min/1.73 m^2, (2) progressive deterioration of kidney function, (3) persistent proteinuria, and (4) biochemical or fluid retention or difficulty in diagnosis (to rule out nondiabetic renal disease).[13]

Compilations from Guidelines for Best Practice

A compilation from earlier-mentioned guidelines is required for easy decision making and not to miss any cases. Referral is necessary if the patient fulfils any of the following criteria. A compilation

---

BOX 1: Indications for referral during initial diagnosis.

During initial diagnosis:
- Presence of micro (≥3 RBC/HPF) or macro hematuria
- Absence of retinopathy
- Discordance between albuminuria and eGFR
- Features of systemic involvement (e.g., rash, hair loss, and joint pain)
- Nephrotic range proteinuria (sudden onset)
- Abnormal morphology of kidneys in USG
- Family history of renal diseases
- Renal stone disease
- Suspected AKI
- CKD IV at diagnosis
- Presence of chronic lower urinary tract symptoms.
- Worsening of GFR over days to weeks (RPGN)
- Duration of diabetes not compatible in type 1 diabetic patients.

(AKI: acute kidney injury; eGFR: estimated glomerular filtration rate; RBC/HPF: red blood cells per high-power field; RPGN: rapidly progressive glomerulonephritis; USG: ultrasonography)

BOX 2: Indications for referral during follow-up in the case of probable DKD.

During follow up in the case of probable DKD:
- Worsening of GFR > 30% on start of hemodynamically active therapies (ACE inhibitor/ARB)
- Resistant hypertension
- eGFR 30–60 mL/min + decline of ≥ 5 mL/min over 6 months ARB
- Doubling of the ACR in subsequent visit
- Resistant hyperkalemia or hypokalemia
- 5-year kidney failure risk of 3–5% (assessed by KFRE equation)
- 2-year kidney failure risk of >10%

(ACE: angiotensin-converting enzyme; ARB: angiotensin receptor blocker; ACR: albumin-to-creatinine ratio; DKD: diabetic kidney disease; eGFR: estimated glomerular filtration rate; KFRE: kidney failure risk equation)

BOX 3: Indications for referral in the presence of complications or comorbidities.

Presence of CKD complications:
- Refractory anemia
- Mineral bone disease
- Refractory volume overload/oliguria (urine output <400 mL/day)
- Malnutrition

Presence of comorbidities which can impact GFR:
- Recurrent UTI (Chronic pyelonephritis results in CKD)
- Recurrent foot infections

(CKD: chronic kidney disease; GFR: glomerular filtration rate; UTI: urinary tract infection)

---

of guidelines intended for best clinical practice for the purpose of referral is enlisted in **Boxes 1 to 3**.

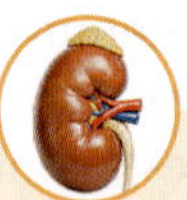

Patients should be referred to a nephrologist when there is:
- *Suspicion of nondiabetic kidney disease*
- *Faster progression of DKD*
- *Complications of CKD*
- *Presence of comorbidities that can affect GFR*

REFERRAL FOR RENAL REPLACEMENT THERAPY

Despite the above guidelines, some patients would require RRT in the initial visit, some follow-up patients would require RRT in case not visiting a nephrologist despite advice and in the event of AKI. There is no absolute eGFR below which RRT to be initiated. Hence, indications for RRT must be known in order to decide on urgent nephrology referral and to initiate RRT in the absence of a nephrologist. The indications for RRT differ in AKI and CKD apart from traditional indications.

Indications for Renal Replacement Therapy in End-stage Renal Disease Patients

Modalities of RRT in ESRD are mHD and CAPD. Decision between modality is based on patient and nephrologist concurrence. The indications for RRT are largely severe manifestations of uremic syndrome, which are refractory to medical management. Decision of RRT can be made by primary-care physician in emergency situation unless traditional indications are present. The absolute and relative contraindications are enlisted in **Boxes 4A and B**.

The presence of relative indications should prompt discussion among the patient, nephrologist, and patient family members and caregivers to carefully weigh the pros and cons of dialysis initiation. Presence of relative indications warrant discussion with nephrologist prior to RRT initiation.

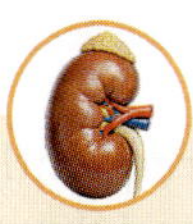

Indications for RRT in CKD–ESRD are largely severe manifestations of uremic syndrome. RRT can be initiated by primary-care physician in the presence of absolute indications whereas nephrologist referral is required in presence of relative indications.

BOX 4: Absolute and relative contraindications for RRT in ESRD patients.

Absolute indications:[14]
- Uremic pericarditis
- Uremic encephalopathy with altered mental status
- Recurrent or persistent hyperkalemia refractory to medical management
- Severe fluid overload leading with pulmonary edema or impaired wound healing
- Refractory nausea with vomiting
- Severe uremic bleeding
- Severe metabolic acidosis

Relative indications:[14]
- Fatigue/lethargy
- Anorexia
- Loss of muscle or fat mass
- Sleep disturbances
- Memory or other neurocognitive dysfunction
- Pruritus
- Musculoskeletal pain
- Sexual dysfunction

(ESRD: end-stage renal disease; RRT: renal replacement therapy)

Indications for Renal Replacement Therapy in Acute Kidney Injury Patients

Definition of AKI:[15] Acute kidney injury can be defined as any of the following—
- Increase in serum creatinine by 0.3 mg/dL within 48 hours or
- Increase in serum creatinine to 1.5 times baseline, which is known or presumed to have occurred within the prior 7 days or
- Urine volume <0.5 mL/kg/h for 6 hours.

The word "or" is important in the definition of AKI.

Acute kidney injury can also be graded based on KDIGO, which is depicted in **Table 2**.

Introduction about Acute Kidney Injury in Diabetes

Acute kidney injury can occur in any individual, while AKI in people with diabetes requires special mention because of already reduced renal reserve (GFR may not return to baseline even after the inciting event of AKI resolves). AKI in people living with diabetes are mostly infection-related or contrast-induced. Multiple episodes of AKI would end up in CKD–ESRD whereas in some individuals, single episode of AKI would end up in patient being dependent on dialysis. Common

TABLE 2: KDIGO staging of AKI.[15]

Stage	Serum creatinine	Urine output
1	1.5–1.9 times baseline (*or*) × 0.3 mg/dL increase	<0.5 mL/kg/h for 6–12 hours
2	2.0–2.9 times baseline	<0.5 mL/kg/h for ≥ 12 hours
3	3.0 times baseline (*or*) increase in serum creatinine to ≥ 4.0 mg/dL (*or*) initiation of renal replacement therapy (*or*), in patients <18 years, decrease in eGFR to <35 mL/min/1.73 m²	<0.3 mL/kg/h for ≥ 24 hours (*or*) anuria for ≥12 hours

(eGFR: estimated glomerular filtration rate; KDIGO: Kidney Disease: Improving Global Outcomes)

conditions resulting in AKI are shown in **Figure 1** and the various causes of AKI are depicted in **Figure 2**. Going into the details of conditions and causes of AKI are beyond the scope of this book. Precautions for prevention of AKI in diabetes are tabulated in **Box 5**.

BOX 5: Precautions for prevention of AKI.

Precautions for prevention of AKI:
- Withholding hemodynamically active agents in the event of AGE
- Primary and secondary prevention of UTI
- Foot care and early control of soft tissue infection
- Judicious use of intravenous contrast
- Drug dosing according to creatinine clearance
- Stopping SGLT2 inhibitors in the event of UTI

(AGE: acute gastroenteritis; AKI: acute kidney injury; SGLT2: sodium-glucose cotransporter-2; UTI: urinary tract infection)

Contrast-induced Acute Kidney Injury[15,16]

Intravenous contrast is used more frequently nowadays for coronary angiography or peripheral computed tomography (CT) angiography or digital subtraction angiography (DSA). Presence of renal dysfunction should not prevent individuals from taking angiography, which could help in clinical decision-making but with some precautions.

Definition: It is defined as a rise in serum creatinine of ≥ 0.5 mg/dL or a 25% increase from baseline value, assessed at 48 hours after a radiological procedure. It has been established that contrast-induced AKI can occur up to 5 days postcontrast exposure.

Risk factors:
- Age > 75 years
- eGFR < 30 mL/min
- High osmolar contrast media
- Concurrent medications such as nonsteroidal anti-inflammatory drugs (NSAIDs) and metformin
- Reduced renal perfused states
- Hyperuricemia
- Albuminuria
- Diabetes

Prevention:
- Judicious use of intravenous iodinated contrast media
- Withholding drugs such as NSAIDs, metformin, and ACE inhibitors

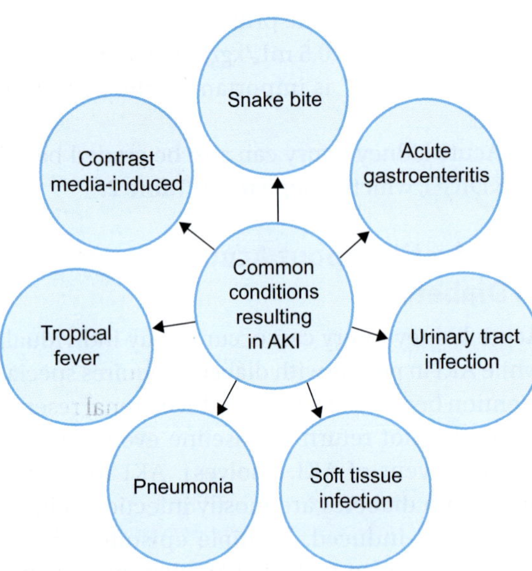

FIG. 1: Common conditions resulting in acute kidney injury (AKI).

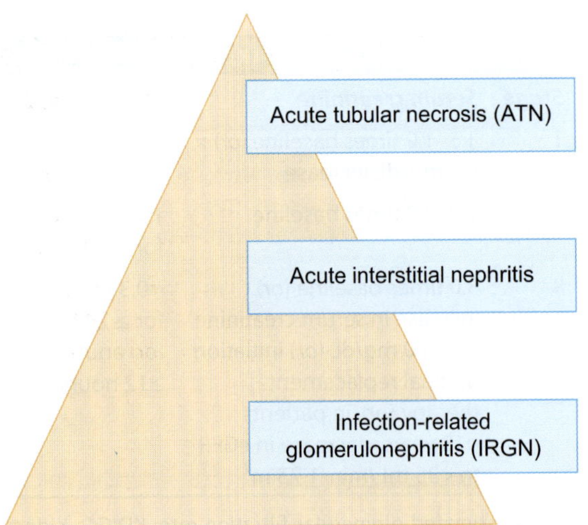

FIG. 2: Common causes of acute kidney injury (AKI).

- Use of low osmolar or iso-osmolar iodinated contrast media
- Use of lowest possible dose
- 1–3 mL/kg isotonic saline 1 hour pre and 12 hours postprocedure
- N-acetylcysteine (NAC) > 1,200 mg/day recommended in KDIGO 2012 AKI guidelines but not proven effective in recent randomized controlled trials (RCTs)
- No use of prophylactic hemodialysis or hemofiltration
- Avoid re-exposure of contrast within 48–72 hours

Indications for Renal Replacement Therapy

The timely initiation of RRT in AKI is important as delay in initiation results in mortality. Frequent clinical assessment is required to decide timing of initiation of RRT. There are many studies comparing early initiation (during KDIGO stage 2 and 3) and late initiation (if there were life-threatening complications or persistent AKI for at least 72 hours). Early initiation brings no benefit in terms of mortality, regardless of septic or nonseptic AKI. On the contrary, it may lead to excess mortality in the absence of oligoanuria and increase the risk of dependence on long-term dialysis, particularly in patients with chronic renal disease. Delayed initiation can avoid up to 49% of RRT (with ~30% attributed to spontaneous renal recovery and the remaining 19% due to other factors, including patient death).[17] Hence timing of RRT initiation is important as are the indications.

The indications for RRT in AKI are controversial apart from traditional indications. The indication of urine output is included in AKI whereas it is not included in CKD. So, nephrologist referral is required for RRT other than conventional indications. There are several conventional, pre-emptive, and nonrenal indications for RRT that are enlisted in **Table 3**.

Options of Renal Replacement Therapy in Acute Kidney Injury

Renal replacement therapy options in the event of AKI include:

- Intermittent hemodialysis (IHD)
- Sustained low efficient daily dialysis (SLEDD)
- Continuous renal replacement therapy (CRRT)
- Acute peritoneal dialysis

TABLE 3: The conventional, pre-emptive, and nonrenal indications for RRT.

Conventional indications[18]	Pre-emptive indications[18]	Nonrenal indications[18]
• Refractory hyperkalemia[a] • Refractory volume overload[b] • Refractory metabolic acidosis[c] • Uremic manifestations (pericarditis and encephalopathy) • Oligoanuria • Progressive increase in azotemia even in the absence of symptoms	• Disrupted fluid electrolyte balance • Disruption of acid base homeostasis • Increased catabolic state (rhabdomyolysis and tumor lysis syndrome)	• Sepsis/removal of cytokines • ARDS • Drug intoxication • Acute liver injury

[a] Serum potassium > 6.5 plus electrocardiogram (ECG) signs and refractory to medical management.

[b] Worsening pulmonary edema, PaO_2/FiO_2 < 200 mm Hg, fluid balance >10% of body weight refractory to maximum dose of diuretics.

[c] pH <7.20 after administration of 250 mL of 4.2% sodium bicarbonate.

(ARDS: acute respiratory distress syndrome; FiO_2: fraction of inspired oxygen; PaO^2: partial pressure of arterial oxygen; RRT: renal replacement therapy)

TABLE 4: Difference between modalities of RRT in AKI.

Mode of RRT	IHD	SLEDD	CRRT
Duration	3–4 h/day	6–12 h/day	24 h/day
Hemodynamic stability	Poor	Fair–good	Good
Efficiency	High	Low	Low-to-moderate
Cost	Low	Moderate	High
Conditions used in AKI	Hemodynamically stable patients	Hemodynamically unstable patients	Critically ill patients, head injury patients, capillary leak syndrome, sepsis, and acute liver injury

(AKI: acute kidney injury; CRRT: continuous renal replacement therapy; IHD: intermittent hemodialysis; RRT: renal replacement therapy; SLEDD: sustained low efficient daily dialysis)

Of the above four, IHD is the most commonly used modality in AKI. The next most commonly used modality is CRRT/SLEDD. Differences between each modality is given in **Table 4**.[19] The advantage of SLEDD is that it can be done with same hemodialysis machine by extending the duration and altering blood flow and dialysate flow whereas CRRT requires separate machine and expensive. The advantage of CRRT is that the machine is mobile and there is no need of reverse osmosis (RO) water connection. Acute peritoneal dialysis is rarely done nowadays other than resource-limited settings.

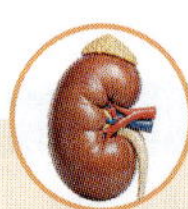

Indications for RRT in AKI are different from that of CKD apart from conventional indications, which include oligoanuria, increased catabolic state, removal of cytokines, and acute liver injury. Available modalities for RRT in AKI are IHD, SLEDD, and CRRT.

STRATEGIES FOR PREVENTING OF DIABETIC KIDNEY DISEASE FROM COMPLICATIONS AND REFERRAL

Prevention of DKD patients from complications and referral include delaying progression of CKD and prevention of AKI in pre-existing CKD–DKD. The strategy that can be followed for delaying CKD progression include adequate glycemic control [glycated hemoglobin (HbA1c) ≤ 6.5%], adequate BP control (BP ≤ 130/80 mm Hg), reducing protein intake in the way that it does not compromise nutrition (≤ 0.8 g/kg/day), adequate physical activity (150 minutes of moderate intensity aerobic activity per week), smoking cessation, control of albuminuria (< 500 mg/day) with the use of RAS inhibitors, SGLT2 inhibitors, glucagon-like peptide-1 (GLP-1) receptor agonists, and nonsteroidal mineralocorticoid receptor antagonists (nsMRA). It is imperative to understand that delaying the progression of CKD can help in delaying the referral to a nephrologist.

Acute kidney injury in pre-existing CKD cannot be prevented altogether but dialysis requirement can be prevented by some strategies. It includes early diagnosis and treatment of the inciting event such as source control and anti-biotics in the event of infection and intravenous fluids in the event of acute gastroenteritis (AGE), judicious use of intravenous contrast, avoiding nephrotoxics during the inciting event and radiographic procedures.

SUMMARY

Diabetic kidney disease is the most common cause of CKD in India, a prompt referral of patients with DKD to a nephrologist plays a major role in delaying the progression of CKD, helps in the management of the patient through the different stages of CKD, discussing the available options of RRT (dialysis and transplantation), planning access for dialysis and timely initiation of RRT, and management of potential RRT complications, if any. Late referral results in increased overall morbidity and mortality, decreased acceptance of RRT initiation, and increased initiation of unplanned dialysis, which results in increased incidence of infection. Early referral causes better long-term outcome; reduced morbidity, mortality, and hospitalization; better uptake of peritoneal dialysis as RRT option; and earlier placement of AVFs for patients with CKD due to diabetes. Referral is decided by two laboratory parameters, namely, albuminuria and eGFR and one risk assessment equation—KFRE. Albuminuria is measured by early morning UACR and graded as moderately (30–299 mg/g) or severely elevated albuminuria (≥ 300 mg/g). eGFR is measured by CKD–EPI 2009 equation. KFRE is calculated from www.kidneyfailurerisk.com, which gives 2 and 5 years risk of disease progression. The 5-year kidney failure risk of 3–5% and 2-year kidney failure risk of >10% calculated using KFRE require referral to a nephrologist. Other indications are when nondiabetic kidney disease is suspected, faster progression of DKD, complications of

CKD, and presence of comorbidities that can impact GFR. Indications for RRT must be known as there is no absolute GFR below which RRT is required. Indications are different in AKI and CKD. In CKD, it is mostly severe manifestations of uremic syndrome and modalities are chronic hemodialysis and CAPD. In AKI, it also includes oligoanuria, fluid electrolyte disorders, and other nonrenal indications. Modalities in AKI include IHD, SLEDD, and CRRT. Referral can be prevented by delaying the progression of CKD and adequate management of inciting event of AKI.

CONCLUSION

Diabetic kidney disease is the most common cause of CKD, appropriate referral to a nephrologist would decrease the prevalence of diabetic patients on mHD. It also decreases the overall morbidity and mortality. It also decreases progression of disease and allows for adequate preparation for RRT—dialysis and transplantation. Referral is decided by albuminuria and eGFR and KFRE. Patient must be referred to a nephrologist when nondiabetic kidney disease is suspected, there is faster progression of CKD, and complications of CKD is present. Indications for RRT must be known for appropriate referral.

TAKE HOME MESSAGES

- Early referral improves long-term outcome.
- Referral is decided by albuminuria, eGFR, and KFRE.
- Refer patients to nephrologist if there is suspicion of nondiabetic kidney disease, faster progression of DKD, and in the presence of complications of CKD.
- Not all proteinuria in diabetic patients are due to DKD.
- Even with regular follow-up, RRT may be suddenly required in the event of AKI.
- Renal replacement therapy can be started by primary care physician in emergency situation unless traditional indications for RRT are present.

REFERENCES

1. Kumar V, Yadav AK, Sethi J, Ghosh A, Sahay M, Prasad N, et al. The Indian Chronic Kidney Disease (ICKD) study: Baseline characteristics. Clin Kidney J. 2021;15(1):60-9.

2. Chan MR, Dall AT, Fletcher KE, Lu N, Trivedi H. Outcomes in patients with chronic kidney disease referred late to nephrologists: A meta-analysis. Am J Med. 2007;120:1063-70.

3. Smart NA, Dieberg G, Ladhani M, Titus T. Early referral to specialist nephrology services for preventing the progression to end-stage kidney disease. Cochrane Database Syst Rev. 2014;(6):CD007333.

4. Yan Y, Ye D, Yang L, Ye W, Zhan D, Zhang L, et al. A meta-analysis of the association between diabetic patients and AVF failure in dialysis. Ren Fail. 2018;40(1):379-83.

5. Creager MA, Lüscher TF, Cosentino F, Beckman JA. Diabetes and vascular disease: Pathophysiology, clinical consequences, and medical therapy: Part I. Circulation. 2003;108(12):1527-32.

6. GołeRbiowski T, Weyde W, Kusztal, M, Porażko T, Augustyniak-Bartosik H, Madziarska K, et al. Vascular access in diabetic patients. Are these patients "difficult"? Postepy Hig Med Dosw. 2015;69:913-7.

7. Brunzel NA. Fundamentals of Urine and Body Fluid Analysis, fifth edition. Amsterdam, Netherlands: Elsevier; 2023.

8. de Boer IH, Khunti K, Sadusky T, Tuttle KR, Neumiller JJ, Rhee CM, et al. Diabetes management in chronic kidney disease: A consensus report by the American Diabetes Association (ADA) and Kidney Disease: Improving Global Outcomes (KDIGO) Diabetes Care. 2022;45(12):3075-90.

9. Kidney Disease: Improving Global Outcomes (KDIGO) CKD Work Group. KDIGO 2024 Clinical Practice Guideline for the Evaluation and Management of Chronic Kidney Disease. Kidney Int. 2024;105(4S):S117-314.

10. National Institute for Health and Care Excellence (NICE). 2021. Chronic kidney disease: Assessment and management (NG203). [online] Available from https://www.nice.org.uk/guidance/ng203 [Last accessed March, 2026].

11. American Diabetes Association Professional Practice Committee. 11. Chronic kidney disease and risk management: Standards of Care in Diabetes—2025. Diabetes Care 2025;48(Suppl. 1):S239-51.

12. Indian Council of Medical Research (ICMR). (2018). Guidelines for Management of Type 2 Diabetes. New Delhi, India: ICMR; 2018.

13. Bajaj S. RSSDI clinical practice recommendations for the management of type 2 diabetes mellitus 2017. Int J Diabetes Dev Ctries. 2018;38(1, Suppl 1):1-115.

14. Nissenson A, Fine RN, Mehrotra R. Allen. Handbook of Dialysis Therapy, 6th edition. Amsterdam, Netherlands: Elsevier; 2023.

15. Kidney Disease: Improving Global Outcomes (KDIGO) Acute Kidney Injury Work Group. KDIGO Clinical Practice Guideline for Acute Kidney Injury. Kidney Int Suppl. 2012;2:1-138.

16. Li Y, Wang J. Contrast-induced acute kidney injury: a review of definition, pathogenesis, risk factors, prevention and treatment. BMC Nephrol. 2024;25(1):140.

17. Barbar SD, Jacquier M, Maldiney T. Timing of initiating renal replacement therapy in acute kidney injury J Intensive Med. 2025;5:246-8.

18. Lerma EV; Weir MR. Henrich's Principles and Practice of Dialysis, 5th edition. Netherlands: Wolters Kluwer; 2017.

19. Fathima N, Kashif T, Janapala R, Jayaraj JS, Qaseem A. Single-best Choice Between Intermittent Versus Continuous Renal Replacement Therapy: A review. Cureus. 2019;11(9):e5558.

Key Research Takeaway

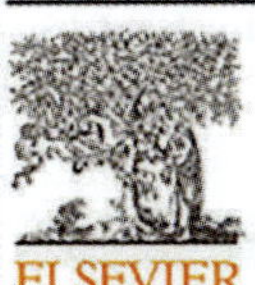

Contents lists available at ScienceDirect

Journal of Intensive Medicine

journal homepage: www.elsevier.com/locate/jointm

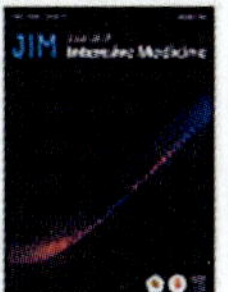

Perspective

Timing of initiating renal replacement therapy in acute kidney injury

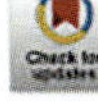

Saber Davide Barbar [1,2,*], Marine Jacquier [3,4], Thomas Maldiney [5,6]

[1] Department of Intensive Care, Nîmes University Hospital, Nîmes, France
[2] Research Unit UR UM 103 "IMAGINE", University of Montpellier, Nîmes, France
[3] Department of Intensive Care, Burgundy University Hospital, Dijon, France
[4] LIPNESS Team, INSERM Research Center LNC-UMR1231 and LabEx LipSTIC, University of Burgundy, Dijon, France
[5] Department of Intensive Care Medicine, William Morey General Hospital, Chalon-sur-Saône, France
[6] LIPNESS Team, INSERM UMR 1231, Center for Translational and Molecular Medicine (CTM), University of Burgundy, Dijon, France

Introduction

Acute kidney injury (AKI) accounts for approximately 15% of all hospital admissions and up to 50% of intensive care unit (ICU) admissions, strongly impacting morbidity (especially increased risks of end-stage chronic kidney disease) and mortality throughout various patient populations.[1] The complexity of AKI in the ICU setting – often involving multi-organ failure and fluid overload – makes the timing of initiating renal replacement therapy (RRT) a crucial decision that may significantly influence patient outcomes. The timing of RRT has been the subject of debate for decades. Several high-level studies[2-6] have recently helped clearly define the timing of RRT initiation for most patients. However, there are still aspects that deserve further exploration, notably the early identification of specific patient groups for whom early initiation might still be beneficial or, *a contrario*, for whom waiting longer might avoid dialysis. This article summarizes the latest research, providing graded recommendations on when and how to initiate RRT in the context of managing AKI in the ICU.

Review of Current Evidence: Timing of Renal Replacement Therapy for Severe Acute Kidney Injury without Life-Threatening Complications

practical insights into management in the subsequent section of this article.

The French multicenter Artificial Kidney Initiation in Kidney Injury (AKIKI) trial[2] found that early RRT initiation in Kidney Disease: Improving Global Outcomes (KDIGO) stage 3 ICU patients did not confer a survival advantage over delayed initiation, which only began upon the manifestation of life-threatening complications or in the event of persistent oligo-anuria for 72 h or if urea levels were >40 mmol/L. However, delayed initiation avoided RRT in nearly 50% of patients.

Reinforcing the findings from its predecessor, the AKIKI-2 trial[3] explored different initiation thresholds and showed that postponing RRT initiation did not confer any additional benefits in terms of RRT-free days but was associated with potential harm. In a multivariate analysis, the hazard ratio for death at 60 days was 1.65 (95% confidence interval [CI]: 1.09 to 2.50, $P = 0.018$) with the more-delayed *vs.* delayed strategy.

The multicenter, randomized controlled Initiation of Dialysis Early Versus Delayed in the Intensive Care Unit (IDEAL-ICU) trial,[4] conducted in France and focusing on patients with septic AKI, concluded that the timing of RRT did not significantly affect mortality in ICU patients with septic shock. In this study, RRT was initiated for KDIGO stage 3 AKI, or delayed for 48 h

Li and Wang *BMC Nephrology*   (2024) 25:140
https://doi.org/10.1186/s12882-024-03570-6

BMC Nephrology

REVIEW   **Open Access**

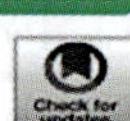

Contrast-induced acute kidney injury: a review of definition, pathogenesis, risk factors, prevention and treatment

Yanyan Li[1] and Junda Wang[2*]

Abstract

Contrast-induced acute kidney injury (CI-AKI) has become the third leading cause of hospital-acquired AKI, which seriously threatens the health of patients. To date, the precise pathogenesis of CI-AKI has remained not clear and may be related to the direct cytotoxicity, hypoxia and ischemia of medulla, and oxidative stress caused by iodine contrast medium, which have diverse physicochemical properties, including cytotoxicity, permeability and viscosity. The latest research shows that microRNAs (miRNAs) are also involved in apoptosis, pyroptosis, and autophagy which caused by iodine contrast medium (ICM), which may be implicated in the pathogenesis of CI-AKI. Unfortunately, effective therapy of CI-AKI is very limited at present. Therefore, effective prevention of CI-AKI is of great significance, and several preventive options, including hydration, antagonistic vasoconstriction, and antioxidant drugs, have been developed. Here, we review current knowledge about the features of iodine contrast medium, the definition, pathogenesis, molecular mechanism, risk factors, prevention and treatment of CI-AKI.

Keywords Contrast-induced acute kidney injury, Pathogenesis, Review, Research progress

Index

Page numbers followed by *b* refer to box, *f* refer to figure, *fc* refer to flowchart, and *t* refer to table.